PEDIATRICS, CHILD AND ADOLESCENT HEALTH

CHILD AND ADOLESCENT HEALTH

SOME RECENT RESEARCH

Pediatrics, Child and Adolescent Health

Joav Merrick - Series Editor

National Institute of Child Health and Human Development, Ministry of Social Affairs, Jerusalem

Child and Adolescent Health: Some Recent Research
Ariel Tenenbaum and Joav Merrick (Editors)
2020. ISBN: 978-1-53617-825-8 (Hardcover)
2020. ISBN: 978-1-53617-826-5 (e-book)

School Health in Asia and Africa
Supa Pengpid, Karl Peltzer and Joav Merrick (Editors)
2020. ISBN: 978-1-53617-868-5 (Hardcover)
2020. ISBN: 978-1-53617-869-2 (e-book)

Chronic Disease and Disability: The Pediatric Liver
Donald E Greydanus, Ransome Eke, Orhan Atay and Joav Merrick (Editors)
2020. ISBN: 978-1-53617-750-3 (Hardcover)
2020. ISBN: 978-1-53617-751-0 (e-book)

Chronic Disease and Disability: The Pediatric Heart, Second Edition
Donald E Greydanus, Premchand Anne, John D. Rowlett and Joav Merrick (Editors)
2020. ISBN: 978-1-53617-656-8 (Hardcover)
2020. ISBN: 978-1-53617-657-5 (e-book)

Adolescence: Behavioural Risk Factors of Non-Communicable Diseases
Supa Pengpid, Karl Peltzer and Joav Merrick (Editors)
2020. ISBN: 978-1-53617-704-6 (Hardcover)
2020. ISBN: 978-1-53617-705-3 (e-book)

Adolescence in Curaçao
Soraya Verstraeten, Supa Pengpid, Karl Peltzer and Joav Merrick (Editors)
2020. ISBN: 978-1-53617-522-6 (Softcover)
2020. ISBN: 978-1-53617-523-3 (e-book)

Building Youth for the Future: Suicide Prevention Aspects
Hatim A. Omar and Joav Merrick (Editors)
2019. ISBN: 978-1-53615-799-4 (Hardcover)
2019. ISBN: 978-1-53616-565-4 (e-book)

Vaccine: Measles and Rubella Vaccination Experience in Zambia
Mazyanga L. Mazaba-Liwewe, Seter Siziya and Joav Merrick (Editors)
2019. ISBN: 978-1-53615-799-4 (Hardcover)
2019. ISBN: 978-1-53615-800-7 (e-book)

The Boko Haram Terror: Adversary to the Wellbeing of Nigerian Kids
Miracle A. Adesina, Kehinde K. Kanmodi and Joav Merrick (Editors)
2019. ISBN: 978-1-53615-443-6 (Softcover)
2019. ISBN: 978-1-53615-444-3 (e-book)

Chronic Disease and Disability: Pediatric Obesity Perspectives
Marisha Agana, Donald E. Greydanus, Manmohan K. Kamboj and Joav Merrick (Editors)
2019. ISBN: 978-1-53615-240-1 (Hardcover)
2019. ISBN: 978-1-53615-241-8 (e-book)

Substance Use Disorders in Adolescents and Young Adults: A Manual for Pediatric and Primary Care Clinicians. Second Edition
Donald E. Greydanus, Gabriel Kaplan, Dilip R. Patel and Joav Merrick (Editors)
2019. ISBN: 978-1-53615-359-0 (Hardcover)
2019. ISBN: 978-1-53615-360-6 (e-book)

Building Youth for the Future: A Path towards Suicide Prevention
Hatim A. Omar and Joav Merrick (Editors)
2018. ISBN: 978-1-53613-768-2 (Hardcover)
2018. ISBN: 978-1-53613-769-9 (e-book)

Soft Skills and Aspirations in Chinese Children and Youth
Daniel T.L. Shek, Janet TY Leung and Joav Merrick (Editors)
2018. ISBN: 978-1-53614-092-7 (Hardcover)
2018. ISBN: 978-1-53614-093-4 (e-book)

Childhood and Adolescence: Tribute to Emanuel Chigier, 1928-2017
Joav Merrick (Editor)
2018. ISBN: 978-1-53613-574-9 (Hardcover)
2018. ISBN: 978-1-53613-574-9 (e-book)

Child Health and Human Development Yearbook 2017
Joav Merrick (Editor)
2018. ISBN: 978-1-53613-628-9 (Hardcover)
2018. ISBN: 978-1-53613-629-6 (e-book)

Child and Adolescent Health Yearbook 2017
Joav Merrick (Editor)
2018. ISBN: 978-1-53613-594-7 (Hardcover)
2018. ISBN: 978-1-53613-595-4 (e-book)

Chronic Disease and Disability: The Pediatric Gastrointestinal Tract
Donald E Greydanus, Orhan Atay, and Joav Merrick (Editors)
2018. ISBN: 978-1-53612-948-9 (Hardcover)
2018. ISBN: 978-1-53612-949-6 (e-book)

Multiple Sclerosis in Children and Adolescents
Hatim Omar and Joshua Chalkley (Editors)
2018. ISBN: 978-1-53612-979-3 (Hardcover)
2018. ISBN: 978-1-53612-980-9 (e-book)

Childhood and Adolescence: Tribute to Emanuel Chigier, 1928-2017
Joav Merrick (Editor)
2018. ISBN: 978-1-53613-574-9 (Softcover)
2018. ISBN: 978-1-53613-575-6 (e-book)

Chronic Disease and Disability: The Pediatric Lung
Donald E Greydanus, Myrtha M Gregoire-Bottex, Kevin W Cates and Joav Merrick (Editors)
2018. ISBN: 978-1-53613-577-0 (Hardcover)
2018. ISBN: 978-1-53613-578-7 (e-book)

Bicycles: Helmet Use of Adolescents at Independent Schools
Ronald Chow, Michael Borean, Drew Hollenberg, Jaclyn Viehweger, Tharani Anpalagan and Anna Rzepka (Editors)
2017. ISBN: 978-1-53612-458-3 (Hardcover)
2017. ISBN: 978-1-53612-459-0 (e-book)

Positive Youth Development: Long Term Effects in a Chinese Program
Daniel TL Shek, Cecilia MS Ma, Janet TY Leung and Joav Merrick (Editors)
2017. ISBN: 978-1-53612-539-9 (Hardcover)
2017. ISBN: 978-1-53612-540-5 (e-book)

Adolescence: Bicycle and Helmet Use of Adolescents and Young Adults
Ronald Chow and Joav Merrick (Editors)
2017. ISBN: 978-1-53612-039-4 (Hardcover)
2017. ISBN: 978-1-53612-060-8 (e-book)

Children and Youth: Post-Traumatic Stress Disorder and Motor Vehicle Crashes
Donald E. Greydanus, Roger W. Apple, Kathryn White, and Joav Merrick (Editors)
2017. ISBN: 978-1-53611-102-6 (Hardcover)
2017. ISBN: 978-1-53611-255-9 (e-book)

Suicide: A Global View on Suicidal Ideation among Adolescents
Mazyanga L. Mazaba, Seter Siziya and Joav Merrick (Editors)
2017. ISBN: 978-1-53611-788-2 (Hardcover)
2017. ISBN: 978-1-53611-799-8 (e-book)

Child and Adolescent Health Yearbook 2016
Joav Merrick (Editor)
2017. ISBN: 978-1-53610-948-1 (Hardcover)
2017. ISBN: 978-1-53610-957-3 (e-book)

Child Health and Human Development Yearbook 2016
Joav Merrick (Editor)
2017. ISBN: 978-1-53610-946-7 (Hardcover)
2017. ISBN: 978-1-53610-958-0 (e-book)

Chronic Disease and Disability: The Pediatric Kidney
Donald E Greydanus, Vimal Master Sankar Raj, and Joav Merrick (Editors)
2016. ISBN: 978-1-63483-793-4 (Hardcover)
2015. ISBN: 978-1-63483-809-2 (e-book)

Child and Adolescent Health Yearbook 2015
Joav Merrick (Editor)
2016. ISBN: 978-1-63484-512-0 (Hardcover)
2016. ISBN: 978-1-63484-543-4 (e-book)

Child Health and Human Development Yearbook 2015
Joav Merrick (Editor)
2016. ISBN: 978-1-63484-513-7 (Hardcover)
2016. ISBN: 978-1-63484-544-1 (e-book)

Pain Management Yearbook 2015
Joav Merrick (Editor)
2016. ISBN: 978-1-63484-515-1 (Hardcover)
2016. ISBN: 978-1-63484-545-8 (e-book)

Children and Childhood: Some International Aspects
Joav Merrick (Editor)
2016. ISBN: 978-1-63484-587-8 (Hardcover)
2016. ISBN: 978-1-63484-594-6 (e-book)

Children and Adolescents: Future Challenges
Daniel TL Shek, Tak Yan Lee, and Joav Merrick (Editors)
2016. ISBN: 978-1-63484-616-5 (Hardcover)
2016. ISBN: 978-1-63484-627-1 (e-book)

Adolescence: Positive Youth Development Programs in Chinese Communities
Daniel TL Shek, Florence KY Wu, Janet TY Leung, and Joav Merrick (Editors)
2016. ISBN: 978-1-63484-044-6 (Hardcover)
2016. ISBN: 978-1-63484-677-6 (e-book)

Growing Up in the Middle East: The Daily Lives and Well-Being of Israeli and Palestinian Youth
Yossi Harel-Fisch, Ziad Abdeen and Miriam Navot
2016. ISBN: 978-1-63484-746-9 (Hardcover)
2016. ISBN: 978-1-63484-765-0 (e-book)

Sexuality:
Some International Aspects
Joav Merrick and Donald E Greydanus (Editors)
2016. ISBN: 978-1-63484-707-0 (Hardcover)
2016. ISBN: 978-1-63484-719-3 (e-book)

Chronic Disease and Disability:
The Pediatric Heart
Donald E Greydanus, Devika Malhotra and Joav Merrick (Editors)
2016. ISBN: 978-1-63484-828-2 (Hardcover)
2016. ISBN: 978-1-63484-842-8 (e-book)

Diabetes Mellitus:
Childhood and Adolescence
Manmohan K Kamboj, Donald E Greydanus and Joav Merrick (Editors)
2016. ISBN: 978-1-53610-095-2 (Hardcover)
2016. ISBN: 978-1-53610-104-1 (e-book)

Chronic Disease and Disability:
Abuse and Neglect in Childhood and Adolescence
Donald E Greydanus, Vincent J Palusci and Joav Merrick (Editors)
2016. ISBN: 978-1-53610-129-4 (Hardcover)
2016. ISBN: 978-1-53610-142-3 (e-book)

Clinical Aspects of Psychopharmacology in Childhood and Adolescence, Second Edition
Donald E Greydanus, Joseph L Calles, Jr, Dilip R Patel, Ahsan Nazeer and Joav Merrick (Editors)
2016. ISBN: 978-1-53610-241-3 (Hardcover)
2016. ISBN: 978-1-53610-253-6 (e-book)

Chronic Disease and Disability:
The Pediatric Pancreas
Donald E Greydanus, Manmohan K Kamboj and Joav Merrick (Editors)
2016. ISBN: 978-1-53610-055-6 (Hardcover)
2016. ISBN: 978-1-53610-065-5 (e-book)

A Pediatric Resident Pocket Guide:
Making the Most of Morning Reports
Arthur N Feinberg
2015. ISBN: 978-1-63482-141-4 (Softcover)
2015. ISBN: 978-1-63482-186-5 (e-book)

Child and Adolescent Health Yearbook 2014
Joav Merrick (Editor)
2015. ISBN: 978-1-63482-162-9 (Hardcover)
2015. ISBN: 978-1-63482-206-0 (e-book)

Tropical Pediatrics: A Public Health Concern of International Proportions Second Edition
Richard R Roach, Donald E Greydanus, Dilip R Patel and Joav Merrick (Editors)
2015. ISBN: 978-1-63463-381-9 (Hardcover)
2015. ISBN: 978-1-63463-404-5 (e-book)

Child and Adolescent Health Issues (A Tribute to the Pediatrician Donald E Greydanus)
Joav Merrick (Editor)
2015. ISBN: 978-1-63463-574-5 (Hardcover)
2015. ISBN: 978-1-63463-576-9 (e-book)

Child Health and Human Development Yearbook 2014
Joav Merrick (Editor)
2015. ISBN: 978-1-63482-163-6 (Hardcover)
2015. ISBN: 978-1-63482-207-7 (e-book)

Behavioral Pediatrics, 4th Edition
Donald E Greydanus, Dilip R Patel, Helen D Pratt, Joseph L Calles Jr, Ahsan Nazeer and Joav Merrick (Editors)
2015. ISBN: 978-1-63483-027-0 (Hardcover)
2015. ISBN: 978-1-63483-052-2 (e-book)

Disability, Chronic Disease and Human Development
Joav Merrick
2015. ISBN: 978-1-63483-029-4 (Hardcover)
2015. ISBN: 978-1-63483-057-7 (e-book)

Caribbean Adolescents: Some Public Health Concerns
Cecilia Hegamin-Younge and Joav Merrick (Editors)
2015. ISBN: 978-1-63483-341-7 (Hardcover)
2015. ISBN: 978-1-63483-343-1 (e-book)

Adolescence and Health: Some International Perspectives
Joav Merrick (Editor)
2015. ISBN: 978-1-63483-791-0 (Hardcover)
2015. ISBN: 978-1-63483-808-5 (e-book)

Youth Suicide Prevention: Everybody's Business
Hatim A Omar (Editor)
2015. ISBN: 978-1-63483-786-6 (Softcover)
2015. ISBN: 978-1-63483-820-7 (e-book)

Human Developmental Research: Experience from Research in Hong Kong
Daniel TL Shek, Cecilia Ma, Yu Lu and Joav Merrick (Editors)
2014. ISBN: 978-1-62808-166-4 (Hardcover)
2013. ISBN: 978-1-62808-167-1 (e-book)

School, Adolescence and Health Issues
Joav Merrick, Ariel Tenenbaum and Hatim A Omar (Editors)
2014. ISBN: 978-1-62948-702-1 (Hardcover)
2014. ISBN: 978-1-62948-707-6 (e-book)

Adolescence and Sexuality: International Perspectives
Joav Merrick, Ariel Tenenbaum and Hatim A Omar (Editors)
2014. ISBN: 978-1-62948-711-3 (Hardcover)
2014. ISBN: 978-1-62948-724-3 (e-book)

Child and Adolescent Health Yearbook 2013
Joav Merrick (Editor)
2014. ISBN: 978-1-63117-658-6 (Hardcover)
2014. ISBN: 978-1-63117-668-5 (e-book)

Adoption: The Search for a New Parenthood
Gary Diamond and Eva Arbel
2014. ISBN: 978-1-63117-710-1 (Hardcover)
2014. ISBN: 978-1-63117-713-2 (e-book)

Adolescence: Places and Spaces
Myra F Taylor, Julie Ann Pooley and Joav Merrick (Editors)
2014. ISBN: 978-1-63117-847-4 (Hardcover)
2014. ISBN: 978-1-63117-850-4 (e-book)

Born into this World: Health Issues
Donald E Greydanus, Arthur N Feinberg, and Joav Merrick (Editors)
2014. ISBN: 978-1-63321-667-9 (Hardcover)
2014. ISBN: 978-1-63321-669-3 (e-book)

Child Health and Human Development Yearbook 2013
Joav Merrick (Editor)
2014. ISBN: 978-1-63117-939-6 (Hardcover)
2013. ISBN: 978-1-63117-958-7 (e-book)

Caring for the Newborn: A Comprehensive Guide for the Clinician
Donald E Greydanus, Arthur N Feinberg and Joav Merrick (Editors)
2014. ISBN: 978-1-63321-760-7 (Hardcover)
2014. ISBN: 978-1-63321-781-2 (e-book)

Environment and Hope: Impoving Health, Reducing AIDS and Promoting Food Security in the World
Leslie Rubin and Joav Merrick (Editors)
2014. ISBN: 978-1-63321-772-0 (Hardcover)
2014. ISBN: 978-1-63321-782-9 (e-book)

Pain Management Yearbook 2013
Joav Merrick (Editor)
2014. ISBN: 978-1-63117-944-0 (Hardcover)
2014. ISBN: 978-1-63117-959-4 (e-book)

Pediatric and Adolescent Dermatology: Some Current Issues
Donald E Greydanus, Arthur N Feinberg and Joav Merrick (Editors)
2014. ISBN: 978-1-63321-853-6 (Hardcover)
2014. ISBN: 978-1-63321-863-5 (e-book)

Adolescence and Behavior Issues in a Chinese Context
Daniel TL Shek, Rachel CF Sun, and Joav Merrick (Editors)
2013. ISBN: 978-1-62618-614-9 (Hardcover)
2013. ISBN: 978-1-62618-692-7 (e-book)

Advances in Preterm Infant Research
Jing Sun, Nicholas Buys and Joav Merrick
2013. ISBN: 978-1-62618-696-5 (Hardcover)
2013. ISBN: 978-1-62618-775-7 (e-book)

Child Health and Human Development: Social, Economic and Environmental Factors
Leslie Rubin and Joav Merrick (Editors)
2013. ISBN: 978-1-62948-166-1 (Hardcover)
2013. ISBN: 978-1-62948-169-2 (e-book)

Children, Violence and Bullying: International Perspectives
Joav Merrick, Isack Kandel and Hatim A Omar (Editors)
2013. ISBN: 978-1-62948-342-9 (Hardcover)
2013. ISBN: 978-1-62948-345-0 (e-book)

Chinese Adolescent Development: Economic Disadvantages, Parents and Intrapersonal Development
Daniel TL Shek, Rachel CF Sun and Joav Merrick (Editors)
2013. ISBN: 978-1-62618-622-4 (Hardcover)
2013. ISBN: 978-1-62618-694-1 (e-book)

Chronic Disease and Disability in Childhood
Joav Merrick
2013. ISBN: 978-1-62808-865-6 (Hardcover)
2013. ISBN: 978-1-62808-868-7 (e-book)

Environmental Health Disparities in Children: Asthma, Obesity and Food
Leslie Rubin and Joav Merrick (Editors)
2013. ISBN: 978-1-62948-122-7 (Hardcover)
2013. ISBN: 978-1-62948-135-7 (e-book)

Environmental Health: Home, School and Community
Leslie Rubin and Joav Merrick (Editors)
2013. ISBN: 978-1-62948-155-5 (Hardcover)
2013. ISBN: 978-1-62948-158-6 (e-book)

Guidelines for the Healthy Integration of the Ill Child in the Educational System: Experience from Israel
Yosefa Isenberg
2013. ISBN: 978-1-62808-350-7 (Hardcover)
2013. ISBN: 978-1-62808-353-8 (e-book)

Internet Addiction: A Public Health Concern in Adolescence
Artemis Tsitsika, Mari Janikian, Donald E Greydanus, Hatim A Omar and Joav Merrick (Editors)
2013. ISBN: 978-1-62618-925-6 (Hardcover)
2013. ISBN: 978-1-62618-959-1 (e-book)

Playing with Fire: Children, Adolescents and Firesetting
Hatim A. Omar, Carrie Howell Bowling and Joav Merrick (Editors)
2013. ISBN: 978-1-62948-471-6 (Softcover)
2013. ISBN: 978-1-62948-474-7 (e-book)

Promotion of Holistic Development of Young People in Hong Kong
Daniel TL Shek, Tak Yan Lee and Joav Merrick (Editors)
2013. ISBN: 978-1-62808-019-3 (Hardcover)
2013. ISBN: 978-1-62808-040-7 (e-book)

University and College Students: Health and Development Issues for the Leaders of Tomorrow
Daniel TL Shek, Rachel CF and Joav Merrick (Editors)
2013. ISBN: 978-1-62618-586-9 (Hardcover)
2013. ISBN: 978-1-62618-612-5 (e-book)

Break the Cycle of Environmental Health Disparities: Maternal and Child Health Aspects
Leslie Rubin and Joav Merrick (Editors)
2013. ISBN: 978-1-62948-107-4 (Hardcover)
2013. ISBN: 978-1-62948-133-3 (e-book)

Child and Adolescent Health Yearbook 2012
Joav Merrick (Editor)
2012. ISBN: 978-1-61942-788-4 (Hardcover)
2012. ISBN: 978-1-61942-789-1 (e-book)

Child Health and Human Development Yearbook 2011
Joav Merrick (Editor)
2012. ISBN: 978-1-61942-969-7 (Hardcover)
2012. ISBN: 978-1-61942-970-3 (e-book)

Child and Adolescent Health Yearbook 2011
Joav Merrick (Editor)
2012. ISBN: 978-1-61942-782-2 (Hardcover)
2012. ISBN: 978-1-61942-783-9 (e-book)

Tropical Pediatrics: A Public Health Concern of International Proportions
Richard R Roach, Donald E Greydanus, Dilip R Patel, Douglas N Homnick and Joav Merrick (Editors)
2012. ISBN: 978-1-61942-831-7 (Hardcover)
2012. ISBN: 978-1-61942-840-9 (e-book)

Child Health and Human Development Yearbook 2012
Joav Merrick (Editor)
2012. ISBN: 978-1-61942-978-9 (Hardcover)
2012. ISBN: 978-1-61942-979-6 (e-book)

Developmental Issues in Chinese Adolescents
Daniel TL Shek, Rachel CF Sun and Joav Merrick (Editors)
2012. ISBN: 978-1-62081-262-4 (Hardcover)
2012. ISBN: 978-1-62081-270-9 (e-book)

Positive Youth Development: Theory, Research and Application
Daniel TL Shek, Rachel CF Sun and Joav Merrick (Editors)
2012. ISBN: 978-1-62081-305-8 (Hardcover)
2012. ISBN: 978-1-62081-347-8 (e-book)

Understanding Autism Spectrum Disorder: Current Research Aspects
Ditza A Zachor and Joav Merrick (Editors)
2012. ISBN: 978-1-62081-353-9 (Hardcover)
2012. ISBN: 978-1-62081-390-4 (e-book)

Positive Youth Development: A New School Curriculum to Tackle Adolescent Developmental Issues
Hing Keung Ma, Daniel TL Shek and Joav Merrick (Editors)
2012. ISBN: 978-1-62081-384-3 (Hardcover)
2012. ISBN: 978-1-62081-385-0 (e-book)

Transition from Pediatric to Adult Medical Care
David Wood, John G Reiss, Maria E Ferris, Linda R Edwards and Joav Merrick (Editors)
2012. ISBN: 978-1-62081-409-3 (Hardcover)
2012. ISBN: 978-1-62081-412-3 (e-book)

PEDIATRICS, CHILD AND ADOLESCENT HEALTH

CHILD AND ADOLESCENT HEALTH

SOME RECENT RESEARCH

ARIEL TENENBAUM, MD
AND
JOAV MERRICK, MD, MMEDSCI, DMSC
EDITORS

nova
Medicine & Health
New York

Library of Congress Cataloging-in-Publication Data

Names: Tenenbaum, Ariel, editor. | Merrick, Joav, 1950- editor.
Title: Child and adolescent health: some recent research / [edited by] Ariel Tenenbaum, Joav Merrick.
Identifiers: LCCN 2020016366 (print) | LCCN 2020016367 (ebook) | ISBN 9781536178258 (hardcover) | ISBN 9781536178265 (adobe pdf)
Subjects: LCSH: Children--Health and hygiene. | Teenagers--Health and hygiene.
Classification: LCC RJ101 .C5174 2020 (print) | LCC RJ101 (ebook) | DDC 618.92--dc23
LC record available at https://lccn.loc.gov/2020016366
LC ebook record available at https://lccn.loc.gov/2020016367

Published by Nova Science Publishers, Inc. † New York

CONTENTS

Introduction **1**

Chapter 1 Youth, cannabis, alcohol and more **3**
Ariel Tenenbaum and Joav Merrick

Section one: Infancy and early childhood **7**

Chapter 2 Infant mortality in Indiana: Perceived beliefs and attitudes of individuals living in the State **9**
Cecilia Obeng, Priscilla A. Barnes, Theresa Hunter and Melissa Weinstein

Chapter 3 Growth of the craniofacial complex and its relationship to common first and second pharyngeal arch malformations: A narrative review **23**
Kazlin N Mason, John W Stockstill and Jamie L Perry

Chapter 4 Pediatric immunizations: Review and discussion on protection of our children and adolescents **45**
Donald E Greydanus and Marisha G Agana

Chapter 5 Ingestion of a hickory tussock caterpillar: A case report **105**
Anna Jain, Patrick Jones and Dilip R Patel

Chapter 6 A multilevel modeling analysis of predictors of neonatal hypoglycemia among diabetic and non-diabetic mothers **111**
Brook T Alemu, Matthew Hoch, Bonnie Van Lunen and Muge Akpinar-Elci

Chapter 7 Identifying factors associated with autism spectrum disorder based on a comprehensive national survey **129**
Kotwoallama R Zerbo, Chen Mo, Jingjing Yin and Hani M Samawi

Section two: From cannabis to food **157**

Chapter 8 Medical cannabinoids in treatment resistant epilepsy disorders **159**
Yasmeen Razvi, Stephanie Chan, Angelo Fefekos, Henry Lam, Carlo DeAngelis and Edward Chow

Chapter 9 The mechanistic role of cytoadherence in thalassemia's protection against malaria **171**
Leena Elbedour, Salman Elbedour and Mohammed Hassan Almasudi

Chapter 10 Food insecurity and BMI for children and adolescents across six grade levels **199**
Oliver W Edwards and Whitney Shipman

Chapter 11 Food for thought: A review of severe acute malnutrition research in the 21st century **215**
Michael T Kody and Shannon Elizabeth Kody

Chapter 12 Food additives: An overview of health implications and regulation and control in the United States **229**
Sharmeen Samuel, Kelly Brown and Dilip R Patel

Section three: Adolescent health **243**

Chapter 13 The relationship between bilingualism and cognitive development among Saudi Arabian school-aged children **245**
Salman Elbedour, Manal Ahmad Sawan, Joseph A Bawalsah, Anan Abu Mariam, Hussien Tarawneh and Gregory Reed

Chapter 14 School psychology: A case study and needs assessment in Riyadh, Saudi Arabia **263**
Mona I Alsoqaih, Salman Elbedour, Gregory Reed, Kamilah Woodson and Joav Merrick

Chapter 15 Exploring physical activity engagement in secondary school students in Montevideo, Uruguay: A qualitative study **293**
Irene Parobii, Andrew E Springer, Melissa B Harrell, Lucía Martinez Gomensoro, María Traversa Fresco, Nianest Alers, Cheryl L Perry and Diego Estol

Chapter 16 Cyberbullying in colleges and universities: A survey of student experiences and attitudes about cyberbullying **313**
Salihah Alqahtani, Salman Elbedour, Kimberley Freeman, Gregory Reed, Kamilah Woodson Reed and Joav Merrick

Chapter 17 Adolescent confidentiality concerns and use of sensitive health services: A retrospective cohort study of AddHealth participants **361**
Kenesha Smith Barber and Larissa R Brunner Huber

Chapter 18 Self-efficacy of overweight and obese youth participating in a multidisciplinary after-school program **377**
Victoria N Ivy, Karen L Gaudreault and Timothy Baghurst

Chapter 19 Anti-doping knowledge of junior international racquetball athletes **405**
Timothy Baghurst

Section four: Acknowledgments **415**

Chapter 20 About the editors **417**

Chapter 21 About the Center for Children with Chronic Diseases and Down Syndrome Center Jerusalem, Israel, Department of Pediatrics, Mt Scopus Campus, Hadassah Hebrew University Medical Center, Jerusalem, Israel **419**

Chapter 22 About the National Institute of Child Health and Human Development in Israel **423**

Section five: Index **427**

Index **429**

INTRODUCTION

In: Child and Adolescent Health
Editors: A Tenenbaum and J Merrick
ISBN: 978-1-53617-825-8

Chapter 1

YOUTH, CANNABIS, ALCOHOL AND MORE

Ariel Tenenbaum[1-3], MD
and Joav Merrick[2-5,*], MD, MMedSci, DMSc
[1]Center for Children with Chronic Diseases and Down Syndrome Center Jerusalem, Israel, [2]Department of Pediatrics, Mt Scopus Campus, Hadassah Hebrew University Medical Center, Jerusalem, Israel, [3]National Institute of Child Health and Human Development, Jerusalem, Israel, [4]Kentucky Children's Hospital, University of Kentucky, Lexington, Kentucky, United States of America and [5]Center for Healthy Development, School of Public Health, Georgia State University, Atlanta, Georgia, United States of America

ABSTRACT

Tobacco, alcohol, cannabis and adolescence are all going together and should be of a public health concern now that many states have legalized the sale and use of cannabis. More thought and research is needed to identify which programs and prevention strategies are most effective in reducing youth use and initiation of marijuana. In this book we have

* Corresponding Author's Email: jmerrick@zahav.net.il.

gathered work by international researchers and present papers on infant mortality in Indiana, discussion of pediatric immunizations, medical cannabis for epilepsy, issues concerned with food insecurity, food additives, various aspects of adolescent health, cyberbullying and much more that we hope will be of interest to the reader.

INTRODUCTION

There are several substances inhaled for the development of euphoria, like marijuana (cannabis, pot), methamphetamine, heroin, crack cocaine, phencyclidine and nitrites (amyl and butyl) (1). Marijuana has been known to Homo sapiens for thousands of years and concern has been raised over the past two centuries regarding its potential adverse effects – leading to various laws in the United States and other countries to control its production and use (1). The psychoactive chemical, delta-9-tetrahydrocannabinol (THC) was isolated in the mid-1960s, while other aspects of the endocannabinoid system [cannabinoid receptors (CB1 and CB2) and key endogenous cannabinoids (2-arachidonoyl glycerol and anandamide)] were identified over 20 years later. Though use of phytocannabinoids are being increasing linked to improvement of some health conditions, frequent users of cannabis are at increased risk for adverse effects, which can lead to additional health problems (1). Research is identifying components of cannabis which are not psychoactive and may become established parts of the pharmacopeia as the twenty-first century continues.

LEGAL ASPECTS

Since the year 2012, purchase of recreational or retail marijuana has become legal for persons aged over 21 years in the District of Columbia, Alaska, California, Colorado, Maine, Massachusetts, Nevada, Oregon and Washington (2). The law taxing and regulating recreational or retail marijuana was approved by Washington voters in 2012 and the first retail licenses were issued in July 2014, while medical marijuana use has been legal since 1998 (2).

WASHINGTON STATE

In order to examine the prevalence, characteristics and behaviors of marijuana users among 10th grade students, the Washington State Department of Health analyzed data from the state's 2014 Healthy Youth Survey (HYS) (2).

In 2014, 18.1% of 10th grade students (age 15-16 years) reported using marijuana during the preceding 30 days and 32% reported using it for more than 10 days (2). So how did these young kids receive the marijuana? 65% reported attaining marijuana through their peer networks, like friends, older siblings or at a party.

The use of marijuana for this group of teenagers differed by race, ethnicity and school performance and the prevalence was highest among American Indian or Alaska Native students. The survey also showed that youths who used marijuana also were more likely to report alcohol and e-cigarette use than youths who did not use marijuana (2).

SOME THOUGHTS

Generalized consumption of the unprocessed marijuana plant can lead to considerable public health risks including increased schizophrenia, psychosis, dependence, and other risks (1). A medical role for specific cannabinoid compounds remains under active medical research, but what is well-known is that there are many potential medical and psychiatric adverse effects to smoking cannabis and its synthetic derivatives. Links between use of alcohol, cannabis and other illicit drugs continues to be unveiled by research (1).

Regular marijuana use in adolescence is associated with impaired school performance and an increased risk for early school dropout and preventing marijuana initiation and use can avoid harms associated with marijuana (1,2). As more states move to legalize marijuana for medical use or retail purchase, concerns about new and broader access to marijuana by youths are increasing.

Tobacco, alcohol, cannabis and adolescence are all going together and should be of a public health concern now that many states have legalized the sale and use of cannabis. More thought and research is needed to identify which programs and prevention strategies are most effective in reducing youth use and initiation of marijuana.

Finally, treatment of an individual with cannabis dependence is very difficult and requires more research and indeed this controversial plant known for thousands of years, remains disputatious and contentious even in the twenty-first century (1).

This Book

In this book we have gathered work by international researchers and present papers on infant mortality in Indiana, discussion of pediatric immunizations, medical cannabis for epilepsy, issues concerned with food insecurity, food additives, various aspects of adolescent health, cyberbullying and much more that we hope will be of interest to the reader.

References

[1] Gredydanus DE, Hawver EK, Greydanus MM, Merrick J. Marijuana: Current concepts. Front Public Health 2013;1:42. doi.org/10.3389/fpubh.2013.00042.

[2] Shah A, Stahre M. Marijuama use amomng 10th grade students: Washington, 2014. MMWR 2016;65(5051):1421-4.

SECTION ONE: INFANCY AND EARLY CHILDHOOD

In: Child and Adolescent Health
Editors: A Tenenbaum and J Merrick
ISBN: 978-1-53617-825-8

Chapter 2

INFANT MORTALITY IN INDIANA: PERCEIVED BELIEFS AND ATTITUDES OF INDIVIDUALS LIVING IN THE STATE

Cecilia Obeng*, PhD,
Priscilla A. Barnes, MPH, PhD, MCHES,
Theresa Hunter, MPH, MS, PhD, CHES
and Melissa Weinstein, MPH, PhD
Indiana University Bloomington School of Public Health,
Bloomington, Indiana and Curry College,
Milton, Massachusetts, United States of America

ABSTRACT

The state of Indiana has one of the highest infant mortality rates in the United States. Although state level assessments suggest that numerous social, economic, and environmental factors are the root causes of death for infants, individuals in local communities may have a different

* Correspondence: Cecilia S Obeng, PhD, School of Public Health, Indiana University, 1025 E 7th St, suite 116, Bloomington, IN 47405, United States. Email: cobeng@indiana.edu.

perspective of the issue. *Objective*: The purpose of this study was to explore what individuals currently living in Indiana perceive as important for deceasing infant mortality in Indiana. Study Groups: Two hundred and twenty-one (n=221) participants from Indiana participated in the research. *Methods*: A self-administered eight-item survey was used asking participants to provide a brief definition of infant mortality, if Indiana's infant mortality rate was higher than the national average, and their thoughts and ideas for decreasing it. *Results*: Participants (41.3%) were not aware of Indiana's infant mortality problem. Healthcare organizations were perceived to be the "ideal" space in the community to educate young mothers and families about infant mortality to help decrease it. *Conclusion*: Understanding knowledge and attitudes can help health educators create strategic alliances in local communities as well as with the state health department to: 1) develop health communication campaigns and 2) improve healthcare policies that influence the health of Indiana's most vulnerable population.

INTRODUCTION

Historically, Indiana has had a higher infant mortality rate than other states in the United States, especially those in the Midwest region. In particular, for over a century, Indiana has reported an infant mortality rate of greater than 6.9 and has consistently been ranked among the worst in the nation (1). In 2013, there were 594 infant deaths across the state creating an alarming infant mortality rate of 7.1 (1). This rate was higher than the national average of 5.96 and the Healthy People 2020 goal of 6.0.

Recent state-level assessments revealed that the primary causes of infant mortality include: preterm births, congenital malformations, disorders related to short gestation and low birth rate, sudden infant death syndrome (SIDS), maternal complications during pregnancy, and injuries such as suffocation (1). These factors have been known to account for more than half of all infant deaths, with preterm birth being the most frequent cause (2). Lifestyle factors, such as smoking during pregnancy and obesity also influence the state's infant mortality (1). Indiana smoking rate during pregnancy of 15.7% nearly doubled that of the national average of 8.5% (1). This ranks Indiana among the top 10 worst states in the nation. Secondhand smoke also has a strong correlation with infant mortality.

Infants who die from SIDS have higher concentrations of nicotine in their lungs and higher levels of cotinine than infants who die from other causes (3). Overall, Indiana ranks last (50th) among all states for adult smoking rates (4). Although there are numerous smoke-free initiatives being implemented across the state. Indiana also has a high ranking of adults who smoke indoors, as well as outdoors, and in the workplace (4).

While data suggest that social, economic, and environmental factors are the root causes of these disparities, individuals in local communities who are directly or indirectly impacted by infant mortality may have a different perspective of the issue. In order for individuals to come together in local communities to address these issues related to infant mortality, they must be aware that infant mortality is a problem. Exploring community members' perceptions about infant mortality can assist in the development of educational initiatives and community interventions that are tailored for specific populations. Another area of interest is identifying the most influential and appropriate 'spaces and places' of dispersing educational materials and disseminating information to the public. Understanding the causes of infant death provides a perspective on a population's need for resources, policies, and healthcare that influence the health of Indiana's most vulnerable population.

Aim

The purpose of this study was to explore what individuals currently living in Indiana perceive as important for disseminating information about infant mortality. Specifically, the research questions under examination are:

- Are individuals living in Indiana aware of the state's infant mortality rate?
- What places/networks do these individuals consider as most effective in delivering information about maternal and child health?

- In what ways do individuals think infant mortality should be addressed?

OUR STUDY

A self-administered eight-item survey was used in this study. The survey included demographic information such as gender, age, race/ethnicity, and current city. Participants were also asked if Indiana's infant mortality rate was higher than the national average, and their thoughts and ideas for decreasing it. In addition, participants rated the places/networks that may be ideal to provide education about infant mortality. These places/networks were: faith based organizations, hospitals, community health centers, doctor's offices, schools, local health departments, TV/radio, social media, posters, and word of mouth. Questions were a mixture of categorical (yes/no), ordinal (Likert scale ranging from 1 to 5), and open-ended questions. A pilot study was completed by two of the authors and two research assistants. The main aim of the pilot study was to check whether participants would have problems understanding how the research questions were worded and the content of the questions. None of the participants (n=25) who participated in the pilot study were invited to participate in the main study because we did not want those who had previous knowledge on the questions to participate.

Sample and data collection

Individuals were eligible to participate in this study if they lived in Indiana at the time the survey was administered and were at least 18 years old. Surveys were administered in various places including university/college classrooms, the YMCA, grocery stores, and places of worship. Data were collected from March – May 2015. The survey was also administered online using Qualtrics. An email explaining the purpose and the rationale for the research was sent to points of contact affiliated with community coalitions, local health departments, health professional associations, and community-based providers. The survey link was also posted on Facebook. Using the Internet to collect quantitative, and especially, qualitative data collection is not a new practice; the above approach can yield "in-depth, effectively rich, creative, detailed responses" (5-6). Furthermore, using the internet to collect data is seen by scholars who use them as the most efficient way to collect data, because of the privacy that participants have in internet data collection (7).

Data analysis

Data were analyzed using SPSS statistical software version 22.0. Overall, 230 surveys were collected. Researchers first reviewed responses in the dataset to ensure that the eligibility criteria for sampling was met. Nine responses were removed because participants reported not living in Indiana at the time of the survey. Once cleaned, percentages were calculated for sex, age, education, and race/ethnicity, awareness about Indiana's infant mortality rate, and suggested places/networks to educate individuals about infant mortality.

Narrative approach (8) was used to solicit participants' attitudes and beliefs about infant mortality. This approach was deemed appropriate in this study because knowledge transferred through people's discourses is known to be useful in providing information about their (participants') views and thoughts about the subject-matter as well as what they believe will work in their communities. Content analysis was used in which units of the data deemed important were read several times by two researchers and were compared in order to generate categories (9). These two approaches were used to determine how infant mortality could be reduced in Indiana.

FINDINGS

Participants' age ranged between 18 and 68 years old (see Table 1). The majority of participants were female (89.1%) and between 18 and 25 years old. About 80.5% of participants identified as White, 9.5% identified as Black, and 5% identified as Hispanic. Five percent did not report their race. Over half of participants (55.2%) reported having an undergraduate or graduate degree and 36.5% reported having at least some college education. Additionally, 32.6% of participants were currently enrolled as an undergraduate college student at a university in the state of Indiana.

Table 1. Descriptive profile of participants by sex, age, education, and race/ethnicity, (n=221)*

Characteristics	**(n)%**
Sex	
Males	24 (10.4))
Females	205 (89.1)
Age	
18-29	113 (51.1)
30-39	35 (15.8)
40-49	35 (15.8)
50-59	22 (10.0)
60+	13 (6.3)
Education	
High school graduate or G.E.D.	15 (6.8)
Some college	65 (29.4)
Technical school/Associate's Degree	5 (2.3)
College degree (4 years or more)	72 (32.6)
Graduate/Professional degree	56 (25.3)
Race/Ethnicity	
Asian American	1 (0.5)
Native American/American Indian	3 (1.4)
Two or more races	3 (1.4)
Hispanic/Latino	11 (5.0)
African American/Black	21 (9.5)
Caucasian/White	178 (80.5)

*Missing data for sex (n= 1) age (n=2); race(n=4); and education (n=8).

Awareness of infant mortality and preferred networks

In regards to knowledge related to Indiana's infant mortality issue, only 58.7% of participants were aware that Indiana has a higher infant mortality rate than the national average. Participants viewed primary care provider offices (44.3%) and community health centers (40.3%) as the most effective places/networks to consider in promoting infant mortality initiatives. Posters (31.7%) were viewed as somewhat effective (see Table 2).

Table 2. Community Organizations and Information Networks to Promote Infant Mortality Initiatives, Number (Percent) Responses (n=221)

	Least effective	Somewhat Effective	Average	Effective	Most Effective
Community Organizations					
Faith-Based Organizations	30 (13.6)	36 (16.3)	75 (33.9)	50 (22.6)	29 (13.1)
Hospitals	7 (3.2)	16 (7.2)	43 (19.5)	70 (31.7)	85 (38.5)
Community health centers	1 (0.5)	6 (2.7)	45 (20.4)	78 (35.3)	89 (40.3)
Primary care provider offices	5 (2.3)	9 (4.1)	44 (19.9)	64 (29.0)	98 (44.3)
Schools	8 (3.6)	38 (17.2)	54 (24.4)	71 (32.1)	50 (22.6)
Information Networks					
Local health departments	6 (2.7)	18 (8.1)	66 (29.9)	75 (33.9)	55 (24.9)
TV/Radio	25 (11.3)	36 (16.3)	62 (28.1)	61 (27.6)	34 (15.4)
Social media	10 (4.5)	22 (10.0)	57 (25.8)	71 (32.1)	55 (24.9)
Posters	26 (11.8)	70 (31.7)	77 (34.8)	36 (16.3)	10 (4.5)
Word of mouth	16 (7.2)	50 (22.6)	52 (23.5)	54 (24.4)	46 (20.8)

Proposed implementation strategies

Concerning the question regarding what participants think Indiana should do to decrease infant mortality, four prominent themes emerged from our coding. The themes included: (a) increasing education to prevent infant mortality; (b) increasing health care for pregnant women and their children; (c) developing effective policies; and (d) addressing social determinants contributing to infant mortality.

Increasing education to prevent infant mortality

The majority of participants (n= 108, 48.9%) indicated that public health programs should focus on three areas: preconception health care, prenatal care, and care after baby's birth. For preconception health care, it was mentioned that mothers should receive information and resources about living a healthier lifestyle that includes increasing nutritional, alcohol, and tobacco education/outreach for new and expecting mothers. Participants recommended that education about risks associated with infant mortality and community resources should be emphasized to new parents during the prenatal period. Decreasing early elective deliveries by carrying babies full term (40 weeks) was another recommendation. Some participants noted that all first time parents should be required to take a course before their child is born and the course should be offered in hospitals, as well as in the communities to expectant mothers (families) on the health and care of their infants. They also noted that it is important to educate women and parents on the importance of going to doctors during pregnancy.

It was indicated that the sleeping practices of children (children sleeping on their stomach) and awareness of the dangers of co-sleeping were crucial to prevent infant mortality. They also called for more breastfeeding education and support for all mothers. Some participants stated that all schools should be required to educate Indiana residents about infant mortality. Participants also asked for word to be spread about infant mortality via advertisements and public service announcements.

Increasing health care access for pregnant women and their children

Participants (n= 50, 22.6%) indicated that affordable and accessible prenatal care as well as postnatal and parenting support should be provided for families, especially in rural areas. They suggested for better financial support for postnatal care for all at-risk babies, and a very close following of such children during their first year. Research participants also suggested for an increase in social services for low-income Indiana residents, especially food stamps to ensure that both mothers and babies have sufficient food nutrients. In this regard, they suggested that stake holders make certain that after each birth, the mother had available, is offered, and also aware of all resources, and help that are available for her new baby such as nutrition education for mothers and their children, physicians' names and appointment schedules, housing assistance, and child care resources. They suggested providing emotional support to families during pregnancy and the postpartum period through community-based programs. Participants recommended that financial incentives should be provided to health care providers that utilize evidence-based practices. In addition, more funding opportunities should be available to organizations dedicated to providing care to at-risk populations. Travel vouchers should also be available for pregnant women and families with young children to go to clinics or hospitals.

Developing effective policies

Participants (n=23, 10.4%) recommended that more funding be allocated to for programs like Women, Infant, and Children (WIC) and to specifically look at what other states with low rates are doing. They noted that it was important and necessary for there be more support to encourage mothers to graduate from high school, which would help to increase prospects for mothers to better themselves economically and socially. Participants also suggested offering doula services to low-income mothers/families. The need for more midwives in hospitals and at home was greatly amplified, as was the need to address socioeconomic stressors that affect health outcomes. Additionally, participants called for an increase of funding for mother-baby services and birth prevention services as well as affordable healthcare for economically challenged citizens.

Addressing social determinants contributing to infant mortality

A smaller percent of participants (n=15, 6.8%) acknowledged the fact that drug use is a problem in Indiana and that it is essential to come up with strategies to decrease smoking rates, stop smoking around children, quit using substances while pregnant and decrease prenatal smoking. They also suggested drug testing parents, and for an expansive testing on prenatal patients in general. Participants also recommended having more follow-up resources specifically for mothers. Some of them felt special attention should be given to furthering exploring root causes of health inequity in an effort to reduce rates of pregnancy among teenagers as well as people from low socioeconomic backgrounds.

DISCUSSION

The main focus of this research was to examine the views of individuals living in Indiana as well as explore the most appropriate avenues to disseminate information related to challenges in reducing the state's infant mortality rate. In considering participants' views of infant mortality, this study revealed that some participants were not aware of Indiana's infant mortality problem. Healthcare organizations were perceived to be the "ideal" space in the community to educate young mothers and families by sharing information (e.g., brochures, in-person counseling) and facilitating small group support groups and interventions. This exploratory study provides a "grassroots" perspective from individuals who may or may not be directly impacted by a health issue that impacts vulnerable populations. These populations include persons of low socioeconomic status, racial and ethnic minorities, young mothers, and women living in communities with limited access to healthcare. Understanding knowledge and attitudes can help health educators create strategic alliances in local communities as well as with the state health department to: 1) develop health communication campaigns and 2) improve healthcare policies that influence the health of Indiana's most vulnerable population.

While this study cannot be generalized to represent all individuals currently living in Indiana, these findings do support the need for increased awareness and education regarding infant mortality throughout the state. The participants' call for improvements in education in this study aligns with current efforts coordinated by the ISDH in cooperation with several public and private organizations. Sometime ago, Labor of Love, a public awareness campaign, was created to educate the public as well as health care professionals on issues that impact infant mortality. Overall, the venture focuses on the importance of early and regular prenatal care; safe sleep practices, avoidance of tobacco, drugs, and alcohol before, during, and after pregnancy, and breastfeeding (10). Each year, a state-wide summit is held in which health care professionals, community residents, and policy makers convene with renowned experts in maternal and child health, health disparities, health information technology, health care access to talk about and create strategies to address infant mortality.

A state-wide website (http://www.in.gov/laboroflove/) (11) is also available to key stakeholders that strategically markets resources throughout the state for women, new mothers, and expectant parents. The overall goal is to connect women and new parents with resources to maximize opportunities for infants to live at the highest quality of life possible (1). The results of this increased presence has yet to be evaluated. Future studies can explore the impact of this state-wide public awareness campaign in further facilitating use of information and human resources to organizations among mothers and new parents. Cleland (12) as well as Lindenbaum (13) and Bicego (14) study that found maternal education is an important predictor of childhood mortality. Studies may also examine differences health seeking information behavior based on maternal education.

Some individuals believed that drug use was an underlying cause for the infant mortality. Most the state's data points to tobacco use as a primary cause. Since this study was carried out in only one state (Indiana), the results and/or findings cannot be generalized to all states (residents) in the United States. Furthermore, in view of the fact that the surveyed participants had to be able to speak English, potential participants who could not speak English were excluded from the study. Thus, our sample was relatively homogeneous with regard to linguistic ability (ability to speak English) and that other key variables that could be related to infant mortality causation and curtailment may have been overlooked. Our partial reliance on email also suggests that some people without access to email who could not meet face-to-face with the research members had to be excluded from the study.

It is recommended that future researchers explore the interconnectedness between social and environmental issues and infant health. In particular, it is recommended that researchers examine the close connection between environmental toxins and infant mortality given the concern raised by the respondents about Indiana's drugs problem. Second, future studies should look at more states with the view in helping to generate ideas that is culturally relevant and appropriate for local communities. The above recommendation may be one initiative that could help tackle the infant mortality problem that is bedeviling Indiana and other states in the United States, and rest of the world.

Translation to health education practice

The findings from this study emphasize the need for a multi-faceted approach to address infant mortality. While it is important to educate expectant mothers, it is also essential to educate the general population on the risk factors related to infant mortality and the ways in which they can help address these health problems. Fathers, grandparents, family members, and caregivers need to be educated on the risks of infant mortality and steps they can take to help decrease the associated risk factors. Future studies in Indiana should examine the impact of other drugs including methamphetamine and other recreational drugs and its impact on infant mortality.

Identification of "access points" in local communities that can promote maternal and child services can significantly improve the use of effective services and programs. In this study, participants believed that primary care provider offices, community health centers and hospitals are important places to deliver infant mortality initiatives. Healthcare institutions primarily focus on early access to prenatal care. Prenatal care is essential to track fetal development, screen for abnormalities and complications, promote vitamin use for proper fetal growth and maternal health, and to decrease the risks that may threaten a healthy birthing process. Adequate use of prenatal care has been associated with improved birth weight and the reduction of the risk of preterm delivery, while inadequate use of prenatal care has been associated with increased risks of low-birth-weight births, premature births, and ultimately, infant mortality (3). Unfortunately only 67.3% of pregnant women in Indiana received prenatal care in the first trimester compared to a national average of 74.2% (1). This finding underscores that strategic partnerships to bridge the gap between population need and clinical services. Faith-based organizations and schools serve as key "access points" where family centered interventions can be administered. In addition, healthcare institutions can work in collaboration with these entities to create a unified message aimed at increasing awareness of infant mortality in Indiana.

REFERENCES

[1] Indiana State Department of Health [ISDH]. Indiana Mortality Report- 2013, 2015. URL: http://www.in.gov/isdh/reports/mortality/2013/index.htm.

[2] Callaghan WM, MacDorman MF, Rasmussen SA, Qin C, Lackritz E. The contribution of preterm birth to infant mortality rates in the United States. Pediatrics 2006;118:1566-73.

[3] Centers for Disease Control and Prevention. Health effects of secondhand smoke, 2014. URL: http://www.cdc.gov/tobacco/data_statistics/fact_sheets/secondhand_smoke/health_effects/index.htm.

[4] Indiana Perinatal Quality Improvement Collaborative. Addressing infant mortality in Indiana: A report to the IPQIC Governing Council 2007. URL: http://www.in.gov/isdh/files/Addressing_Infant_Mortality_in_Indiana.pdf.

[5] Suzuki L, Ahluwalia M, Arora A, Mattis J. The pond you fish in determines the fish you catch. Couns Psychol 2007;35(2):295-327.

[6] Shields C. Giving voice to students: Using the internet for data collection. Qual Res 2003;3(3):397-414.

[7] Hessler RM, Downing J, Beltz C, Pelliccio A, Powell M, Vale, W. Qualitative research on adolescent risk using e-mail: A methodological assessment. Qual Sociol 2003;26:111-24.

[8] Connelly F, Clandinin D. Stories of experience and narrative inquiry. Educ Res 1990:19(5):2-14.

[9] Mayring P. Qualitative content analysis. Forum Quai Soc Res 2000:1(2): 20.

[10] Indiana University Health. Labor-of-love, 2015. URL: http://iuhealth.org/blog/detail/labor-of-love-campaign-to-reduce-infant-deaths-in-indiana/#.VgiEJJfweK8.

[11] Indiana State Department of Health. Winter Newsletter, Public health matters. Labor of Love Campaign focuses on saving infants, 2015. URL: http://www.state.in.us/isdh/files/Winter_2015_newsletter.pdf.

[12] Cleland J, van Ginneken J. Maternal education and child survival in developing countries: The search for pathways of influence. Soc Sci Med 1988;27(12):1357-68.

[13] Lindenbaum S, Chakraborty M, Elias M. The influence of maternal education on infant and child mortality in Bangladesh. Dhaka: International Centre Diarrhoeal Disease Research, 1985.

[14] Bicego GT, Boerma JT. Maternal education and child survival: A comparative analysis of DHS Data. Proceed Demographic and Health Surveys World Conference, Vol. 1. Columbia, MD: IRD/Macro International, 1991:177-204.

In: Child and Adolescent Health
Editors: A Tenenbaum and J Merrick ISBN: 978-1-53617-825-8

Chapter 3

GROWTH OF THE CRANIOFACIAL COMPLEX AND ITS RELATIONSHIP TO COMMON FIRST AND SECOND PHARYNGEAL ARCH MALFORMATIONS: A NARRATIVE REVIEW

Kazlin N Mason[1,*], PhD, CCC-SLP, John W Stockstill[2], DDS and Jamie L Perry[1], PhD, CCC-SLP

[1]Department of Communication Sciences and Disorders, East Carolina University, Greenville, North Carolina, United States of America

[2]Center for Orthodontics, Seton Hill University, Greensburg, Pennsylvania, United States of America

---

* Correspondence: Ms Kazlin Mason, PhD, 2310B Allied Health Sciences Building, Department of Communication Sciences and Disorders, East Carolina University, Mail Stop 668 Greenville, NC 27834, United States.
Email: masonka14@students.ecu.edu; perryja@ecu.edu.

ABSTRACT

Craniofacial development is a complex progression that necessitates the assimilation of numerous dedicated embryological processes. This review provides an integration of the genetic underpinnings, craniofacial development, and clinical features related to deficiencies of the first and second pharyngeal arches. A focus on Pierre Robin Sequence (PRS) is presented. Review of the literature included searches of Medline, PubMed, Google Scholar, and online sources using search terms related to craniofacial development, specific gene patterns, neural crest development, and pharyngeal arch malformations. Associated terms in craniofacial biology, craniofacial physiology, and syndromic conditions were also used. This review serves as an introduction to current research regarding the genetic basis of craniofacial development and its relationship to pharyngeal arch development and PRS. Given the substantial influence of genetics in the development of the pharyngeal arches, craniofacial anomalies can frequently be traced to embryological deviations within these structures. Interruption in the embryological processes secondary to chromosomal abnormalities, genetic disorders, teratogenic effects, or mechanical factors can result in the mandibular deficits and subsequent lingual, airway, and palatal issues observed in pharyngeal arch malformations.

INTRODUCTION

Craniofacial development is a complex progression that necessitates the assimilation of numerous dedicated embryological processes and tissues. The first and second branchial or pharyngeal arches characterize the embryologic origin of early developing craniofacial structures. Interruption in the development of the pharyngeal arches can lead to a variety of anomalies. Thus, distinctive embryologic patterns result secondary to incremental progressions which produce a subtle anatomic pattern that can be observed clinically.

Craniofacial and auditory anomalies are traditionally associated with malformations of the first and second pharyngeal arches and have a common embryonic origin as well as similar periods of vulnerability that lead to speech, swallowing, masticatory, and hearing deficits throughout the lifespan. Understanding of the anatomic and embryological foundation is central in understanding anomalies in development. This narrative review uniquely synthesizes the embryological and genetic underpinnings of disorders related to the first and second pharyngeal arches. A specific focus on the craniofacial features of Pierre Robin sequence and its clinical considerations for surgical, dental and speech-language outcomes are presented.

SEARCH

Review of published literature involved searches of major databases including Medline, PubMed, Google Scholar, and online sources using search terms related to craniofacial development, specific gene patterns, neural crest development, and pharyngeal arch malformations. Associated terms in craniofacial biology, craniofacial physiology, and syndromic conditions were also used. Titles and abstracts were reviewed and relevant full text articles retrieved for inclusion. Additional articles were identified from reference lists of identified articles. Results are presented in a narrative form.

FINDINGS

Primary germ layers involved in embryological development include the ectoderm, mesoderm, endoderm, and neural crest cells. These create the central and peripheral nervous systems as well as the axial skeleton, connective tissue, and musculature, and have their primary origin within the pharyngeal arches. Past research has cited the importance of the neural crest cells in the embryological development process (1). However, recent studies have found that growth and the development of the craniofacial complex and pharynx is organized by the integration of the patterning systems of both the neural crest and endoderm (2). Prior to the development of the neural crest and patterning of the endoderm, embryogenesis must take place. During this time, crucial gene mapping occurs that controls the organization of the embryonic cell structure. Research utilizing serial analysis of gene expression (SAGE) and microarray identification has identified nearly 7,000 genes that are expressed in the first pharyngeal arch during the fourth and fifth weeks of gestation (3). Key gene families involved in craniofacial embryological development are described below.

Homeobox (HOX) Genes

The homeobox (HOX) genes are involved in the segmental organization of the anterior-posterior direction of the embryo and production depends on the combinatorial expression of the SHH and FGF genes, among others. The HOX genes establish the spatial identity of prospective craniofacial compartments as well as the rhombencephalon and are some of the key genes responsible for initiating craniofacial development (4). Within the HOX gene family, Msx genes play a significant role in craniofacial growth and odontogenesis (5). Expression of Msx1 in the mandibular mesenchyme additionally specifies patterning events for tooth formation (6). HOX genes play a role in neural crest specification and specific HOX genes pattern distinct subpopulations of the neural crest (7). Mutations in the HOX genes (specifically the Msx1 gene) can cause orofacial clefting and tooth agenesis (8, 9).

SHH genes

The sonic hedgehog (SHH) gene is involved in the patterning of the anterior-posterior axis for the embryonic development of limbs, gut formation, somites, and the establishment of the midline central nervous system. DeRobertis and colleagues (10) found that development of the craniofacial complex relies on the inductive activities of the prosencephalic and rhombencephalic organizing centers regulated by the SHH genes through a signaling protein in the neural floor plate cells. Mutation of the SHH pathway can result in disorders such as holoprosencephaly, a defect caused by a failure of the early forebrain to divide in distinct halves (11).

FGF genes

The fibroblast growth factor (FGF) genes are responsible for the stimulation of mitosis and differentiation of the underlying mesoderm. In the craniofacial region, the FGF gene family is involved in development of craniofacial structures through early patterning to growth regulation. With that, this gene provides for lengthening of the limbs, somite segmentation, angiogenesis, and axon growth. It additionally controls the anterior and posterior neural tube patterning (12). In craniofacial skeletogenesis, the FGF signal pathway assists in suture and synchondrosis regulation (7). Mutations of FGF receptors can result in syndromatic and non-syndromatic craniosynostosis (13). The Fgf10/Fgfr2b signal loop is crucial for palatogenesis and submandibular gland formation and interruption of the FGF signal is a possible mechanism of palatal clefting (7). The FGF signal is also a key regulator of tooth formation (14) and, in the absence of *Fgfr2b,* tooth development is arrested at the bud stage (15). Fgfr4 is additionally reported to be a key signal mediator in myogenesis (15).

Embryogenesis and the neural crest cells

During embryogenesis, the ectoderm and endoderm signal the facial mesenchyme which is composed of mesoderm and neural crest. The mesodermal component gives rise to the voluntary craniofacial muscles and endothelial cells, whereas the neural crest-derived mesenchyme forms the bulk of the craniofacial skeleton.

The neural crest cells are a significant contributor to craniofacial development and formation. Specification of the neural crest occurs at the early stages of embryonic development via transcription of the PAX7 gene (16). The neural crest cells travel from the dorsal site above the early developing brain to ventral locations that are determined by the HOX genes (17). Segmentation of the rhombencephalon results in the creation of the pharyngeal arches and facial prominences secondary to the sequencing and migration of the ectomesenchyme. During the fourth week of development, the neural crest mesenchyme migrates across the prosencephalon to develop the frontonasal prominence. Additionally, neural crest tissue from the first two rhombomeres migrates in a ventral direction, developing the first pharyngeal arch, which will create the maxillary and mandibular prominences (18). Neural crest tissue from the fourth rhombomere assists in the formation of the second pharyngeal arch. Many pharyngeal derivatives, including facial bones, are of neural crest origin (19). Thus, as neural crest cells migrate caudally and ventrally to encounter the pharyngeal endoderm, the formation of the branchial or pharyngeal arches is induced. The pharyngeal arches play a significant role in the development of the craniofacial morphology.

Given the substantial influence of the neural crest to the development of the pharyngeal arches, craniofacial anomalies can frequently be traced to deviations in the neural crest. Thus, as the craniofacial complex advances during this critical phase, deviation from normal development can result in craniofacial anomalies and/or syndromic conditions such as clefting or other hypoplasias.

Pharyngeal arch development

Neural crest cells migrate to the pharyngeal arches and serve an important role in the structural development of all arch derivatives. The pharyngeal arches are a series of tissues that give rise to structures of the face, ear, and neck. As described by Szabo-Rogers et al. (18), patterning of the pharyngeal arches is complex and requires cranial neural crest signaling, reciprocal signals from the arch mesoderm, as well as contributions from the underlying pharyngeal pouch endoderm and overlying ectoderm. The first pharyngeal arch appears during the fourth week of development, during which time an additional five arches form (Figure 1). The pharyngeal arches, also known as branchial arches, are structures that consist of an outer ectodermal layer and an inner endodermal layer. Between these two layers are mesodermal cores surrounded by mesenchyme derived from the neural crest. These paired structures contribute to the lower face, upper neck, and ear (19). Additionally, the somatic mesoderm contributes to the arch artery as well as the development of skeletal muscle tissue within each arch. The neural crest mesenchyme will become the bone, cartilage, and connective tissue within each arch.

Cranial nerves are additionally associated with each of the pharyngeal arches. Arch one is innervated by the trigeminal nerve. The facial nerve is associated with arch two and the glossopharyngeal nerve is associated with pharyngeal arch three. The superior branch of the vagus nerve is associated with arch four and the recurrent laryngeal branch of the vagus is associated with arch six (Table 1).

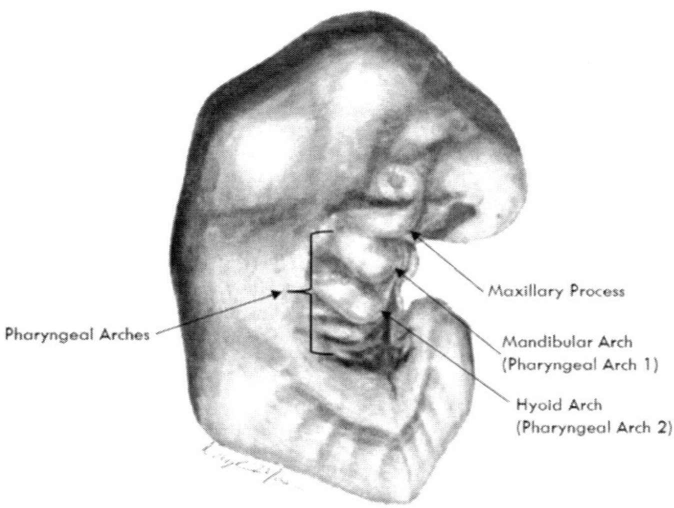

Figure 1. Illustration of the pharyngeal arches during the embryonic period of development.

Table 1. Pharyngeal arch derivatives

Arch	Cranial Nerve (CN)	Muscular Contribution	Cartilaginous Contribution	Associated Anomalies
1	CN V Mandibular branch of Trigeminal	Muscles of mastication Tensor tympani Tensor veli palatini Anterior belly of the digatric Mylohyoid	Incus Malleus	Developmental facial and masticatory muscle discrepancies; Aplasia/hypoplasia of inner ear and mandibular structures
2	CN VII Facial	Muscles of the face	Body of the hyoid Lesser cornu of hyoid Stapes Styloid process of temporal bone	Auditory and facial muscle discrepancies Dysplasia of stapes
3	CN IX Glossopharyngeal	Stylopharyngeus	Greater cornu of hyoid	Deformities of the hyoid bone Aplasia of thymus
4	CN X Pharyngeal branch of Vagus	Extrinsic laryngeal musculature Levator veli palatini	Thyroid cartilage Corniculate and cuneiform cartilages	Abnormalities of the faucial muscles Cervical clefts, cysts, or fistulae
5	*Exists only transiently and no structures are derived from this arch during embryogenesis*			
6	CN X Recurrent laryngeal branch of Vagus	Intrinsic laryngeal musclulature	Cricoid cartilage Arytenoid cartilage	Laryngeal anomalies, cysts, fistulae, or clefts

Pharyngeal arch 1

The first pharyngeal arch is the precursor to the maxillary and mandibular structures and plays a substantial role in facial development (20). The myogenic elements, condensed by the mesodermal core of the first pharyngeal arch, are innervated by the motor branch of the trigeminal nerve (21). Once fully developed, these muscles become responsible for masticatory and swallowing function (20). Additionally, Meckel's cartilage arises from the first pharyngeal arch which leads to the development of two auditory ossicles: the malleus and the incus. Interactions between the oral epithelium and the mesenchyme of the first arch regulate early tooth formation as well (7). The musculature that stems from the development of the first pharyngeal arch includes the muscles of mastication, anterior belly of the digastric, the mylohyoid muscle, the tensor tympani, and the tensor veli palatini.

Interruption in development of the first pharyngeal arch can lead to conductive and sensorineural hearing deficits secondary to underdevelopment of the auditory ossicles. Chronic middle ear infections can arise from deficits of the tensor veli palatini and palatal clefting that are associated with disruption of this early embryologic process. Speech disorders can additionally arise from underdevelopment of the mandible if interruptions in development of the first pharyngeal arch occur. Micrognathia and posterior tongue displacement can lead to the compensatory speech pattern of backing. Glossoptosis, related to micrognathia, may additionally cause upper airway obstruction. These deficits can be traced to early interruptions or disruptions in the formation of the first pharyngeal arch.

Pharyngeal arch 2

The second pharyngeal arch is innervated by the facial nerve which consists of the occipital, temporal, zygomatic, mandibular, and cervical branches. These branches migrate through the milieu of facial prominences to establish the foundations for the facial musculature (21). The second pharyngeal arch forms the basis of the stapes, the styloid process of the temporal bone, and the lesser horn and body of the hyoid bone. The stapedial artery originates from the second pharyngeal arch and breakdown of this artery can result in midface discrepancies of the maxilla and mandible. Muscles that develop from the second pharyngeal arch include the muscles of facial expression, posterior belly of the digastric, stapedius, and stylohyoid. Reduced facial expression and difficulties with swallowing and intelligibility of *speech can arise from the second pharyngeal arch, stemming from deficits of CN VII.*

The third, fourth, and sixth pharyngeal arches

The third pharyngeal arch develops into the caudal portion and greater cornu of the hyoid bone. The stylopharyngeus muscle is innervated by the glossopharyngeal nerve and the sensory innervation of the posterior tongue is additionally derived from the third arch. The fourth pharyngeal arch is associated with development of the thyroid cartilage. The cricothyroid and pharyngeal constrictor muscles along with the palatopharyngeus, musculus uvula, palatoglossus, and levator veli palatini are additionally developed from the fourth pharyngeal arch (20, 21). These latter muscles are the primary muscles of velopharyngeal closure. The sixth pharyngeal arch is further responsible for the cricoid and arytenoid cartilages within the larynx. The recurrent laryngeal branch of the vagus is also involved within the sixth arch. Additionally, the pulmonary arteries are created via patterning of the sixth pharyngeal arch (22). Voice and resonance disorders can arise secondary to deficits in the cartilage and musculature developed from these pharyngeal arches.

Development of the face, lips, and palate

Formation of the face occurs between the fourth and eighth weeks of development and requires multifaceted morphogenetic changes. Facial structures are primarily derived from five prominences which are comprised of the frontonasal prominence along with paired maxillary and mandibular prominences.

During the fourth week, nasal placodes appear alongside the frontonasal prominence and optic discs appear. The first three pharyngeal arches are developed and the first arch forms into its maxillary and mandibular prominences. Between the first arches and frontonasal prominence, openings across the buccopharyngeal membrane appear.

Nasal pits develop from the nasal placodes during the fifth week and the rims of the placodes develop into the median and lateral nasal prominences. Mandibular arch mesenchyme migrates medially and the caudal end of the medial nasal prominence fuses with the maxillary prominence. As the sixth week progresses, the medial and lateral nasal prominences begin to fuse. The maxillary prominence continues to assist with the formation of the maxilla while the medial nasal prominence develops into the nasal septum. The nasal septum has been found to significantly control outgrowth of the midface (18, 23). Across the seventh week, the nasal tip becomes elevated between the medial nasal prominences, and eyelids begin to take shape along with the pinna. Following this, the development of the lower face occurs in two stages including a phase for labial and maxillary development and a phase for secondary palatogenesis.

As the maxillary prominences and lateral and medial nasal processes meet, fusion of these structures assists in the formation of the upper lip. The lateral nasal prominences do not directly contribute to formation of the upper lip, but failure of fusion of the lateral prominence appropriately with the medial nasal prominence frequently results in clefts of the lip that may extend through the nostril (24).

Secondary palatogenesis occurs as the palatal shelves develop from the bilateral projections of the maxillary prominence. As the eighth week progresses, the palatal shelves grow vertically and border the tongue. Inferior migration of the tongue is needed for the palatal shelves to move from a vertical alignment to a horizontal orientation. As the tongue descends, the palatal shelves are able to rotate towards the midline (25). Horizontal growth then occurs which allows the individual palatal shelves to elevate, approximate one another, and fuse. The shelves contact one another at midline. Fusion begins at approximately one third of the way from the primary palate and migrates both anteriorly and posteriorly. The palatal shelves fuse with the nasal septum and primary palate. However, the posterior palatal shelf, or area of the soft palate, does not fuse with the septum and therefore sustains the ability to remain mobile for later speech production. A small area additionally remains unfused between the primary and secondary palate, known as the incisive foramen, which acts as an opening for vascularization and nerves to pass. The palatal mesenchyme experiences differentiation and ossification following the fusion process. This then forms the secondary hard palate, thus separating the oral and nasal cavities. Palatal fusion is hypothesized to occur due to epithelial apoptosis, epithelial to mesenchymal transformation, or epithelial cell migration (26). Failure of the palatal shelves to fuse, however, results in palatal clefting along with any number of conditions that can arise during this critical time of morphogenetic changes.

Failure to thrive conditions related to the growth and development of arches 1 and 2

The adequate development of the craniofacial complex primarily depends upon genetic factors, environmental factors, and mechanical factors. Any interruption in the expression of the inherited genotype, nutritional or biochemical interactions, extrinsic or intrinsic forces of muscle action, growth expansion, and/or atrophic attenuation can affect the outcome of normal development.

Syndromic conditions can be identified according to the pharyngeal arch involved. First arch syndromes are most common and the frequency of deficient development is less common as the arch number increases. Additionally, deficiencies occurring in the lower arches are typically more severe. Sperber (20) cites agnathia, synotia, and microstomia as examples of first arch anomalies. Mandibulofacial dysostosis (Treacher Collin's syndrome), micrognathia (associated with Pierre Robin sequence), and cleft palate are additional first arch malformations that commonly occur. Further, Stickler's syndrome and 22Q11.2 deletion syndrome have been found to be associated with deficient development of the pharyngeal arches (27). External ear defects are also seen as a result of disruptions in the development of the first arch. Isolated anomalies involving only the second arch and laryngeal mechanism are less common, but can include laryngeal clefting. Additional lower arch anomalies can result in midline deficiencies.

COMMON FIRST AND SECOND PHARYNGEAL ARCH MALFORMATIONS AND ASSOCIATED GENETIC COMPONENTS

Hemifacial microsomia involves a range of morphogenic anomalies derived from the first and second pharyngeal arches (28). The main facial features of hemifacial microsomia include unilateral underdevelopment of craniofacial structures that are associated with the first two pharyngeal arches. This comprises mandibular hypoplasia, orbital asymmetry, a malformed or absent pinna with accessory tags, and, at times, facial clefts (29, 30). Prevalence rates are reported to occur in approximately 1 in 3,500 to 1 in 15,000 (31, 32). Data from experimental mouse models indicate that this pattern of malformation may be caused by hemorrhaging of the stapedial artery which supplies a portion of the embryonic second pharyngeal arch (33). Genetic reports have additionally linked chromosome 14q32 to hemifacial microsomia and the first arch abnormalities associated within this malformation (34).

Treacher Collins syndrome

Treacher Collins syndrome is an autosomal dominant condition that arises from a single-gene and is associated with significant abnormalities of facial development. This syndrome is reported to occur with an incidence of 1 in 50,000 live births (35). The primary clinical features include underdeveloped facial bones (particularly the mandible and zygomatic arches), downward slanting palpebral fissures, microtia, malformed ossicles, and middle ear anomalies. Cleft palate can additionally be associated with this disorder, although it is not as common. Treacher Collins syndrome has been mapped to chromosome 5q32-5q33 and is associated with the TCOF-1 gene which is reported to be expressed at the edges of the neural folds in the first two pharyngeal arches (36).

Stickler syndrome

Stickler syndrome is an autosomal dominant condition that results in underdevelopment of the mandible and is characterized by distinctive facial features and palatal anomalies as well as deficits in connective tissue throughout the musculoskeletal system. Sticker syndrome occurs secondary to mutations on the COL2A1 gene on chromosome 12q13.11 (37). Radiographic evaluation of children with Stickler syndrome reveals a flat midface appearance with a depressed nasal bridge and micrognathia (27). Additionally, palatal clefting in the form of an isolated cleft of the soft palate to a more severe presentation of Pierre Robin sequence is frequently associated with this syndrome and related to deficits of the first and second pharyngeal arches.

The above common syndromic conditions all include some form of Pierre Robin sequence or under-development of the mandible secondary to disruption in development of the first two pharyngeal arches. In syndromes involving micrognathia or oromandibular abnormalities, clinical intervention is often warranted. Severe cases of mandibular hypoplasia may result in airway obstruction, feeding difficulties, and failure to thrive conditions. Malocclusion can additionally result in dental deviations that require orthodontic treatment and/or orthognathic surgery and speech therapy may be warranted should articulation defects occur. Thus, the remainder of this review focuses on deficiencies of the first two pharyngeal arches as they relate to the clinical presentation of Pierre Robin sequence.

Deficiencies in pharyngeal arches 1 and 2 and the relationship to Pierre Robin sequence

Pierre Robin sequence (PRS) was first described as a condition involving the presence of micrognathia, glossoptosis, and respiratory distress in newborns (38). Nearly a decade later, the occurrence of cleft palate was included within this description leading to the establishment of a triad of symptoms (micrognathia, glossoptosis, and cleft palate) as the hallmark indicators of PRS (39). A sequence, such as PRS, results from the occurrence of multiple anomalies during development where one specific irregularity, such as micrognathia, leads to the sequential development of additional anomalies. The primary anomaly may have multiple etiologies and PRS is not unique in this regard.

The etiology of PRS can vary based on environmental, genetic, teratogenic, and mechanically induced factors, or a multifactorial combination of these factors (40). Gorlin et al. (41) attributed the development of PRS to arrested embryonic development. In contrast, others have suggested that micrognathia may arise from mechanical constraints which limit the growth of the mandible prior to palate closure (42, 43). Additionally, recent research has indicated that deletions in 4p16-14, 4q31-35, 6q25-27, and 11q23 and duplications in 10q24 and 18q12-23 may interfere with mandibular development (44). Changes in the *SOX9* gene disrupt protein regulation of tissues that control the development of the mandible and most commonly result in isolated Pierre Robin sequence. Thus, a multifactorial theory is commonly accepted in which the occurrence of mandibular hypoplasia appears between 7th and 11th weeks of gestation secondary to factors listed above, resulting in deficits on the first pharyngeal arch during embryological development.

As the palate begins to form during the embryological period, the vertically oriented palatal shelves flank the embryonic tongue which rests against the base of the early skull. During typical development, the mandibular processes grow and the oral cavity expands following fusion of the primary palate. The mandibular growth spurt allows for the tongue to descend to the floor of the mouth which provides the palatal shelves space to move into their horizontal orientation. Following this, outward growth from the midline and fusion of the palatal shelves can occur (secondary palatogenesis). In infants with PRS, however, the genesis of mandibular development, or lack of mandibular development (micrognathia), prevents the mandible from growth. Inadequate growth of the mandible leads to protracted descent of the tongue and the inability for the palatal shelves to orient horizontally at the appropriate time. When the tongue ultimately descends, the palatal shelves are unable to adequately fuse, leading to a cleft of the secondary palate.

The diagnosis of PRS is complex due to the many underlying etiologies that contribute to the clinical findings. Isolated PRS is reported in approximately 17% of cases (40). However, there are discrepancies for non-syndromic incidence rates which reach as high as 60% (45). The variability in reported incidence rates of non-syndromic diagnoses may be indicative of the many factors that may cause PRS unrelated to a syndromic condition. However, clinical findings of PRS are often present in a number of syndromic conditions. Shprintzen (40) reported that PRS-related anomalies and characteristics were present in approximately 83% of other syndromes or malformations being identified or diagnosed. Of these cases, 34% were associated with Stickler's syndrome, which has subsequently been found to have the highest association with PRS. Stickler's syndrome can be associated with deficiencies of the first pharyngeal arch during embryological development, as symptoms include deficits of the eyes, ears, and palate along with the joints and heart. One third of children diagnosed with Stickler's syndrome present the symptoms associated with PRS along with hearing loss, a flattened midface and flat nasal bridge, and epicanthal folds (40). Velocardiofacial syndrome (22Q11.2 deletion syndrome) is also reported to coincide with PRS in approximately 11% of cases.

The consequences of mandibular hypoplasia or micrognathia, along with the resulting sequence of pathologies reported in PRS, are well described (40, 46-48). Airway compromise and/or airway obstruction are the primary concerns for patients with PRS soon after birth. Micrognathia and the posteriorly displaced tongue are catalysts for airway obstruction. As such, is it suspected that the mandibular growth disturbance during embryological development prevents elongation of the genioglossus fibers leading to this clinical presentation (49, 50). The retrusive mandible creates susceptibility for the posteriorly positioned tongue to fall against the posterior wall of the oropharynx during swallowing and inspiration (47, 51). Feeding difficulties in infancy are also reported as a consequence of PRS. An infant with PRS experiences feeding disorders similar to those exhibited by an infant with an unrepaired isolated cleft palate. However, feeding is made more complex with the presence of glossoptosis (47). Additionally, class II malocclusions are common for children with PRS in their primary dentition and mixed (primary and permanent) dentitions. However, this typically resolves, to some extent, as the child grows, unless the diagnosis of PRS is associated with a syndromic condition (49). In syndromes such as Stickler's or Treacher Collin's, the disproportion between the mandible and the maxilla becomes more apparent with growth (52). This can affect speech production and difficulties with cuspid alignment for mastication.

Developmental, cognitive, and communication issues are also reported to occur in patients with PRS as well (45, 53). Reports have cited deficits leading to learning disabilities in children with cleft palate, and research is needed within this area to more clearly define the role of cognitive developmental issues in patients with PRS. Recent investigations have found differences in the cerebellar and cerebral anatomy in individuals with isolated cleft palate (54-56). Speech and language deficits are additionally related to the midline deficits associated with clefting secondary to variations in brain structure that may be present in some individuals with cleft palate (55). Delayed onset of speech and language is often present in children with PRS when associated with a syndromic condition (48).

Airway management is typically the initial focus for infants born with PRS. In the supine position, infants often demonstrate labored breathing, stridor, sternal retractions, and cyanosis. Positioning of the infant in the prone position may resolve these issues and improve the airway (57). In mild cases of PRS, positioning alone can often resolve airway symptoms. However, monitoring for the presence of apneic periods during sleep is recommended. For infants who continue to demonstrate episodes of airway obstruction, or consistent airway obstruction regardless of positioning, additional airway management, such as intubation, should be considered (57). Prior to intubation, detailed assessment of the airway is crucial to determine the exact locus of airway obstruction (58). In addition to glossoptosis as a primary obstructer, additional levels of obstruction may be present at the nasopharyngeal or laryngeal level (choanal atresia, subglottic stenosis, laryngomalacia, etc.) which may indicate the need for a management other than intubation, such as a tracheostomy (58). Surgical management options may additionally include a tongue-lip adhesion or mandibular distraction (59-61). Additional surgical treatment for patients with PRS, unrelated to the airway, can include palatoplasty, myringotomy with PE tube placement, gastrostomy placement if issues with weight gain are present, Nissen fundoplication when reflux is present, and pharyngoplasty for secondary palatal management if needed (62, 63). The timing of procedures should be determined with careful multidisciplinary planning and with consideration of the child's overall medical status.

CONCLUSION

The deficits seen in children with PRS can be attributed to deficiencies present during embryological development within the first two pharyngeal arches. The clinical presentation of PRS can differ in severity levels and have numerous underlying etiologies. Interruption in the embryological process secondary to chromosomal abnormalities, genetic disorders, teratogenic effects, or mechanical factors can result in the mandibular deficits and subsequent lingual, airway, and palatal issues that are observed in PRS. Therefore, it is important that the embryological connection that exists between the pharyngeal arches and the long term sequelae of PRS be identified as soon as possible in order to develop and facilitate appropriate management strategies for these patients. Furthermore, it is essential for practitioners to be familiar with the anatomic and embryological foundation of craniofacial development so that differential and diagnostic considerations may be identified.

REFERENCES

[1] Lumsden AG. Spatial organization of the epithelium and the role of neural crest cells in the initiation of the mammalian tooth germ. Development 1988;103(Suppl):155-69.

[2] Graham A, Smith A. Patterning the pharyngeal arches. Bioessays 2001;23(1):54-61.

[3] Cai J, Ash D, Kotch LE, Jabs EW, Attie-Bitach T, Auge J, et al. Gene expression in pharyngeal arch 1 during human embryonic development. Hum Mol Genet 2005;14(7):903-12.

[4] Trainor PA, Krumlauf R. Hox genes, neural crest cells and branchial arch patterning. Curr Opin Cell Biol 2001;13(6):698-705.

[5] Alappat S, Zhang ZY, Chen YP. Msx homeobox gene family and craniofacial development. Cell Res 2003;13(6):429-42.

[6] Francis-West P, Ladher R, Barlow A, Graveson A. Signalling interactions during facial development. Mech Dev 1998;75(1):3-28.

[7] Wilkie AO, Morriss-Kay GM. Genetics of craniofacial development and malformation. Nature Rev Genetics 2001;2(6):458-68.

[8] Lidral AC, Romitti PA, Basart AM, Doetschman T, Leysens NJ, Daack-Hirsch S, et al. Association of MSX1 and TGFB3 with nonsyndromic clefting in humans. The Am J Hum Genetics 1998;63(2):557-68.

[9] Lidral AC, Reising BC. The role of MSX1 in human tooth agenesis. J Dent Res 2002;81(4):274-8.

[10] De Robertis EM, Morita EA, Cho KW. Gradient fields and homeobox genes. Development 1991;112(3):669-78.

[11] Nanni L, Ming JE, Bocian M, Steinhaus K, Bianchi DW, Die-Smulders C, et al. The mutational spectrum of the sonic hedgehog gene in holoprosencephaly: SHH

mutations cause a significant proportion of autosomal dominant holoprosencephaly. Hum Mol Genet 1999;8(13):2479-88.

[12] Nie X, Luukko K, Kettunen P. FGF signalling in craniofacial development and developmental disorders. Oral Dis 2006;12(2):102-11.

[13] Marie P, Coffin J, Hurley M. FGF and FGFR signaling in chondrodysplasias and craniosynostosis. J Cell Biochem 2005;96(5):888-96.

[14] Neubüser A, Peters H, Balling R, Martin GR. Antagonistic interactions between FGF and BMP signaling pathways: a mechanism for positioning the sites of tooth formation. Cell 1997;90(2):247-255.

[15] Niswander L, Martin GR. Fgf-4 expression during gastrulation, myogenesis, limb and tooth development in the mouse. Development 1992;114(3):755-768.

[16] Basch ML, Bronner-Fraser M, García-Castro MI. Specification of the neural crest occurs during gastrulation and requires Pax7. Nature 2006;441(7090):218-22.

[17] Le Douarin NM, Creuzet S, Couly G, Dupin E. Neural crest cell plasticity and its limits. Development 2004;131(19):4637-50.

[18] Szabo-Rogers HL, Smithers LE, Yakob W, Liu KJ. New directions in craniofacial morphogenesis. Dev Biol 2010;341(1):84-94.

[19] Le Douarin N, Kalcheim C. The neural crest. Cambridge: Cambridge University Press, 1982;2.

[20] Sperber GH, Guttmann GD, Sperber SM. Craniofacial development. Shelton, CT: People's Medical Publishing House, 2001.

[21] Noden DM, Francis- West P. The differentiation and morphogenesis of craniofacial muscles. Dev Dynamics 2006;235(5):1194-1218.

[22] Kirby ML, Waldo KL. Neural crest and cardiovascular patterning. Circ Res 1995 Aug;77(2):211-5.

[23] Howe A, Hawkins J, Webster W. The growth of the nasal septum in the 6–9 week period of foetal development—warfarin embryopathy offers a new insight into prenatal facial development. Aust Dent J 2004;49(4):171-6.

[24] Jiang R, Bush JO, Lidral AC. Development of the upper lip: morphogenetic and molecular mechanisms. Dev Dynamics 2006;235(5):1152-66.

[25] Greene RM, Pratt RM. Developmental aspects of secondary palate formation. J Embryol Exp Morphol 1976;36(2):225-45.

[26] Gritli-Linde A. Molecular control of secondary palate development. Dev Biol 2007;301(2):309-26.

[27] Johnson JM, Moonis G, Green GE, Carmody R, Burbank HN. Syndromes of the first and second branchial arches, part 2: syndromes. Am J Neuroradiol 2011;32(2):230-7.

[28] Murray JE, Kaban LB, Mulliken JB. Analysis and treatment of hemifacial microsomia. Plast Reconstr Surg 1984;74(2):186-99.

[29] Beddington RS, Robertson EJ. Axis development and early asymmetry in mammals. Cell 1999;96(2):195-209.

[30] Vento AR, LaBrie RA, Mulliken JB. The OMENS classification of hemifacial microsomia. Cleft Palate-Craniofacial J 1991;28(1):68-77.

[31] GRABB WC. The first and second branchial arch syndrome. Plast Reconstr Surg 1965;36(5):485-508.

[32] Poswillo D. The pathogenesis of the first and second branchial arch syndrome. Oral Surg Oral Med Oral Pathol 1973;35(3):302-28.

[33] Cousley R, Wilson D. Hemifacial microsomia: developmental consequence of perturbation of the auriculofacial cartilage model? Am J Med Genet 1992;42(4):461-6.

[34] Kelberman D, Tyson J, McInerney A, Malcolm S, Winter R, Bitner-Glindzicz M. Mapping of a locus for autosomal dominant hemifacial microsomia. J Med Genet 2000;37:618.

[35] Fazen LE, Elmore J, Nadler HL. Mandibulo-Facial Dysostosis:(Treacher-Collins Syndrome). Am J Dis Child 1967;113(4):405-10.

[36] Dixon J, Hovanes K, Shiang R, Dixon MJ. Sequence analysis, identification of evolutionary conserved motifs and expression analysis of murine tcof1 provide further evidence for a potential function for the gene and its human homologue, TCOF1. Hum Mol Genet 1997;6(5):727-37.

[37] Annunen S, Körkkö J, Czarny M, Warman ML, Brunner HG, Kääriäinen H, et al. Splicing mutations of 54-bp exons in the COL11A1 gene cause Marshall syndrome, but other mutations cause overlapping Marshall/Stickler phenotypes. Am J Hum Genetics 1999;65(4):974-83.

[38] Robin P. A fall of the base of the tongue considered as a new cause of nasopharyngeal respiratory impairment. Bull Acad Natl Med 1923;89:37.

[39] Robin P. Glossoptosis due to atresia and hypotrophy of the mandible. Am J Dis Child 1934;48(3):541-7.

[40] Shprintzen RJ. The implications of the diagnosis of Robin sequence. Cleft Palate-Craniofacial J 1992;29(3):205-9.

[41] Gorlin RJ, Pindborg JJ. Cohen MMJr. Syndromes of the head and neck. New York: McGraw-Hill, 1976.

[42] Smith D. Recognizable patterns of human malformation, 3rd ed. Philadelphia, PA: WB Saunders, 1982.

[43] Jones K. Smith's recognizable patterns of human malformation. Philadelphia, PA: WB Saunders, 1988.

[44] Brewer C, Holloway S, Zawalnyski P, Schinzel A, FitzPatrick D. A chromosomal deletion map of human malformations. Am J Hum Genetics 1998;63(4):1153-9.

[45] Williams AJ, Williams MA, Walker CA, Bush PG. The Robin anomalad (Pierre Robin syndrome)--a follow up study. Arch Dis Child 1981;56(9):663-8.

[46] Hong P, McNeil M, Kearns DB, Magit AE. Mandibular distraction osteogenesis in children with Pierre Robin sequence: impact on health-related quality of life. Int J Pediatr Otorhinolaryngol 2012;76(8):1159-63.

[47] Goldberg MH, Eckblom RH. The treatment of the Pierre Robin syndrome. Pediatrics 1962;30:450-8.

[48] Pasyayan HM, Lewis MB. Clinical experience with the Robin sequence. Cleft Palate J 1984;21(4):270-6.

[49] Randall P, Krogman W, Jahina S. Pierre Robin and the syndrome that bears his name. Cleft Palate J 1965;2(3):237-46.

[50] Randall P. The Robin sequence: Micrognathia and glossoptosis with airway obstruction. Plastic Surgery 1990;4(63):3123-34.

[51] Mallory SB, Paradise JL. Glossoptosis revisited: on the development and resolution of airway obstruction in the Pierre Robin syndrome. Pediatrics 1979;64(6):946-8.

[52] Daskalogiannakis J, Ross RB, Tompson BD. The mandibular catch-up growth controversy in Pierre Robin sequence. Am J Orthodontics Dentofacial Orthopedics 2001;120(3):280-5.

[53] Van den Elzen, Annet PM, Semmekrot BA, Bongers EM, Huygen PL, Marres HA. Diagnosis and treatment of the Pierre Robin sequence: results of a retrospective clinical study and review of the literature. Eur J Pediatr 2001;160(1):47-53.

[54] Boes AD, Murko V, Wood JL, Langbehn DR, Canady J, Richman L, et al. Social function in boys with cleft lip and palate: relationship to ventral frontal cortex morphology. Behav Brain Res 2007;181(2):224-31.

[55] Nopoulos P, Langbehn DR, Canady J, Magnotta V, Richman L. Abnormal brain structure in children with isolated clefts of the lip or palate. Arch Pediatr Adolesc Med 2007;161(8):753-8.

[56] van der Plas E, Conrad A, Canady J, Richman L, Nopoulos P. Effects of unilateral clefts on brain structure. Arch Pediatr Adolesc Med 2010;164(8):763-8.

[57] Benjamin B, Walker P. Management of airway obstruction in the Pierre Robin sequence. Int J Pediatr Otorhinolaryngol 1991;22(1):29-37.

[58] Sher AE. Mechanisms of airway obstruction in Robin sequence: implications for treatment. Cleft Palate-Craniofacial J 1992;29(3):224-31.

[59] Kirschner RE, Low DW, Randall P, Bartlett SP, McDonald-McGinn DM, Schultz PJ, et al. Surgical airway management in Pierre Robin sequence: is there a role for tongue-lip adhesion? Cleft Palate-Craniofacial J 2003;40(1):13-8.

[60] Myer CM, Reed JM, Cotton RT, Willging JP. Airway management in Pierre Robin sequence. Otolaryngol Head Neck Surgery 1996;115(2):P63-P64.

[61] Burstein FD, Williams JK. Mandibular distraction osteogenesis in Pierre Robin sequence: application of a new internal single-stage resorbable device. Plast Reconstr Surg 2005;115(1):61-7.

[62] Shprintzen RJ. Pharyngeal flap surgery and the pediatric upper airway. Int Anesthesiol Clin 1988;26(1):79-88.

[63] Dudkiewicz Z, Sekuła E, Nielepiec-Jałosińska A. Gastroesophageal reflux in Pierre Robin sequence—early surgical treatment. Cleft Palate-Craniofacial J 2000;37(2):205-8.

In: Child and Adolescent Health
Editors: A Tenenbaum and J Merrick
ISBN: 978-1-53617-825-8

Chapter 4

PEDIATRIC IMMUNIZATIONS: REVIEW AND DISCUSSION ON PROTECTION OF OUR CHILDREN AND ADOLESCENTS

Donald E Greydanus*, MD, DrHC (Athens) and Marisha G Agana, MD, MPH
Department of Pediatric and Adolescent Medicine,
Homer Stryker MD School of Medicine,
Kalamazoo, Michigan, United States of America

ABSTRACT

Immunizations for all citizens of the world should be an important goal of all clinicians including those dealing with children and adolescents in developing and developed countries. Vaccine preventable diseases continue to take a devastating toll on these vulnerable human beings. This chapter summarizes current concepts of immunizations with the caveat

---

* Correspondence: Donald E Greydanus, MD, DrHC(Athens), Professor and Founding Chair, Department of Pediatric and Adolescent Medicine, Western Michigan University Homer Stryker MD School of Medicine, 1000 Oakland Drive, Kalamazoo, MI 49008-1284 United States. Email: donald.greydanus@med.wmich.edu.

that widespread travel brings many diseases around the globe whether one lives in a tropical or subtropical area or anywhere in the world. After an introduction to vaccinology, this discussion considers individual vaccines and updates progress on maternal immunizations. The current anti-vaccine hysteria, now prevalent in developed countries, threatens to induce an explosion of epidemics of diseases now controlled by vaccinology with significant yet unnecessary and tragic increase in human morbidity and mortality.

INTRODUCTION

Proper immunizations of all children, adolescents, and adults should be a mission of all clinicians (1, 2). Global travel allows easy dispersal of dangerous organisms that can infect and injure persons who have no prior exposure to these microbes and thus, often have limited or no immunity against them. Fortunately, many of these diseases are preventable due to existing vaccines which allow the vaccinated individual to avoid the devastation from a growing list of these vaccine preventable diseases (VPDs).

After millions of years without protection against these microbes, considerable progress has been made since the historic work of Edward Jenner (1749-1823) in 1796 against the smallpox virus. Small pox was one of the deadliest epidemics haunting humans, killing over one-third of those infected for thousands of years. One hundred and eighty one years after Jenner inoculated 8 year old James Phipps with cowpox vaccine in 1796, using what was then called the "Turkish" method, smallpox was eliminated from the world, except for stockpiles of this virus in some countries (3). This monumental achievement in medicine had its beginnings in India in the 800s with oral snake venom experimentation and continued in China in the 1100s. Stimulated by Jenner's work in 1796, the Spanish government embarked on the world's first immunization campaign between 1803 and 1813 (4), and improved greatly with scientific progress in immunology and microbiology in the 20th and now 21st centuries.

Vaccine benefits

As a result of such progress, many diseases have been reduced or even eliminated in some parts of the world, and millions of human lives have been saved worldwide, because of the successful immunization campaigns of the World Health Organization (WHO) and the US Centers for Disease Control and Prevention (CDC) (5-7). For example, smallpox was still seen in the 1960s and 1970s in Africa and Asia but was eliminated by a WHO smallpox campaign starting in 1967; the last case was reported in 1977 (5, 8). Polio has been eliminated in most parts of the world and in many places, diphtheria and congenital rubella syndrome are rarely seen (9).

The CDC estimated that between its establishment in 1994 and 2013, the vaccines for children program (VFC) in the United States, prevented an estimated 322 million illnesses, 21 million hospitalizations, and 732,000 deaths over these childrens' lifetimes with a net savings of $295 billion in direct costs and $1.38 trillion in total cost to society (10). The Expanded Programme on Immunization (EPI) of WHO, started in 1974, prevents two to three million human deaths annually (11). Increased immunization programs in Mexico have resulted in a 34% decreased in mortality in children under 5 years of age from universal immunization for influenza, rotavirus, and pneumococcus (7).

Global issues

Experts recommend increased vaccine research in more countries. The Vaccines for Africa Initiative (VACFA), for example, note that half of immunization research in Africa comes from only six countries: South Africa, The Gambia, Nigeria, Senegal, Guinea-Bissau, and Kenya (12). Increased communication is recommended between health decision-makers and researchers to improve research in vaccines as well as improved vaccine implementation to the public in Africa (13). Attention to proper vaccine storage is an important issue. Modern vaccines vials are equipped with a vaccine viral monitor consisting of an image of a square inside a circle and contain heat-sensitive material noting cumulative exposure. Transporting and storing vaccines at the proper temperature is a major global effort which maximizes vaccine efficacy.

Nearly all countries now have immunization programs with dedicated budgets, vaccine safety protocols, and surveillance systems. These programs have gone beyond the WHO original plans to deal with the six classic childhood vaccines: tetanus, diphtheria, pertussis, measles, poliomyelitis, and tuberculosis. The world's infants are now routinely vaccinated against haemophilus influenza type b, hepatitis B, rubella, rotavirus, and streptococcus pneumoniae. Selected countries also have campaigns to provide vaccines for dengue, yellow fever, and epidemic meningococcal meningitis (5). The human papillomavirus vaccine is also offered in some countries for girls between 9 and 12 years of age.

Unfortunately, many countries are not reaching the goals of the 2020 Global Vaccine Action Plan (GVAP) adopted at the 65th World Health Assembly in 2012 (Geneva, Switzerland). Global immunization coverage was 5% in 1974 and the 2020 target is to reach at least 90% of the world's population (80% or more in all districts). This goal has been reached in 59 countries in 2012 including some low and middle-income countries (5). Unfortunately, one in five children do not receive basic vaccines as recommended by the WHO's Expanded Programme on Immunizations (EPI), now in its 40th year of life-saving efforts. Only one in four children in Ethiopia are fully immunized, and some parts of this country, as noted in many countries, provide better coverage than others. Efforts to improve vaccination rates among children need to target increased education for the mothers of these children (14). Neglect in covering children with CDC and WHO recommended immunizations remains in some countries as well as sex inequality with regard to vaccination rates (15, 16).

Anti-vaccine movement

Unfortunately, controversy surrounding vaccines arose as soon as vaccinology began, with a number of people in the 19th century mounting an anti-vaccine campaign. Vaccine controversy all began in 1763 when the French Parliament banned inoculation because of improper quarantine procedures. There was a general distrust of Medicine and doctors at that time especially coming from clergymen who believed that smallpox was "God's punishment and should not be treated." Then against the backdrop of the United Kingdom Vaccination Act of 1853 which mandated vaccination against smallpox for infants 3 months and older associated with severe penalties for vaccine refusal, the anti-vaccination league was formed (17). The Leicester Demonstration March of 1885 wherein 80,000 to 100,000 demonstrators protested the imprisonment of seven anti-vaccine activists facilitated the creation of the new Vaccination Act of 1898 that removed the penalties associated with vaccine refusal. Through the centuries, England and the United States had to quell the pockets of anti-vaccine campaign that arose from unfortunate incidences of vaccine-derived crises like the Cutter incident in Berkeley, California in 1955 secondary to polio cases and the Great Ormond Street hospital fiasco of DTP-vaccine in England in 1974 (17).

Despite gains in safety and vaccine technology, the anti-vaccine movement remains strong in the 21st century (4, 18). The publication of the research paper linking MMR vaccination with the development of autism by a British doctor in 1998 (which was later debunked as fraudulent research in 2011) fueled the birth of anti-vaxxer movements across the United States with celebrity endorsements by Jenny McCarthy who blamed MMR vaccination for her son's autism diagnosis (17). Such controversy has reduced the number of people around the globe who have received immunization against vaccine preventable diseases (VPDs). In the United States a survey of parents published in 2011 noted that 83% had vaccinated their children, 11% were planning on such an action, 5% agree to have their children take some but not all vaccines, and 2% refused to have their children vaccinated (19). Measles which is a disease that was reportedly eradicated in 2000 in the US has now come back with a vengeance with cases of measles rising to 668 in 27 states in 2014 (17).

Incomplete immunizations

In addition to parental refusal, other issues with regard to providing comprehensive coverage of VPDs to the public have continued. Some families do not have access to immunizations because of poverty, others have limited access to clinicians, or have clinicians who do not emphasize the important role that vaccinations play in health care. Despite World Health Organization's (WHO, Geneva, Switzerland) and the Centers for Disease Control and Prevention's (CDC, Atlanta, Georgia, US) guidelines, immunization schedules and recommendations can be vary from country to country. Barriers to full implementation include lack of access to comprehensive preventive health care, vaccinations that were administered at the wrong time, or given at incorrect intervals because of clinician error.

Estimates in the United States note that over 35 million American adolescents are missing one or more recommended vaccinations (20, 21) Some may have been vaccinated at the wrong time or with an incorrect schedule because of error by the busy health care system (22). Sometimes an opportunity to vaccinate an individual is missed because the health care system utilizes incorrect contraindications for vaccinations. Some vaccines (such as hepatitis B and varicella) were not part of the recommended vaccine schedule when current youth or college students were younger; in some cases, immunity has waned from earlier vaccinations (23).

Some of the VPDs considered in this discussion are listed in Table 1. More vaccines are being developed and their safety must be demonstrated to a sometimes skeptical public that may receive the wrong information from the media (8, 24) (www.cdc.gov/od/science.iso/). In this discussion, the immunization schedule used in the United States is considered (25, 26). Specific recommendations and schedules will vary from country to country depending on the issues within that country and the precise recommendations of local public health experts—as for example, in Argentina (27).

Table 1. Available vaccines for preventable diseases (partial list)

1)	Tetanus, Diphtheria, Pertussis (DTaP/Td/Tdap)
2)	Measles, Mumps, Rubella (MMR)
3)	Meningococcal Vaccine (MCV4, MPSV4)
4)	Haemophilus influenza b (Hib)
5)	Human Papillomavirus (HPV)
6)	Hepatitis A vaccine
7)	Hepatitis B vaccine
8)	Varicella vaccine
9)	Influenza vaccine (IIV, LAIV)
10)	Pneumococcal (polysaccharide): PPV23, (conjugate) PCV13
11)	Rotavirus vaccine
12)	Cholera vaccine
13)	Rabies vaccine
14)	Japanese encephalitis vaccine
15)	Typhoid vaccine
16)	Yellow fever vaccine
17)	Lyme disease vaccine

Precautions and contraindications

Clinicians should pay close attention to the contraindications or precautions for the use of vaccines (28). Sometimes *precautions* are noted for a person who has a condition in which the vaccine might increase the chance or the severity of an adverse reaction, or compromise the ability of the vaccine to produce immunity. Absolute or permanent *contraindications* are rare and include known anaphylactic reaction to a vaccine or a component of the vaccine. Temporary contraindications include moderate or severe illness; additional contraindications for live, attenuated vaccine include pregnancy and immunosuppressive disorders. Clinicians should note that contraindications do not include low grade fever, upper respiratory infections, ear infections, or mild gastroenteritis.

Consultation with experts may be necessary for immunosuppressive conditions. In general, these vaccines are acceptable for use in those with HIV/AIDS who have an adequate CD4 count (at or over 25%), those with leukemia or other cancers if healthy and 3 to 6 months post-chemotherapy, those taking less than 2 mg/kg/day of corticosteroids, and those prescribed a dose of steroids of 2 or more mg/kg/day if less than 2 weeks duration. If two or more live viral vaccines are needed they should be given at the same time; if one vaccine is missed, they must be, separated by 28 days to avoid possible interference from circulating antibodies to the first vaccine.

Adult vaccinations

Children are not the only ones at risk for morbidity and mortality from vaccine preventative diseases. Many adults are at considerable risk because of low vaccination rates. For example, the combination of influenza and pneumococcal disease represent the 5th leading cause of death in adults in the US over 65 years of age. Annual adult US mortality statistics include as many as 48,000 deaths (average over 23,000) annually from influenza, 6,000 from hepatitis B, and over 5,000 from invasive pneumococcal disease (21, 26). If clinicians caring for adults to not provide these vaccines, death rates for vulnerable adults will remain high.

Future developments

Recent advances in vaccinology include the production of new vaccines and combination vaccines. New products in development include vaccines against cytomegalovirus, herpes simplex virus, *Mycoplasma pneumoniae, Neisseria gonorrhoeae, Chlamydia trachomatis*, malaria, HIV, tuberculosis, and others (29). Unfortunately, Immunization against HIV remains elusive at present (30-34). New vaccine delivery systems are under development including patch vaccines, nasal vaccines, microencapsulation, and use of bioengineered plants. This discussion now turns to providing information on specific vaccines.

Polio Immunization

Infectious poliomyelitis was a public health problem at the turn of the 20th century and with the widespread application of polio immunization there was elimination of this infection from the Western Hemisphere and in the United States in the early 1970s (9). In the United States inactivated polio vaccine (IPV) is given at 2, 4, 6-18 months, and 4-6 years; it is not routinely given at or after age 18 years in the U.S. If a 4th dose is given before age four, a 5th dose is recommended. IPV is found as component in multiple combination vaccines: DTap/IPV/Hib, DTap/IPV/Hep B, and DTaP/IPV. Oral polio vaccine (OPV) continues to be used in some developing countries.

In 1988, the forty-first World Health Assemby adopted a resolution for the worldwide eradication of polio by launching the Global Polio Eradication Initiative (GPEI). Since the GPEI was launched, the number of polio cases has been reduced by over 99% (35). WHO launched a vigorous anti-polio campaign in Africa (Polio Eradication Initiative: "Kick Polio Out of Africa") from 1993 to 2002 that reduced the number of countries with endemic polio from 34 to 2 (5). By March 2014, the WHO South-east Asia region was certified polio-free, meaning that transmission of wild poliovirus has been interrupted in this bloc of 11 countries from Indonesia to India marking a significant advancement in global eradication with 80% of the world's population living in certified polio-free areas (35).

WHO recommends at least one dose of inactivated polio vaccine (IPV) as part of routine immunization protocols in order to reduce the possibility of type 2 polio development since Sabin type 2 strains have been withdrawn from oral polio vaccine (OPV) (36). Those travelling to areas with endemic polio must receive polio vaccination, if indicated, based on their current vaccine status (37). With further push of a worldwide polio immunization program, polio can be removed from the world and placed in the same elimination status solely occupied by smallpox (9).

HAEMOPHILUS INFLUENZA B IMMUNIZATION

Haemophilus influenza type b is an encapsulated gram negative coccobacillus. Prior to the availability of the vaccine, it was the leading cause of meningitis in the US and caused a wide range of other infections including bacteremia, pneumonia, cellulitis and epiglottis. The introduction of the Hib conjugate vaccine saw a significant decrease in the cases of invasive Hib disease. The Hib conguate vaccine remains available as a single agent. It is also available in two different combination products: combined with DTaP and IPV (3-dose primary series at 2,4, 6 months with a booster at 12-15 months) (39), or combined with hepatitis B vaccine in another combination vaccine in a three dose plan (primary series at 2 and 4 months with a booster dose at 12-15 months). In countries where the Hib vaccine is not routinely provided, there is an increase in *hemophilus influenzae* type b infections such as epiglottis and meningitis. It is not routinely recommended to give the Hib vaccine after 59 months of age.

TETANUS IMMUNIZATION

Tetanus (Greek word for taut or stretch) is caused by the Clostridium tetani exotoxin and there are about 40 to 50 cases of tetanus in the United States each year, ranging from a low of 34 in 2004 to a high of 601 in 1948. It is usually found in the elderly adult whose immunization never occurred or was many years in the past. Clostridium tetani is a gram-positive, rod-shaped, obligate, anaerobic bacterium that lives in the soil as well as the intestinal tract. It causes the classic tetanus disorder with skeletal muscle spasms and lockjaw in generalized tetanus; other forms include neonatal, local, and cephalic tetanus (40).

Tetanus remains a major etiologic agent in disease and death in developing countries (30). The WHO estimates 59,000 newborns died from neonatal tetanus around the world in 2008 (21). Neonatal tetanus can develop if the mother does not have antibodies to this organism. The mortality rate from tetanus varies between 48% to 75%. The tetanus vaccine was first introduced in the US in 1927 and this tetanus toxoid vaccine develops serum IgG antibodies to prevent tetanus. Protection against this organism is noted with a serum tetanus antitoxin level of 0.1 IU/ml or more as measured by ELISA technology. Coverage for tetanus in pregnant women (including adolescents) can dramatically reduce the incidence of neonatal tetanus in tropical regions (41, 42).

DIPHTHERIA IMMUNIZATION

Diphtheria is caused by the corynebacterium diphtheriae toxin produced by this Gram positive, pleomorphic, facultative, anaerobic bacterium also known as the Klebs-Loffler bacillus. It gains entry into the person via the respiratory tract and induces a severe infection with local inflammatory membrane involvement (pseudomembrane), myocarditis, and distal neuritis. The mortality rate is 10%-20% and the highest number of cases recorded in the US was 206,939 in 1921, with 15,520 deaths; between 1980 and 2000 there were 53 cases and only two have been reported in the first part of the 21st century.

The diphtheria toxoid vaccine was introduced in the United States in 1923 and develops both serum IgG and mucosal IgG antibodies to prevent diphtheria. Diphtheria is common in various parts of the world including Latin America and the Caribbean countries. Cases increased dramatically in the USSR after its breakup in 1989; by 1998, there were 200,000 cases with 5,000 deaths (43).

PERTUSSIS IMMUNIZATION

Pertussis is caused by *Bordetella pertussis*, a gram-negative, aerobic, coccobaccillus in which humans are the only hosts (44). It was isolated by the Belgian microbiologist, Jules Bordet, in 1906. It causes a highly contagious infection of the respiratory tract with a classic cough lasting over two weeks and up to 180 days; the classic cough is characterized by coughing paroxysms, post-tussive emesis, and/or a respiratory whoop (45, 46). Pertussis diagnosis is confirmed with a nasopharyngeal swab via culture or polymerase chain reaction (PCR) technology. There are over 300,000 pediatric deaths worldwide each year due to pertussis (45).

The highest number of pertussis cases in the United States was 256,269 in 1934, though the first pertussis vaccine (whole cell vaccine) was developed in the early part of the 20th century. Dr. Louis Sauer developed an inactivated whole cell vaccine in the 1920s in Evanston, Illinois, and the Danish scientist, Dr. Thorvald Madsen, accomplished the first large scale test of the pertussis vaccine in the Faroe Islands of the North Sea in 1925 (43). In 1942, Pearl Kendrick produced the first combined DTP vaccine with tetanus toxoid, as well as diphtheria vaccine and an inactivated whole cell pertussis compenent. Before the pertussis vaccine was developed, 10,000 persons were dying each year in the United States from this infection.

Though cases of pertussis and numbers of infant deaths dropped dramatically after widespread use of the DPT vaccine in the United States, anti-vaccine forces launched an assault on this vaccine with a charge that the whole cell pertussis vaccine produced encephalopathy in infants. The power of the media was witnessed by a one-hour television documentary that aired on April 19, 1982, in the Washington, DC area called "DTP: Vaccine Roulette"; it alleged that pertussis vaccine induced severe neurological damage in infants (47) Though these charges were later noted to be spurious, the damage was done and many parents withheld this vaccine from their children leading to increase in pertussis infections and increase in infant deaths (48).

While pertussis infections reached a nadir in 1976 with 1,020 cases in the United States, importation of unvaccinated persons to the US along with a decrease in DTP vaccinations lead to a rise of pertussis cases with over 25,000 reported cases in 2004, and 48,277 in 2012. Cases are often to adolescents and adults who have lost their immunity to this infection. Experts suggest there are over 600,000 cases of pertussis each year in the US, and perhaps over three million (43, 49). Unfortunately adolescents and adults without full immunity to pertussis can transmit this infection to infants, often resulting in severe consequences. Approximately half of infants under one year of age who develop pertussis are hospitalized, one in twenty develops pneumonia, one in 100 develops seizures, and death can occur. In the United States there are 10-20 infant deaths each year, and 195,000 annual deaths worldwide in children.

Pertussis immunity from natural infection or vaccine can begin to wane within a few years after an infection or vaccine dose (including the 5 dose DTaP childhood series) (50). This drop in protection from the natural disease or vaccine may be due to genetic changes in *Bordetella pertussis,* representing an ability that other organisms possess in the evolutionary dance for survival. An inactivated acellular pertussis vaccine was developed by Dr. Yuji Sato in 1981, and an acellular vaccine received FDA approval in 2005. This acellular pertussis technology resulted in the Tdap vaccine that is recommended as a one-time dose for adolescents and adults who need a booster (44, 51-55).

It is important to protect ("cocoon") young infants by vaccinating those around them until they can complete their own primary pertussis series (56). This includes persons living with an infant less than 12 months of age and health care personnel. Coverage of pregnant females is discussed in the maternal immunization section (*vida infra*). A 2012 study investigating the effectiveness of the pertussis vaccine during a pertussis epidemic noted a range from 95% (92%-97%) in those who were 15 to 47 months of age, to 47% (19%-65%) in those who were 13 to 16 years of age; in this study the incidence of pertussis was higher in the unimmunized versus immunized group (57).

TETANUS/DIPHTHERIA/PERTUSSIS (DTAP/TDAP/TD) IMMUNIZATION

Children are usually protected against tetanus, diphtheria, and pertussis as recommended by the Centers for Disease and Control (CDC) and the WHO. The CDC recommends that young children receive a combination vaccine which covers all three diseases and is administered in a series of immunizations (DTaP at 2, 4, 6, and 15 to 18 months). Globally the number of children protected from these diseases has increased due to continued efforts to educate physicians, governments, and society.

In 1980 world vaccine coverage for the first dose of diphtheria-tetanus-pertussis vaccine (DTP) was 30%, and 20% for the third dose; it was 88% and 76% respectively in 1990, and 91% and 83% in 2012 (5). The third dose (DTP3) reached 77% in 2010 by 12 months of age, as measured by the WHO African Region and more vaccine research as well as immunization policy implementation in Africa is recommended by experts of the Vaccines for Africa Initiative (VACFA) (12).

The US CDC notes that the fourth dose of DTaP may be given as soon as 12 months of age if the interval between doses 3 and 4 doses is at least 6 months, and the child is at risk for not returning for a visit at the recommended age of 15 to 18 months. The CDC recommends that a DTaP booster be given at 4 to 6 years of age, and a Tdap booster between 11 and 12 years, usually five years after the primary childhood series. The Td immunization used to be given for the early adolescent booster, but now a combination of all three is recommended in the United States (i.e., Tdap) because of a recent rise in pertussis. After the adolescent dose, a booster for tetanus and diphtheria (Td) is recommended every 10 years. If one is over 7 years of age and did not receive the recommended primary childhood series, the primary series is started as soon as possible utilizing Tdap for the first dose, and completing the series with Td. A second dose is given 4 weeks after the first, a third primary dose 5 to 12 months later, and then a booster every 10 years.

Children between 7 and 10 years of age who did not complete a DTaP series can receive the Tdap. Those 11-12 years who have received a full DTaP series can receive a Tdap vaccine and those who are 13-18 years of age can receive a Tdap if not given at 11-12 years. Older persons who are due for a tetanus-diphtheria booster can be given a Tdap booster if they have never received one. Only one immunization for all three diseases (Tdap) is recommended after the primary series at this time (38). It is not currently recommended to give more than one lifetime Tdap for males and non-pregnant females.

The Food and Drug Administration (FDA) has licensed 11 combination vaccines for use in the United States to date to help protect against diptheria and tetanus with eight of these vaccines also providing protection against whooping cough. These combination vaccines contain two or more vaccines in a single shot in order to decrease the number of shots given at any one time. Some of these combination vaccines include protection against other diseases like polio, H. influenza type b disease and Hepatitis B. These are:

1) DT (generic) and Td (Tenivac and generic)
2) DTaP (Daptacel, Infanrix, Kinrix, Pediarix, Pentacel and Quadracel)
3) Tdap (adacel and Boostrix)

MEASLES, MUMPS, RUBELLA (MMR) IMMUNIZATION

Measles, mumps, and rubella are well-known contagious viral infections that are spread via the respiratory tract with episodic outbreaks. Measles (rubeola or morbilli) has been described since the 9th century and is caused by a paramyxovirus of the genus Morbillivirus that can lead to major complications and death. Unfortunately 900,000 persons die from measles annually around the world. Two doses of this live viral vaccine (MMR—Edmonston-Enders strain) are given to children with recommendations in the US since 1989; the first one is given at or after 12 months of age (12-15 months) and the second one at 4 to 6 years of age (58).

It can be given between 6 and 11 months if the infant is traveling to or living in an endemic area; this early dose does not count for the recommended two dose series. Children and adolescents given separate MMR doses that are not separated by at least four weeks need to get caught up with the two-dose series. Being born before 1957 is not in itself proof of measles immunity for those who might be pregnant; those wishing to become pregnant should have evidence of appropriate measles vaccination or serologic results indicating immunity to measles. Fortunately, measles and rubella are rare in the United States due to the high coverage of children with vaccination.

Failure to vaccinate individuals leads to increase in measles. In 2005, a 17 year old unvaccinated female returned to the US from a visit to Romania; during that time she attended a family gathering of 500 people. After she returned from visiting relatives, 34 cases of measles were confirmed and traced back to her (58). Such examples are increasing because of the failure to immunize among all ages, with an increase in the number and percentage of measles cases in those over age 20.

In 1973, only 3% of the measles cases occurred in those over 19 years of age. This increased to 34% in the year 2000. Measles elimination was declared by the CDC in the United States in 2000 since there was interruption of endemic transmission of measles for the year. Reduction in measles vaccination rates since then has increased the prevalence of this disease, with 222 cases reported in the US in 2011, and 288 cases between January 1, 2014 and May 23, 2014 (59). This is in contrast to over 600 cases in 1996 (one-third of which were in adolescents) and a high of 894,000 in 1941. In order to ensure that measles epidemics do not recur, we should strive for a vaccination rate as close as possible to 100%.

Measles is the leading vaccine-preventable disease studied by researchers in Africa between 1991 and 2010 (12). Failure of the measles vaccine to provide protection can arise from ineffective vaccine cold chain system. A report of Nigeria vaccine effectiveness noted a low, 68.6% sero-conversion rate (61). Failure to maintain a high measles vaccination rate leads to measles epidemics with death in some infected individuals. For example, In 2011 India recorded 36% of global measles deaths that included 28 deaths from a group of 3,670 measles cases (62). There is an increase in post-vaccination seizures for children given delayed versus on time MMR vaccinations in the second year of life; this is increased with MMRV (MMR with varicella vaccine) (63).

College students who leave their countries to study in the U.S. are advised to be fully vaccinated against measles to protect them from a potential outbreak at their university and also prevent them from staring the epidemic (64). Adults born in the United States in 1957 or later can receive one MMR dose while adults who need 2 doses are those at high risk for disease and include health care workers, international travelers, and college students. Though measles has been targeted by the Centers for Disease Control and Prevention (CDC) for eradication from the United States and beyond, the recent surge has put this goal on hold for now (65, 66).

Rubella

Rubella was reported at its highest level in the US at 57,000 cases in 1969, and vaccination with the MMR vaccine has practically removed it from the U.S. with very few if any cases reported each year; the few cases noted are mostly in adults with no immunity. No endemic rubella cases have been reported in the U.S. since 2009. Unfortunately, rubella cases are seen around the world where vaccination rates are low, leading to over 100,000 rubella cases and 100,000 cases of congenital rubella syndrome (CRS) being reported (67). Congenital rubella syndrome (CRS) is a serious condition in which rubella infection during pregnancy results in an infant with many congenital defects including mental retardation, deafness, cardiac defects, cataracts, encephalitis, and others.

The U.S. had a high of 20,000 CRS cases in the 1964 to 1965 period, and now has none thanks to the official rubella vaccination program that began in the US in 1969. It is a tragic result when an infant is born into the world with CRS when it is a preventable condition. Waiver of the rubella vaccine may be acceptable in a female who may become pregnant and who either has a positive serological test for rubella or has documentation of acceptable vaccination. Ironically, though the MMR vaccine has been falsely linked with an increase in autism, its use has been shown to reduce autism in addition to measles, mumps, rubella, and CRS (18, 58, 68).

Mumps

Mumps is caused by a paramyxovirus that can lead to classic parotitis but also orchitis, epididymitis, spontaneous miscarriage, meningitis (usually mild), oophoritis, pancreatitis, and even rare encephalitis. It reached its highest 20th century level in the US at over 152,000 cases in 1968, and vaccination reduced its prevalence to less than one case per 1 million population in the early 2000s. The mumps vaccine was introduced in the US in 1976 with one dose and then 2 doses (MMR) as of 1989.

A resurgence of mumps is noted in the US since the early 2000s with over 250 cases per year and a number of outbreaks in many states (69). In 2006 there were 6,500 mumps cases in the middle of the US, with the state of Iowa as the epicenter. The outbreak eventually involved 45 states and the District of Columbia (2). During this epidemic, mumps cases occurred in greater than 2 per 100,000 in eight Midwestern states, with over 6 per 100,000 in those 18 to 24 years of age. In this epidemic, complications included orchitis (9.6%), meningitis (0.5%), encephalitis (0.4%), and deafness (0.4%); 2.1% of these students were hospitalized. Failure for some to have received two MMR vaccinations was the cause for some students, but decreasing immunity to the mumps vaccine may have been the main factor in this epidemic. The vaccine seems to be 80 to 85% effective and thus, vaccine failure, played a part in this outbreak (2, 58).

The MMR vaccine has been proven to be efficacious at protecting people against measles, mumps and rubella as well as preventing the complications caused by these diseases. A newer vaccine MMRV is a combination vaccine that also protects against chicken pox that is licensed for use in children 12 months through 12 years of age (58). The CDC recommends that children get one dose of MMRV vaccine between 12-15 months with the second dose at 4-6 years of age just like the MMR vaccine.

Antivaccine Concerns

Perhaps a much greater problem than limited vaccine failure is the growing movement in the United States and Europe against vaccinations including the MMR vaccine. The movement against vaccines began as soon as vaccinology began with the work of Edward Jenner on smallpox (vida infra) (8). As previously noted, concerns with vaccines over the past two centuries have focused on a myriad of issues such as claims of greater efficacy with natural infection versus vaccination, anger at compulsory vaccine programs, concerns with mercury in vaccines, worries about side effects from vaccines, worries about the low efficacy of vaccines, and others.

The MMR vaccine has been the epicenter of current antivaccine angst due to false claims linking it with causing autism (18). The first salvo in this current movement was fired by the 1982 television documentary falsely alleging brain damage from the pertussis vaccine (8). Then Bernhard Rimland, PhD (1928 to 2006), a highly respected psychologist in the field of developmental-behavioral disorders (i.e., autism, ADHD, learning disorders, and learning disorders) asserted that the mercury-containing vaccine preservative thimerosal was linked to what he saw was an epidemic rise in autism. In 1965, Dr. Rimland founded the Autism Society of America and shortly thereafter, in 1967 he founded and directed the Autism Research Institute in San Diego, California, USA.

Adding to this belief was the work of Andrew Wakefield who is a medical researcher and surgeon from England, but moved to the United States. In 1998 he authored a highly-publicized study in the well-known medical journal, *Lancet*, claiming a link between the MMR vaccine and what he called "autistic enterocolitis" (70). Though this research was later discredited and his article recalled by the journal that published it, the pebble-in-the-pond effect continued, as increasing numbers of alarmed mothers stopped and/or delayed allowing their children to receive the MMR vaccination resulting in increased numbers of infections such as measles (18, 71-75). The public remains concerned even though science has clearly shown there is no link between autism and vaccines or mercury (76-80).

Even so, the lawsuits continue in the United States, the media continues to pursue such stories, and some choose to ignore the remarkable science of vaccinology as in the past (81-85). Globally cases of death from measles have continued; mortality in some countries is about 1 in 1,000 with about 450 deaths in children each day in sub-Saharan Africa (86). Mumps is increasing and children remain at risk to be born with preventable congenital rubella syndrome estimated, as previously noted, at 100,000 infants per year. This remains a poignant and tragic consequence of the failure to vaccinate and the global anti-vaccine hysteria in developed countries.

> **Alice in Alice in Wonderland, 1865**
> *If I had a world of my own, everything would be nonsense.*
> *Nothing would be what it is because everything would be what it isn't.*
> *And contrary-wise; what it is it wouldn't be,*
> *and what it wouldn't be, it would. You see?*
> Lewis Carroll [Charles Lutwidge Dodgson]

MENINGOCOCCAL IMMUNIZATION

There are approximately 3,000 meningitis cases of meningitis each year due to *Neisseria meningitidis* in the United States, and it has a mortality rate of 14% in addition to a high risk for complications in the survivors that include deafness, mental retardation, and loss of limbs (87-89). *N meningitidis* is a leading cause of meningitis and bacterial sepsis in the US and the world, especially among adolescents and young adults. In a 2009 meningococcal epidemic in 14 African countries, there were 88,199 reported (suspected) cases that included 5,352 deaths; this was the highest number of reported since an epidemic in 1996.

Infectious rates can range from 0.5 to 1.3 per 100,000 in the U.S. and 1.4 in selected young adults in a college or university setting (90). Those immunized at 11-12 years of age may have decreased protective immunity when 16 to 21 years of age and thus, a booster dose of the meningococcal immunization is recommended. If a dose is given at 16 years of age or older, a booster is not needed later unless the person remains at high risk for this infection (see Table 2) (91). MCV4 (meningococcal conjugate vaccine: vida infra) contains 48 micrograms of diphtheria toxoid but does not provide any protection against diphtheria.

Table 2. Persons at increased N meningitidis risk

Adolescents and young adults (aged 11 through 21); including living in crowded college dormitory conditions and military recruits
Persons exposed during an acute epidemic or outbreak
Those traveling to Mecca during annual Haij
Those traveling to West Africa or other areas with high rates of infection
Individuals with some conditions that lower immunity
-Functional or anatomical asplenia
-Terminal complement component deficiency
Persons (i.e., microbiologists) working in labs with *N. meningitidis*

In the US, most cases of meningococcal infection (98%) are sporadic and 62% involve those over 11 years of age. Thus, a university with 40,000 students in the U.S. can expect one case of invasive meningococcal disease every 1 to 2 years unless these students are protected through meningococcal vaccination (92). Table 2 notes those at high risk for *N. meningitidis* meningitis, including university students in crowded dormitory situations with increased smoking and nasopharyngeal carriage of this microbe (93-99). Those in college who are 21 years of age and younger should have received an MCV4 dose within the past 5 years; if not, they can be given this vaccine. Those who are 22 or older do not need a routine MCV4 vaccination. Meningococcal immunization is recommended for those traveling to high risk areas such as the meningitis belt in Sub-Saharan Africa (98, 99). Those getting an MCV4 for travel only need one primary dose while those with medical indications (i.e., asplenia) need two primary doses, 8 weeks apart.

There are two types of meningococcal vaccines available: Meningococcal conjugate or MenACWY and the serogroup B meningococcal or MenB vaccines (99). All 11-12 year olds should get the MenACWY vaccine with a booster dose at 16 years old (99). The CDC also recommends the MenACWY for children between 2 months and 10 years old if they have the following: a rare type of immune discorder called complement component deficiency, are taking a complement inhibitor (Soliris or Ultomiris), have a damaged spleen or has had splenectomy, have HIV, are traveling to countries in which disease is common and are part of a population identified to be at increased risk for serogroup ACW or Y disease outbreak (99). MenACWY is also recommended for adults with the the same risk criteria like the younger children. MenB is recommended for all teens between 16-18 years old, children 10 years or older and adults with certain immunocompromised conditions such as complement component deficiency, damaged spleen or splenectomy (99). There is also a bivalent meningococcal polysaccharide protein conjugate vaccine providing protection for meningococcal serogroups C and Y added to Haemophilus influenzae type b (Hib-MenCY-TT) licensed for use in children aged 6 weeks to 18 months (101,102).

The polysaccharide vaccine produces (MPSV4) a less effective T-cell independent immune response but can be used if the conjugate vaccine is not available and for those at or over age 56. Conjugate vaccine technology was developed in the 1980s and utilizes chemical conjugation to carrier proteins that leads to an induced T-cell dependent response for improved protection against this organism. This vaccine (MVC4) was first licensed by the U.S. Food and Drug Administration (FDA) in 2006. Both the polysaccharide and conjugate meningitis vaccine protect against 4 subtypes: A, C, Y, and W-135. MCV4 is given intramuscularly and MPSV4 is given subcutaneously. Vaccine for the protection from the B subtype is available in some countries outside the US, and serotype B can cause 20% of invasive meningococcemia in the US (103).

Human papillomavirus (HPV) immunization

The human papillomavirus (HPV) is the most common sexually transmitted disease microbe that infects over 20 million individuals in the United States with over 6 million new cases each year (88). Prevalence data for adolescent females can range up to 65%; additionally, up to 75% of new infections are found in those between ages 15 and 24 years. Over half of sexually active persons are infected with at least one subtype of HPV, with over 80% of the exposure occurring before 50 years of age. New infections typically develop soon after sexarche (i.e., onset of coital activity).

Over 100 HPV serotypes are classified including 40 that affect the genitals and 15 that are listed as being oncogenc—particularly types 16,18,31,33, and 45. HPV is a global infection and found throughout the world (104). Chronic HPV infection can lead to cervical cancer with over 10,000 cases diagnosed in adult females each year in the US and over 4,000 deaths annually. Globally there are over 250,000 deaths annually from cervical cancer.

HPV-associated cancers in males include oropharyngeal, penile, and anal cancers due to HPV 16 (105-107). There are an estimated 22,000 HPV 16- and HPV 18-associated cancers each year in the United States that include approximately 7,000 HPV 16- and 18-associated cancers in males. In males oropharyngeal cancers increased 1% per year from 1973 to 2007 and 3% per year for anal cancers. There are an estimated 250,000 cases of genital warts each year among sexually active males in the U.S. due primarily to HPV 6 and 11. Males having sex with males have an increased prevalence of HPV types 6, 11, 16, and 18.

The first infection in females usually occurs soon after sexual behavior initiates (sexarche) and infection with more than one HPV type often occurs. Use of condoms is not fully protective and rare genital infection may develop from non-penetrative sexual contact as well as underclothes transmission and even surgical gloves as agents of transmission. Though HPV infection is typically cleared from the female within two years after initial infection, it can become a persistent infection in about 10% of females leading to an increased risk for cervical and other anogenital cancers.

Recombinant DNA technology led to the development of the HPV vaccine (HPV4) that includes VLPs (viral-like particles) of the oncogenic types 16 and 18 and in one vaccine, the addition of two types causing over 90% of anogenital warts—6 and 11 (108). Serotypes 16 and 18 are responsible for over 70% of cervical cancers and cross-over immunogenicity may lead to proposed protection from up to 80% of cervical cancer cases (109). The HPV vaccine contains the L1 protein that self-assembles into VLPs that are immunogenic but non-infectious by mimicking the HPV virion. Despite low HPV vaccine uptake (*vida infra*) the prevalence of the covered HPV types (i.e., 6, 11, 16, 18) dropped 56% among females aged 14 to 19 years—i.e., from 11.5% in 2003-2006 to 5.1% in 2007-2010 (110).

There are three HPV vaccines licensed by the FDA which protect against serotypes 16 and 18 that are known to cause majority of HPV cancers. Gardasil is the quadrivalent HPV vaccine (containing serotypes 6,11,16, and 18) and the Gardasil-9 which is nine-valent HPV vaccine containing the 4 previous serotypes 6,11,16, and 18 plus serotypes 31, 45, 52 and 58 (109). Either form is given in three intramuscular injections at 0, 2, and 6 months with minimal intervals between doses 1 and 4 at 4 weeks and 12 weeks between doses 2 and 3 with the first dose recommended to be given at 11-12 years of age. Vaccination with the two-dose series can be initiated at age 9 and through 14 years (109). It is FDA-approved for females and males between 9 and 26 years of age; it is recommended to give this vaccine before the initiation of any sexual behavior. The vaccine effectiveness for one dose is 82%. Even if one is infected with one HPV, the vaccine is recommended since it is unlikely the person has been exposed to both cancer promoting types. Providing the HPV vaccine does not replace the recommendation for cervical cancer screening for females (111). Though there is no evidence of teratogenicity, it is not given to pregnant females since data on this is still limited. Contraindications to the HPV vaccine include history of allergic reaction to a previous HPV vaccine injection, Baker's yeast, or other vaccine components.

In light of the new evidence from scientific literature published during January 1, 2006 through October 18, 2018 in terms of the efficacy of HPV vaccination preventing occurrence of ano-genital cancers, catch-up HPV vaccination has been recommended to be a shared clinical decision-making for adults aged 27 through 45 years who are not adequately vaccinated (112).

HPV vaccination has not been as well accepted by the public as the classic childhood vaccines, partly because of fear of side effects promoted by anti-vaccine forces. One manner to counter this reluctance is clear clinician endorsement that this is a safe, effective, and CDC as well as clinician-recommended immunization (113-115). Side effects are minimal and based on 21,194 VAERS reports in females from 56 million doses given between June of 2006 and March of 2013. Reported side effects include 92.1% that were listed as "non-serious": dizziness, fever, hives, local injection site reactions (i.e., pain, redness, swelling), nausea, and headache (116).

There were 7.9% of side effects listed as "serious" that included headache, nausea, vomiting, fatigue, dizziness, syncope, and generalized weakness (116). In addition to prophylactic immunization protocols, research is occurring on therapeutic strategies for HPV-associated disorders including cancers (116). Other anti-STD vaccines under research include vaccines against *Neisseria gonorrhoeae*, herpes simplex virus, *Chlamydia trachomatis*, and the HIV virus (118, 119).

HEPATITIS A IMMUNIZATION

In 2006 the CDC recommended that all children 12 to 23 months of age receive two doses of the hepatitis A vaccine 6 months apart. Hepatitis A vaccine also comes in combination form containing both hepatitis A and B that can be given to anyone over 18 years of age as 3 shots over 6 months (119). Data revealed it was widespread in the United States and was capable of causing significant morbidity with increased health care costs and loss of days from work or school. Rates of hospitalization from

Hepatitis A infection vary from 11 to 22%, and adults lose an average of 27 days from work. Those older than 23 months who were not vaccinated earlier can be covered through 18 years of age. The CDC Healthy People 2020 goal is 85% for those 19-35 months of age.

High-risk conditions for this virus include traveling to countries with a high Hepatitis A prevalence, those using illegal drugs, those with chronic liver disease, and men having sex with men (119). Pre-vaccination serologic testing may be useful for some adults, such as those over 40 years of age, those born or living for a prolonged time in places with high hepatitis A infection, and certain populations in the US (such as Hispanics, native Americans, or Alaskan natives). There are an estimated 1.4 million cases of Hepatitis A in the world, and research notes that 90.8% of developing world children with chronic liver disease are exposed to Hepatitis A; thus, Hepatitis A vaccination is recommended to protect these children (121).

Table 3. Risk factors for hepatitis B infection

Multiple sex partners (including more than one partner in last 6 months)
History of sexually transmitted diseases
Male-male sexual behavior
Intravenous drug use
Use of contaminated needle (body piercing, tattooing)
Requiring hemodialysis or clotting factor
Person from a country where Hepatitis B infection is common
Caring for or living with a person with Hepatitis B infection
Health care workers

HEPATITIS B IMMUNIZATION

Annually there are approximately 140,000 cases of hepatitis B infection, with 70% noted in adolescents and young adults in the US; overall there are 1.2 million persons infected in the US and the incidence is about 2.8 per 100,000 population (122). There are over 5,000 new carriers each year and 5,000 deaths each year from hepatitis B in the United States. There are approximately 350 million persons with chronic hepatitis B infection in the world.

Hepatitis B infection leads to hepatitis of various types: acute, chronic, and fulminant. Table 3 lists known risk factors for infection from this DNA virus, although 25% of infected persons do not have any of these risk factors. Faulty screening of donated blood and injection of illegal drugs accounts for many cases of hepatitis B infections in the world—the latter resulting in 16 million annual cases.

Research notes that 39.1% of developing world children with chronic liver disease are exposed to Hepatitis B and universal hepatitis B vaccination is recommended to protect these children (121). The CDC recommends that the hepatitis B vaccine be given a birth, 1-2 months, and 6 to 12 months of age. Hepatitis B vaccine is a recombination of antigenic groups (hepatitis B incorporated into plasmids) and has been available in the US since the mid-1980s. One of the doses should be given at or after 6 months of age to ensure lifelong immunity. There is a two-dose vaccine series that is only available for adolescents between 11 and 15 years of age.

Most adults with diabetes mellitus will become high risk conditions hepatitis B infection due to the development of chronic liver disease and end stage renal disease; thus, those with diabetes are at risk for increased morbidity and mortality from hepatitis B. All three doses of the recommended 3-dose vaccine series are required to provide maximum protection as noted by various studies including a recent study in India that recorded a seroprotection rate of 49.1% after the first dose, 86.9% after the second dose, and 96.7% after the third dose; the rate was 89% by the end of the second year and 85.5% by the end of the third year post-vaccination (123). The importance of providing a birth dose of hepatitis B vaccine has been shown by studies around the world (124). There is no proven link between hepatitis B vaccination and the development of multiple sclerosis (125).

Coverage should insure protection of newborns by beginning the hepatitis B series within 12 hours of birth. If a mother is positive for HBsAg and HBeAg, 70%-90% of her infants will become infected without post-exposure prophylaxis; the risk of perinatal transmission is 10% if the mother is positive only for HBsAg. An infant born to an HBsAg+ mother should receive the hepatitis B vaccine and also hepatitis B immune globulin (HBIG) within 12 hours of birth. Up to 90% of infected infants develop a chronic infection with HBV. Pregnant women should be tested for Hepatitis B (i.e., HBsAg) with each pregnancy since their hepatitis B status can change.

VARICELLA IMMUNIZATION

Varicella (chickenpox) is the most common vaccine preventable disease in the United States and immunization begins with the 12 to 15 month old and the routine second dose is recommended for all children 4 to 6 years of age. The vaccine (*Oka-Merck strain*) is also suggested for all adolescents and adults who have not been infected with the varicella virus in a schedule of 2 doses, with a minimal interval of 3 months if under age 13 years and 4 weeks if over 13 years of age (126). Antibodies develop after the first dose in 78% and 99% after the second dose.

There are two types of chicken pox vaccines licensed in the United States and they are: Varivax which contains only chickenpox and ProQuad which is a combination of measles, mumps, rubella and chicken pox. Varivax can be used for children 12 months and older and adults while ProQuad is recommended for use in children 12 months through 12 years old (126).

Table 4. Criteria for evidence of varicella immunity

1)	Born in the US before 1980 (not used as criteria if pregnant or for health care personnel)
2)	Documentation of appropriate vaccination
3)	Laboratory documentation of immunity
4)	Clinician report of herpes zoster history
5)	Others

Infection can develop after immunization, though it is much milder with fewer than 50 lesions that are mainly maculopapular and not vesicular. It has not been shown that the risk of breakthrough infection rises the longer one is from vaccination. Risk of breakthrough infection can be lowered with a second varicella dose. A natural infection without immunization protection can lead to 300 to 500 blisters.

Efficacy of the vaccine is up to 90% against infection, 95% against moderate to severe disease and over 90% retain effective antibody levels for at least 6 years. Criteria for evidence of immunity to varicella are noted in Table 4 (127). Prior to the introduction of this varicella vaccine in the United States in 1995, 11,000 persons were hospitalized each year from varicella infection (2-3 per 1,000 healthy children and 8 per 1,000 adults) with one child and one adult dying each week from this infection, 80% of deaths occurred in previously "healthy" individuals (126). Unfortunately countless millions of infections occur in the world each year, secondary infection with group A Streptococcus may occur, and varicella can be teratogenic in pregnancy.

The fatality rate of varicella infection is 1 per 100,000 for those 1 to 14 years of age, 2.7 per 100,000 if 15 to 19 years of age, 8 per 100,00 for those 20 to 29 years of age, and 25.2 if 30 to 49 years of age (126). Persons over 19 years of age account for only 5% of varicella cases in the United States, but 35% of the deaths. The implementation of the varicella vaccine program in the United States resulted in a 97% decrease in deaths from this virus in persons under age 20 years and 96% decrease in those under age 50 years (128).

Table 5. Conditions with Increased streptococcus pneumoniae risk

Age (at or over 65 years)
Alcoholism
Asplenia (anatomical or functional)
Cancer
Chronic cardiovascular disorders
Chronic pulmonary disorders
Chronic renal failure
Diabetes mellitus
HIV infection
Nephrotic syndrome
Sickle cell disease
Others

PNEUMOCOCCUS IMMUNIZATIONS

Streptococcus pneumoniae is a bacterium that can causes serious infection in individuals of all ages, especially in those with chronic illness (129-132) (see Table 5). All children should receive the pneumococcal conjugate vaccine (PCV13 or Prevnar 13) at 2,4,6, and 12-15 months of age; PCV-13 has replaced the PCV-7 in which only 7 serotypes are covered versus the current 13 (133). Use of the PCV vaccine at age 2 through 64 years old is dependent on the underlying chronic illness that is present and all adults 65 years and older should receive PCV13 (133). Those who are 6 to 18 years and adults 19 years and older should receive one PCV (if there is no previous PCV history) for cochlear implants, cerebrospinal fluid leakage, and immunosuppression due to HIV, asplenia (anatomic or function [i.e., sickle cell disease]), malignancy, and others (134-136). Use of PCV vaccine has led to less invasive pneumococcal disease in children who are less than 5 years of age with 99 cases/100,000 persons in 1998-1999 dropping to 21 cases per 100,000 in 2008. There is an increased risk of febrile seizure with simultaneous use of PCV 13 and inactivated trivalent influenza vaccine (II3).

The *pneumococcal polysaccharide vaccine* (PPSV23 or Pneumovax23) is recommended for persons (2 years of age through 64 years) at high risk of S. pneumonia infections, adults 19 through 64 years who are cigarette smokers and all adults 65 years and older, as noted in Table 5 (133, 134). It reduces the rate of drug-resistant *Streptococcus pneumoniae* (especially type 19A) and provides coverage for 23 of the 90 pneumococcal serotypes (129). One dose is given to persons 2 to 18 years of age with cardiac or kidney disease, diabetes mellitus, chronic pulmonary disease, alcoholism, CSF leaks, or cochlear implants. Two doses are given to those 2 to 18 years of age with immunosuppression caused by HIV, asplenia, sickle cell, and malignancy; the two doses are separated by a minimum of 5 years. It is not contraindicated because of pregnancy (see the Maternal Immunization section—vida infra).

Introduction of the pneumococcal conjugate vaccine into the South African public immunization program has resulted in less pneumococcal morbidity and mortality (137). PPSV-23 is 60-70% effective in preventing invasive disease. It appears to be less effective in preventing non-bacteremic pneumococcal pneumonia and also is less effective in those with significant underlying illness (see Table 5).

Those at high risk for pneumococcal infection can receive the PPSV-23 vaccine including those 19 to 64 years of age who have asthma or smoke cigarettes and all those 65 years of age and older. One dose is given and a second dose can be given 5 years or more after the first dose; no more than 2 lifetime doses are recommended for those at high risk for complications from infection with *Streptococcus pneumonia* (129, 132). Efficacy of PPSV23 is about 60% to 70% in preventing invasive pneumococcal disease. Implementation of pneumococcal vaccines around the world will improve global health because of reduced health consequences of this devastating infection (138).

INFLUENZA VACCINES

Influenza is caused by an enveloped RNA orthomyxovirus with two main types (A and B) that annually leads to millions of symptomatic infections globally. Type A is subdivided using two surface proteins: **H**emagglutinin and **N**euraminidase; the most common A strains are H1N1 and H3N2. There have been four influenza pandemics in the world over the past century, including the infamous Spanish influenza pandemic of 1918-1920 (see Table 6) (139). Public health officials remain vigilant for the possibility of H and N strains that come from animals (i.e., pigs, birds, others) and may cross over to humans with hybrid strains. Currently three hybrid strains are being watched in the US: H5N1 (pathogenic avian strain from southeastern Asia), H7N9 (strain from poultry in China), and H3N2v (pig strain in the US).

In the Northern Hemisphere a seasonal pattern of influenza occurs annually starting in the fall and ending in April. There are typically four different influenza viruses circulating and produce epidemics lasting 8 to 10 weeks. Though laboratory testing is not necessary in most mild cases, lab testing is available, and depending on local medical capabilities as well as recommendations, consists of culture-based tests, antigen-based tests (direct fluorescent antibody, enzyme immunoassays), nucleic acid amplification tests (Singleplex, Multiplex), and serology.

The highest prevalence rates usually occur in children, and the highest rates of complications (i.e., hospitalizations, deaths) are usually seen in those under age 5 (especially infants), those over 65 years of age ("seniors"), and those with immunocompromised states. During each influenza season in the United States, 200,000 are hospitalized with over 35,000 deaths, mostly in the elderly and those under 5 years of age. Mortality rates are 2.7% higher when H3N2 is predominant. H1N1 tends to have a higher attack rate in those over age 25 but not over age 65 years.

Table 6. Influenza type A pandemics

Year	Subtype	Severity of Pandemic
1889	H3N2	Moderate
1918	H1N1	Severe
1957	H2N2	Severe
1968	H3N2	Moderate
1977	H1N1	Mild

Viral changes from genetic reassortment (i.e., antigenic drift or shift) alters one's immunity to influenza each year, particularly the ability to deal with the changing hemagglutinin antigen. The vaccine-induced immunity does not last from year to year and thus, a new vaccine is introduced each year in attempts to deal with these viral changes. Unfortunately, millions of humans avoid this yearly vaccine with potentially devastating results in some. Starting with the 2011 to 2012 influenza season, allergy to eggs is a precaution and not a contraindication to the influenza vaccine. People with egg allergies can receive any licensed, recommended age-appropriate influenza vaccine that is deemed appropriate. People who have a history of severe egg allergy should be vaccinated in a medical setting, supervised by a health care provider who is able to recognize and manage severe allergic reactions (139). Those with a history of anaphylactic reaction to the influenza vaccine should be under the care of an allergist if further influenza immunization is given (140). Vaccination of pregnant females is recommended to protect infants under 6 months who are too immunologically young to receive the influenza vaccine (141).

Table 7. High risk groups for influenza complications

1. Diabetes mellitus and other metabolic disorders
2. Cardiovascular disorders (not hypertension)
3. Asthma and other chronic pulmonary disorders
4. Nephrotic syndrome and renal failure
5. HIV infection and other immunosuppressive disorders
6. Those with spinal cord injuries that increase aspiration risks
7. Sickle cell disease; other hemoglobinopathies
8. Pregnancy
9. Children and adolescents (to 18 years of age) on long term aspirin management

Table 7 lists conditions that place individuals at high risk for morbidity and mortality from influenza infection, though anyone can become very ill from this infection, with death a potential risk (142-144). Current CDC recommendations include universal influenza vaccination each year for all those over 6 months of age, since all are at potential risk from this infection. This is in addition to recommendations covering those at high risk which have been in place since the early 1960s in the United States.

Pregnant females, even without other high-risk conditions, carry a 3 to 4 times increased risk for hospitalization and even death from influenza infection because of the pregnancy (see the maternal immunization section—vida infra). This high-risk situation is substantially lowered with receiving the intramuscular influenza vaccination. In the United States, coverage of pregnant females with annual influenza vaccine is less than 50% (range: 33.7% to 49.2%) (145). Though fears have increased for an Avian influenza (H5N1) epidemic or pandemic in the United States and the world, there is no evidence that such an event is imminent—though certainly possible (146). Recent improvements in the preparedness for pandemic influenza have been noted in eight Central American countries between 2008 and 2012 (147).

Influenza vaccines

The CDC recommends use of any licensed, age-appropriate influenza vaccine during the 2018-2019 influenza season, including inactivated influenza vaccine [IIV], recombinant influenza vaccine [RIV] or live attenuated influenza vaccine (LAIV) without any preference expressed for any type over another. Both trivalent (4-component) and quadrivalent (4 component) flu vaccines will be available (139). A quadrivalent cell-based flu shot (Flucelvax) contains virus grown in egg-free cell culture that is approved for 4 years and older (139).

Inactivated influenza vaccine is recommended for pregnant females in the last trimester (vida infra). Recent studies have noted the higher-induced mortality from pandemic H1N1 influenza in pregnant females and their fetuses in contrast to the healthy, non-pregnant population (148, 149). Vaccination during pregnancy lowered the risk of being diagnosed with influenza, did not increase fetal deaths, and may have lowered the risk of fetal deaths from the 2009 Influenza A (H1N1) pandemic in Norway (149). As there is substantial risk to the pregnant female as well as the fetus (infant), influenza vaccination should occur at the start of the influenza season (26).

Immunity from the influenza vaccine wanes after 8 to 10 months. It is up to 80% effective in healthy individuals under 65 years of age. Among sickly elderly individuals, the influenza vaccine is less effective: 80% effective in prevention of death, up to 60% effective in prevention of hospitalization, and up to 40% overall efficacy (143).

Each influenza season results in changes in the types of strains that are predominant and population groups at most risk. For example, the influenza vaccine for the 2011 to 2012 season in the U.S. was the same for the previous year: A/California/7/2009 (H1N1)-like virus, an A/Perth/16/2009 (H3N2)-like virus, and a B/Brisbane/60/2008-like virus. Influenza A (H1N1) predominated but H3N2 (influenza A) and influenza B viruses were also seen in the 2013-2014 influenza season in the US;

increased hospitalization rates were reported in those 50 to 64 years of age (150). H3N2 (influenza A) was dominant during the 2012-13 influenza season in the United States. The flu strains in the 2014-2015 vaccine are the same as found in the 2013-2014 season in the United States.

ROTAVIRUS VACCINES

Rotavirus is a viral infection that is the leading cause of severe diarrhea in those under 5 years of age leading up to 70,000 hospitalizations in infants and young children in the U.S. with 20 to 60 deaths annually (151, 152). It leads to over 500,000 deaths in children under age 5 years each year in developing countries (153, 154). Rotavirus infection causes a viral gastroenteritis with severe emesis, diarrhea, and dehydration. It is the most common case of diarrheal diseases in young children in the world. Prior to the current rotavirus immunization program that was begun the US in 2006, 95% of children had this infection by age 5 (151).

Introduction of rotavirus vaccines into the South African public immunization program has resulted in less rotavirus related morbidity and mortality (154). Success has also been seen in other countries, such as recently noted in Nicaragua where other main viral causes (i.e., norovirus, sapovirus) as well as Giardia lamblia are found in children with diarrhea) (154). Use of rotavirus provides up to 85% to 90% protection against rotavirus-induced hospitalization and is 80% protective in preventing emergency department treatment. Also, use of a live rotavirus vaccine appears to be safe when utilized to protect infants hospitalized in the NICU (156).

Table 8. Contraindications to the rotavirus vaccines

Demonstrated history of hypersensitivity to the vaccine or any of its components
History of intussusception
History of uncorrected congenital gastrointestinal tract malformation that may lead to intussusception
History of SCID (severe combine immunodeficiency)

Two live oral rotavirus vaccines (RV5 or RotaTeq and RV1 or Rotarix) are currently available in the U.S. and many other countries (151, 153,157). One is derived from an attenuated human strain (89-12) rotavirus (RV1) and the other contains five bovine-human reassortant strains (RV5) (153). Both vaccines have high efficacy rates and are not associated with increased rates of intussusceptions that were noted in 1999 with the previous vaccine. Contraindications to these vaccines are noted in Table 8, and include a history of intussusception. Prior to the vaccine availability intussusception occurred in 44 per 100,000 (1 in 2300) by one year of age, 37% required surgery, and 0.2% (4 infants) died (158). The risk of intussusception increases to 1 extra case in 20,000 to 100,000 vaccinated infants.

The vaccines are given to young infants, beginning at two months of age. RV1 Is given at 2 and 4 months of age versus RV5 which requires three doses at 2,4, and 6 months. The first dose of the rotavirus vaccine should be given before the child is 15 weeks of age and children must receive all doses before they turn 8 months old (153). Unfortunately most countries, including those with the highest burden of rotavirus disease, have not placed the rotavirus vaccines as part of their national vaccine programs (152). Ways to improve this situation in tropical countries include addressing the cost of these vaccines, continued education of governments as well as clinicians, and use of zinc supplementation to improve the performance of oral rotavirus vaccines in developing countries (152). Expansion of age limits for this vaccine are also proposed (159).

TYPHOID FEVER VACCINES

Typhoid fever is a historical global disease due to consumption of water or food that contains feces from a person with typhoid; the etiologic bacterium is *Salmonella enterica enterica*, serovar Typhi. Infection can lead to high fever, weakness, abdominal pain, anorexia, fatigue, rash, and other symptoms. Approximately 30% of infected persons die if not treated with hydration, and antibiotics. Prevention is with sanitation, hygiene, and in endemic areas—vaccination. Two vaccines are currently available—an inactivated vaccine (ViCPS) and a live, attenuated oral vaccine (Ty21a). The inactivated vaccine is an injection given once two weeks before travel and can be given to two years and older while the oral form is given as a capsule by mouth for a total of 4 doses every other day 1 week before travel (160). Typhoid vaccination is effective and recommended if one is traveling to or living in an endemic typhoid fever area (160).

YELLOW FEVER VACCINE

Yellow fever is an acute viral illness due to the yellow fever virus leading to fever, anorexia, nausea, chills, headaches, back pain, and other muscular pain. It is spread via a female mosquito (i.e., Aedes aegypti) and can lead to involvement of the liver and kidneys. It appeared in Africa and spread to South America in the 17th century, eventually leading to epidemics in the Americas and Europe in addition to Africa. Widespread vaccination programs decreased yellow fever infestation from the 1940s to 1960s while reduced funding for immunization lead to an increase in this infection since 2006 (161). Currently yellow fever is found in tropical areas of Africa and South America with over 200,000 global infections and 30,000 deaths each year—mostly in Africa (162). This is yet another piece of data that serves to remind us that all countries must never let up in the constant war on vaccine preventable diseases.

The yellow fever vaccine (17DD sub-strain of yellow fever vaccine: YEL-AND) is available and recommended for those living in endemic countries as well as those traveling to endemic areas. One dose of the live, weakened form of the virus given as a single shot can confer lifelong immunity and a booster dose is not recommended (161). Adverse effects from the vaccine are infrequent but include neurological (neurotropic, neurological autoimmune disease) that is highest in 5 to 9 years olds (2.66 per 100,000 vaccine doses), with a national analysis in Brazil finding 0.83 cases per 100,000 vaccine doses (163). These neurological adverse events usually have a favorable outcome and do not negate the need for nor the safety of the yellow fever vaccine (164).

Japanese Encephalitis Vaccine

Japanese B encephalitis is due to the Japanese encephalitis virus spread by mosquitoes (*Culex tritaeniorhynchus, Culex vishnui*) and found especially in east Asia and southeast Asia (165). Most infections are without symptoms but one in 250 infections can cause acute encephalitis which can lead to death, deafness, hemipariesis and other adverse effects. Three vaccines are available on the global market: SA14-14-2, ChimeriVax-JE, and IC51 but the inactivated Vero cell culture-derived Japanese encephalitis (JE) vaccine manufactured as IXIARO is the only vaccine licensed and available in the United States (166). The US CDC recommends vaccine protection for children (2 months through 16 years) at risk for this potentially serious infection (165, 166).

Immunizations for Pregnant Females

Pregnant females should be fully protected from vaccine preventable disorders (VPDs) both for the health of the mother and her offspring (167). Immunologic protection in the pregnant mother can confer protection for her newborn to various diseases, including influenza, tetanus, pertussis, diphtheria, hepatitis B virus, respiratory syncytial virus, group B streptococcus, and *haemophilus influenzae* type b (41, 124, 126). Very low risk is conferred to the pregnant female or offspring by use of killed vaccines. According to the CDC: "Benefits of vaccinating pregnant women usually outweigh potential risks when the likelihood of disease exposure is high, when infection would pose a risk to the mother or fetus, and when the vaccine is unlikely to cause harm (168)."

Studies of pregnant women given influenza and poliomyelitis vaccines in the 1950s and 1960s noted that these vaccines were not harmful to the mother nor the fetus/infant; studies looking at the offspring up to seven years of age noted no increase in teratogenicity, learning disorders, nor malignancy (169,170). Influenza vaccination to pregnant females decreases influenza morbidity and mortality in both the mother and the infant (148, 149). One study in Bangladesh giving inactivated influenza vaccine (TIV) to pregnant females reported a 63% vaccine efficacy and a lowering of influenza-like illness in infants by 29% and mothers by 36% (171). Studies in other countries have consistently revealed the safety and efficacy of influenza vaccine (TIV) with reduction in maternal as well as fetal/infant morbidity and mortality (170).

Though there is no evidence of teratogenicity using US FDA approved, attenuated, live viral vaccines (i.e., MMR, Varivax, LAIV), they should be avoided on a theoretical basis, one month prior to and during pregnancy. Women should be advised to avoid conception for one month after receiving live vaccines. Neither killed nor live vaccines are contraindicated for breast-feeding females. Breastfeeding is not a contraindication for any vaccine except for smallpox vaccine.

Maternal immunization is used to improve passive immunity of infants to microbes that can severely harm them, and has been recommended by leading national health care organizations in the U.S. since 1957. The key is to protect both mother and infant. Most maternal IgG antibody crosses the placenta in the third trimester, but the best timing seems to be when the vaccine is given at least 6 weeks prior to delivery; vaccination of the mother has not been shown to be detrimental to primary infant immunization (172).

The CDC ACIP currently recommends two vaccines for pregnant females: inactivated influenza and Tdap (tetanus toxoid, reduced diphtheria toxoid, and acellular pertussis) (170, 172). Females given influenza (TIV) or tetanus toxoid (TT) noted increased IgG antibodies to maternal vaccine antigens in cord and infant serum (173). Since antibody levels drop in subsequent pregnancies, pregnant women should receive 1 dose of Tdap during every pregnancy with the best timing between 27 and 36 weeks of gestation to best provide maternal antibody placental transfer to the fetus. Vaccination during the third trimester confers the highest antibody concentrations to the fetus/newborn. It takes about 2 weeks after maternal vaccination to reach maximal immune response in the infant. Active transport of maternal immunoglobulin G does not significantly occur before 30 weeks of gestation (174).

Death from pertussis occurs primarily in infants under 2 months of age. Infant cord blood reveals increased pertussis antibody if their mothers received Tdap during pregnancy, and in 2012, the CDC recommended that all pregnant women receive Tdap during the third trimester regardless of previous Tdap history (175). Tdap given before the third trimester does not result in transfer of sufficient pertussis antibody for the fetus (176). A 2012 study in England has noted the safety and efficacy of Tdap given in the third trimester with reduction of infant deaths due to pertussis (177).

A randomized, double-blind, placebo-controlled crossover study of the effects of Tdap given during pregnancy from 2008 to 2012 noted that the vaccine was safe for mother as well as infant, that it was immunogenic for the mother, and that there was effective transplacental antibody transfer (178). Interference with infant vaccination was not seen, though more research is needed to see if interference with other infant vaccinations does occur (179). The effect of repeated Tdap dosing during subsequent pregnancies is not clear, for example, could it induce reduced antibody production; more research is needed to monitor the effects of this recommendation (179).

Table 9. Issues affecting transport of maternal IgG during pregnancy (170A)

Maternal placental integrity
Vaccination timing
Total concentration of maternal IgG
IgG subtype

A number of issues influence the transport of maternal IgG during pregnancy (see Table 9). For example, maternal IgG transfer mainly occurs after 32 weeks of gestation and thus, a premature infant has low levels in contrast to a full term infant who may have higher levels than the mother at delivery. There are subtypes of maternal IgG such as IgG1 and IgG2; the former is stimulated by tetanus toxoid which induces protein antigens in contrast to pneumococcus vaccine which induces polysaccharide antigens that stimulates IgG2 (167). High levels of maternal IgG can decrease antigen-specific IgG transfer because of competitive binding to Fc receptors (placental) (170). If the mother is infected with HIV or malaria, this can lower maternal IgG placental transfer because of defective Fc receptor ability (180).

Research has shown that other vaccines can be given safely to pregnant females to provide antibodies with immunogenic effects to the infant in a safe manner. These include Haemophilus influenzae serotype b, group B streptococcus, meningococcus, and pneumococcal vaccines (170). Research is currently looking at the use of cytomegalovirus, herpes simplex virus, and respiratory syncytial virus vaccines (170).

Varicella and MMR vaccines should be given to susceptible females immediately postpartum. Subclinical fetal infection has been identified via serology in 1-2% of infants born to susceptible mothers (regardless of the vaccine strain); congenital rubella syndrome has not been found in the babies of 321 susceptible women given rubella vaccine who completed their pregnancies (181).

Hepatitis B

One classic study of pregnant females given hepatitis B immunoglobulin and hepatitis B vaccine noted that passive active immunization can be started safely during pregnancy and that response to the vaccine was "weak"; monitoring of anti-Hep B one month after the initial vaccine series was recommended (182).

Group B streptococcus

Another study looked at giving pregnant women a polysaccharide vaccine to group B streptococcus and provided some passive immunity against systemic Type III group B streptococcus infection in most newborns, though more research was recommended (183). A follow-up report by the same lead author noted immunizing pregnant females with group B streptococcal type III capsular polysaccharide-tetanus toxoid conjugate vaccine was a safe and immunogenic. The vaccine resulted in effective transfer of transplacental antibody to the newborn with good levels until 2 months of age (184). Research is focusing on provision of a global maternal immunization program for group B streptococcus, which is the most common invasive infection in infants less than 3 months of age in the United States (185, 186).

Haemophilus influenza type b

A study in The Gambia noted that maternal immunization with Haemophilus influenzae type b polysaccharide-tetanus protein conjugate vaccine may lower the rates of Hib disease in infants who are too young to receive their own immunization (187). Other research on use of this vaccine for maternal immunization in developing countries has shown it to be safe and immunogenic with protective serum and cord antibody levels (188). The Haemophilus influenza conjugate vaccine is better than the polysaccharide vaccine in raising infant antibody levels at birth and at two months of age; also, immunization of the mother with conjugate vaccine does not reduce the infant's reaction to conjugate vaccine in comparison to infants with mothers who did not receive Haemophilus influenza vaccination. (189).

Streptococcus pneumoniae

Research on the pneumococcal polysaccharide vaccine (PPV23) has shown it to be a safe vaccine for pregnant females and there is good placental antibody transfer (190-192). The actual effect of maternal immunization with PPV23 on protecting infants is unclear at this time. It is known that polysaccharide vaccines do not stimulate a vigorous T-cell with memory B-cell effect and limited studies to date have not demonstrated lowering of neonatal infection nor nasopharyngeal colonization in infants at 2-3 months of age following maternal PPV23 immunization (192).

Neisseria Meningitidis

Limited studies have been conducted on meningococcal vaccines and pregnant females. Use of the polysaccharide vaccine in pregnancy does result in antibody rise in both mother (sera and breast milk) and infant though transplacental antibody levels were not consistent (193). Use of meningococcal vaccine in pregnant women has not been shown to be harmful upon reviewing the US Vaccine Adverse Event Reporting System (194).

Poliovirus vaccine

Though inactivated poliovirus vaccine is not recommended for pregnant females, extensive use of polio vaccine during the 1950s with pregnant females noted it was safe and effective for both mother and infant (195, 196).

Herpes simplex virus (HSV) vaccine

Neonatal herpes is a major infection with a high mortality rate. While no vaccine has been shown to be effective in protecting the newborn from maternal infection, research is currently looking at a number of potential vaccines for the future (197, 198).

Cytomegalovirus vaccine

Cytomegalovirus (CMV) is another serious infection in newborns with many complications, and the pregnant female may acquire CMV infection and transmit it to her newborn. One study of postpartum women susceptible to CMV who were given a CMV vaccine noted a 50% efficacy (199).

Respiratory syncytial virus (RSV) vaccine

RSV is a major cause of respiratory disease (i.e., bronchiolitis and pneumonia) in infants, especially those under 6 months of age; there is minimal treatment and an expensive monoclonal antibody, palivizumab, that can be used prophylactically for infants judged to be at high risk for this infection during RSV season. Research on an RSV vaccine (formalin-inactivated) for infants in the 1960s was not effective and in fact led to increase infection (200). Since infants under 6 months are not good vaccine candidates, maternal vaccination would seem to be a better option to protect the infant. Research in this area is underway with a number of potential vaccines being studied (200, 201).

CONCLUSION

Immunizations for all citizens of the world should be an important goal of all clinicians, including those dealing with children and adolescents in developing and developed countries. Vaccine preventable diseases (VPDs) continue to take a devastating toll on these vulnerable human beings. Failure to provide available vaccines is a common problem in the world for various reasons; poverty, limited health care systems, ignorance on the part of individuals or governments, difficulty in keeping up with ever more complex and changing immunization schedules, failure to fund agencies responsible for immunization policies in specific regions, failure to understand barriers to vaccinations unique to an area, and the growing influence of anti-vaccine movements fueled by false information from the media as well as the internet (126, 201). All countries should carefully review their immunization programs and improve them as needed for the health of their citizens who will benefit greatly from vaccines to control and eliminate VPDs (7, 147, 155, 203, 204).

Despite these issues, vaccinology has been one of the greatest advances in modern medicine in the 21st century that can potentially benefit billions of human beings on earth (205-211). Smallpox has been eliminated from the globe and poliomyelitis has been wiped out in many parts of the world; in addition, diseases such as tetanus and diphtheria have been controlled in some parts of the world (23). Children are now safer from a variety of viral and bacterial infections that were previously devastating. Research is seeking to apply vaccine science in dealing with HIV, tuberculosis, malaria, and various forms of cancer (212).

A key strategy to improve the world's health is lifelong vaccination of VPDs starting in early childhood and continuing throughout life. Those traveling internationally need to receive the recommended vaccines from their own country and as well as those recommended for their destination(s). This is important not only to protect the traveler and but also to protect foreigners who come in contact with the traveler (98, 213). Another strategy is to ensure the immunization of healthcare providers to protect the safety of patients (214). Vaccination of children at high risk for VPDs is also important (22).

The actual impact of vaccines on morbidity and mortality in various countries may take years to verify, but the role of the clinician in this important process remains critical to ensure maximum success in the global campaign to achieve protection against VPDs in over 90% of the world's population. Sometimes the impact is rapid, as noted with decreased deaths from measles, pertussis, and diphtheria; while for other diseases like hepatitis B and HPV, the impact can take years to determine. Effects of vaccines on invasive pneumococcal disease and rotavirus gastroenteritis in developed countries is easily documented by the decrease in disease incidence and hospitalizations (215).

Maternal vaccination (inactivated influenza and Tdap) is recommended for pregnant females to help strengthen maternal and neonatal health since both populations are vulnerable due to a reduced immunological state (172). Indeed, vaccines save lives around the world and clinicians must remain pro-active in educating their patients and their parents in order to aggressively counter-act the pseudo-science of the anti-vaccine proponents (215). Clinicians must be prepared to deal with a public who obtain inaccurate health information from the internet, medical/dental smartphone Apps, anti-vaccine groups, and others (18, 216-221). Research continues to expand our knowledge of vaccines to deal with old infectious agents and new ones (222-225).

REFERENCES

[1] Kaul P, Kaplan DW. Caring for adolescents in the office. In: Greydanus DE, Patel DR, Pratt HD, eds. Essential adolescent medicine. New York: McGraw-Hill Medical, 2006:17-27.

[2] Greydanus DE, Patel DR. Vaccines for adolescents leaving for higher studies in the USA. In: Bhave S, Parthasarathy A, Yadav S, eds. A ready manual for vaccinations: Adult, adolescents, and pediatric. New Delhi, India: Jaypee Brothers Medical, 2010:154-72.

[3] Huygelen C. Jenner's cowpox vaccine in light of current vaccinology. Verh K Acad Geneedskd Belg 1996;58:479-536. [Dutch]

[4] Mark C, Rigau-Pérez JG. The world's first immunization campaign: The Spanish smallpox vaccine expedition,1803-1813. Bull Hist Med 2009;83:63-94.

[5] Reid M, Fleck F. The immunization programme that saved millions of lives. Bull World Health Organ 2014;92(5):314-5.

[6] McCarthy M. US vaccine program will prevent 732,000 deaths, CDC says. BMJ 2014;348:g2978.

[7] Richardson V, Sánchez-Uribe E, Esparza-Aguilar M, Esteves-Jaramillo A, Suárez-Idueta L. Contribution of Mexico's universal immunization program to the fourth millennium development goal. Rev Panam Salud Publica 2014;35(4):248-55.

[8] Okwo-Bele JM, Cherian T. The expanded program on immunization: a lasting legacy of smallpox eradication. Vaccine 2011;29(Suppl 4):D74-9.

[9] Minor P. The polio endgame. Hum Vaccin Immunother 2014 May 8;10(7).

[10] Whitney CG, Zhou F, Singleton J, Schuchat A; Centers for Disease Control and Prevention (CDC). Benefits from immunization during the vaccines for children program era-United States, 1994-2013. MMWR 2014;63(16):352-5.

[11] Cherian T, Okwo-Bele JM. The decade of vaccines global action plan: shaping immunization programmes in the current decade. Expert Rev Vaccines 2014;13(5):573-5.

[12] Machingaidze S, Hussey GD, Wiysonge CS. Trends in the types and quality of childhood immunizations research output from Africa 1970-2010: Mapping the evidence base. BMC Health Serv Res 2014;14:52. Doi:10.1186/1472-6963-14-52.

[13] Wiysonge CS, Uthman OA, Ndumbe PM, Hussey GD. A bibliometric analysis of childhood immunization research productivity in Africa since the onset of Expanded Program on Immunization in 1974. BMC Med 2013;11:66. doi:10.1186/1741-7015-41-66.

[14] Animaw W, Taye W, Merdekios B, Tilahun M, Ayele G. Expanded program of immunization coverage and associated factors among children age 12-23 months in Arba Minch town and Zuria District, Southern Ethiopia, 2013. BMC Public Health 2014;14:464. doi:10.1186/1471-2458-14-464.

[15] Singh PK, Parsuraman S. Sibling composition and child immunization in India and Pakistan, 1990-2007. World J Pediatr 2014;10(2):145-50.

[16] Goldfarb IT, Little S, Brown J, Riley LE. Utilization of the combined tetanus-diphterhia and pertussis vaccine during pregnancy. Am J Obstet Gynecol 2014 May 22. pii:S0002-9378(14)00497-9.

[17] The anti-vaccination movement in Learn Act Resource News. URL: https://measlesrubellainitiative.org/anti-vaccination-movement/

[18] Greydanus DE, Toledo L. Historical perspective on autism: Its past record of discovery and its present state of solipsism, skepticism, and sorrowful suspicion. Pediatr Clin North Am 2012;59(1): 5-12.

[19] Kennedy A, Lavail K, Nowak G, Basket M, Landry S. Confidence about vaccines in the United States: understanding parents' perceptions. Health Aff (Millwood) 2011;30(6):1151-9.

[20] Recommended immunization schedules for persons aged 0-18 years—United States, 2007. MMWR 2007;55(51):Q1-Q4.

[21] Infectious Diseases Society of America. Actions to strengthen adult and adolescent immunization coverage in the United States: policy principles of the Infectious Diseases Society of America. Clin Infect Dis 2007;44(e):104-11.

[22] Kimmel SR, Burns IT, Wolff RM, Zimmerman RK. Addressing immunization barriers, benefits, and risks. J Fam Pract 2007;56:S61-9.

[23] Bonanni P, Sacco C, Donato R, Capei R. Longlong vaccination as a key disease-prevention strategy. Clin Microbiol Infect 2014;20(Suppl 5):32-6.

[24] Ellenberg SS, Foulkes, MA, Midthun K et al. Evaluating the safety of new vaccines: summary of a workshop. Am J Publ Health 2005;95:800-7.

[25] Advisory Committee on Immunization Practices Recommended Immunization Schedules for Persons aged 0 through 18 years-United States, 2014. MMWR 2014;63(05):108-9.

[26] Bridges CB, Woods L, Coyne-Beasley T. Immunization Services Division, National Center for Immunization and Respiratory Diseases, CDC. Advisory Committee on Immunization Practices Recommended Immunization Schedule for adults aged 19 years or older-United States, 2014. MMWR 2014;63(5):110-2.

[27] Calendario National de vacunacion de la republica Argentina, 2011. Congresso del Centenario de la Sociedad Argentina de Pediatría. September, 2011.

[28] Cohen NJ, Laudendale DS. Physician knowledge of catch-up regimens and contraindications for childhood vaccinations. Pediatrics 2003;111:925-32.

[29] Jindal H, Bhatt B, Malik JS, Sk S, Mehta B. Malaria vaccine: A step toward elimination. Hum Vaccin Immunother 2014 Mar 18;10(6).

[30] Chanzu N, Ondondo B. Induction of potent and long-lived antibody and cellular immune responses in the genitorectal mucosa could be the critical determinant of HIV vaccine efficacy. Front Immunol 2014;5:202.

[31] Dutruel C, Thole J, Geels M, Mollenkopf HJ, Ottenhoff T, Gusman CA et al. TRANSVAC workshop on standarisation and harmonization of analytical platforms for HIV, TB and malaria vaccines: 'How can big data help?' Vaccine 2014 June 17. pii:S0264-410X(14)00803-2.

[32] Di Giacomo A. The EFIS-EJI Ruggero Ceppelini Advance School of immunology: Malaria, tuberculosis, and HIV/AIDS: Novel vaccination strategies against the three major killers. Eur J Immunol 2014;44(6):1573-4.

[33] Doll KL, Harty JT. Correlates of protective immunity following whole sporozoite vaccination. Immunol Res 2014 May 14.

[34] Srinivasan P, Ekanem E, Diouf A, Tonkin ML, Miura K, Boulanger MJ et al. Immunization with a functional protein complex required for erythrocyte invasion protects against lethal malaria. Proc Natl Acad Sci USA 2014 Jun 23. pii:201409928.

[35] Poliomyelitis. URL: https://www.who.int/news-room/fact-sheets/detail/poliomyelitis.

[36] WHO. Polio vaccines: WHO position paper, January, 2014. Recommendations. Vaccine 2014 Apr 24. pii:S0264-410X(14)00538-6.

[37] Rutter PD, Donaldson LJ. Mandatory polio vaccination for travelers: protecting global public health. Lancet 2014;383(9930):1695-7.

[38] Updated recommendations for use of Tetanus toxoid, reduced diphtheria toxoid and pertussis (Tdap) Vaccine from the Advisory Committee on Immunization Practices, 2010. 2011 Jan 04.

[39] Prevention and Control of Haemophilus influenzae Type b Disease: Recommendations of the Advisory Committee on Immunization Practices (ACIP) Recommendations and Reports. MMWR 2014;63(RR01):1-14.

[40] Tetanus. URL: Http://en.wikipedia.org/wiki/tetanus.

[41] Orimadegun AE, Adepoju AA, Akinyinka OO. Adolescent girls' understanding of tetanus infection and prevention: implications for disease control in Western Nigeria. Front Public Health 2014;2:24.

[42] Roach RR. Reduction of neonatal tetanus in Madagascar. Personal communication 2014 Sep 20.

[43] Diphtheria. URL: Http://en.wikipedia.org/wiki/diphtheria.

[44] Atkinson W, Wolfe S, Hamborsky J, eds. Epidemiology and prevention of vaccine-preventable diseases, 12th ed. Centers for Disease Control and Prevention. Washington, DC: Public Health Foundation, 2011:215-32.

[45] Crowcroft NS, Pebody RG. Recent developments in pertussis. Lancet 2006; 367:1926-36.

[46] Purdy KW. Pertussis in the United States. Clin Infect Dis 2004;39:20-8.

[47] Adashi EY, Offit PA. Paul Offit on the dangers of the anti-vaccine movement. URL: http://www.medscape.com/viewarticle/741343?src=mp&sponCommittee on.

[48] Cherry J. Pertussis vaccine encephalopathy: It is time to recognize it as the myth that it is. JAMA 1990;263:1679-80.

[49] Cherry JD. The epidemiology of pertussis: A comparison of the epidemiology of the disease pertussis with the epidemiology of Bordetella pertussis infection. Pediatrics 2005; 115:1422-7.

[50] Tartof SY, Lewis M, Kenyon C, White K, Osborn A, Liko J, et al. Waning immunity to pertussis following 5 doses of DTaP. Pediatrics 2013;131(4):e1047-52.

[51] Infectious Diseases: Prevention of pertussis among adolescents: Recommendations for use of tetanus toxoid, reduced diphtheria toxoid, and acellular pertussis (Tdap) vaccine. Pediatrics 2006;117 (3):965-78.

[52] Preventing tetanus, diphtheria among adolescents; Use of tetanus toxoid, reduced diphtheria toxoid, and acellular pertussis vaccines. MMWR 2006;55(Early Release): 1-34.

[53] Pichichero ME, Rennels MB, Edwards KM et al. Combined tetanus, diphtheria, and 5-component pertussis vaccine for use in adolescents and adults. JAMA 2005;293: 3003-11.

[54] Marshall GS, Happe LE, Lunacsek OE et al. Use of combination vaccines is associated with improved coverage rates. Pediatr Infec Dis J 2007;26:496-500.

[55] Preventing tetanus, diphtheria, and pertussis among adults: Use of tetanus toxoid, reduced diphtheria toxoid, and acellular pertussis vaccine. Recommendations of the ACIP, supported by the Healthcare Infection Control Practices Advisory Committee (HICPAC) for use of Tdap among health-care personnel. MMWR 2006;55(RR17):1-43.

[56] Rossman Beel E, Rench MA, Montesinos DP, Healy CM. Acceptability of immunization in adult contacts of infants: possibility of expanding platforms to increase adult vaccine update. Vaccine 2014;32(22):2540-5.

[57] Liko J, Robson SG, Cieslak PR. Pertussis vaccine performance in an epidemic year-Oregon, 2012. Clin Infect Dis 2014 Apr 18. pii:ciu273.

[58] Measles, mumps, and rubella (MMR) vaccination: What everyone should know. URL: https://www.cdc.gov/vaccines/vpd/mmr/public/inde.html#what-i-need-to-know

[59] Parker AA, Staggs W, Dayan GH et al. Implications of a 2005 Measles outbreak in Indiana for sustained elimination of measles in the United States. N Engl J Med 2006; 355:447-55.

[60] Gastañaduy PA. Redd SB, Fiebelkorn AP, Rota JS, Rota PA, Bellini WJ, et al. Measles-United States, January 1-May 23, 2014. MMWR 2014;63(22):496-9.

[61] Fowotade A, Okonko IO, Nwabuisi C, Bakare RA, Fadeyi A, Adu FD. Measles vaccine potency and sero-conversion rates among infants receiving measles immunization in Ilorin, Kawara State, Nigeria. J Immunoassay Immunochem 2014 May 13.

[62] Murhekar MV, Ahmad M, Shukla H, Abhishek K, Perry RT, Bose AS et al. Measles case fatality rate in Bihar, India, 2011-2012. PLoS One 2014;9(5):e96668.

[63] Hambidge SJ, Newcomer SR, Narwaney KJ, Glanz JM, Daley MF, Xu S, et al. Timely versus delayed early childhood vaccination and seizures. Pediatrics Online 2014. doi:10.1542/Peds.2013-3429.

[64] Baughman AL, Williams WW, Atkinson WL. The impact of college prematriculation immunization requirements on risk for measles outbreaks. JAMA 1994;272:1127-32.

[65] Meissner HC, Reef SE, Chochi S. Elimination of rubella from the United States: A milestone on the road to global elimination. Pediatrics 2006;117:933-5.

[66] Progress in global measles control and mortality reduction, 2000-2006. MMWR 2007;56(47):1237-41.

[67] Adam O, Ali AK, Hübschen JM, Muller CP. Identification of congenital rubella syndrome in Sudan. BMC Infect Dis 2014;14(1):305-7.

[68] Berger BE, Navar-Boggan Am, Omer SB. Congenital rubella syndrome and autism spectrum disorder prevented by rubella vaccination—United States, 2001-2010. BMC Public Health 2011;11:340.

[69] Parker AA, Staggs W, Dayan GH. Implications of a 2005 Measles outbreak in Indiana for sustained elimination of measles in the United States. N Engl J Med 2006; 355:447-55.

[70] Wakefield AJ, Murch SH, Anthony A. Ileal-lymphoid-nodular hyperplasia, non-specific colitis, and pervasive developmental disorder in children. Lancet 1998;351: 637-41.

[71] Eggertson L. Lancet retracts 12-year-old article linking autism to MMR vaccines. CMAJ 2010;182:E199-200.

[72] Godlee F, Smith J, Marcovitch H. Wakefield's article linking MMR vaccine and autism was fraudulent. BMJ 2011;342:c7452.

[73] Rapin I. High hopes, shoddy research, and elusive therapies for autism examined and exposed. Neurology Today 2009;9:23.

[74] Offit PA. Autism's false prophets. Bad science, risky medicine, and the search for a cure. New York: Columbia University Press, 2008.

[75] Freed GL, Clark SJ, Butchart AT. Parental vaccine safety concerns in 2009. Pediatrics 2010;125:654-9.

[76] Mrozek-Budzyn D, Kieltyka A, Majewska R. Lack of association between measles-Mumps-rebella vaccination and autism in children: A case-control study. Pediatr Infect Dis J 2010;29:397-400.

[77] Thompson WW, Price C, Goodson B. Early thimersol exposure and neuropsychological outcomes at 7 to 10 years. N Engl J Med 2007;357:1281-92.

[78] DeStefano F, Chen RT. Autism and measles, mumps, and rubella vaccine: No epidemiological evidence for a causal association. J Pediatr 2000;136:125-6.

[79] Institute of Medicine. Immunizaition Safety Review Committee. Immunization safety review: Vaccines and autism. Washington, DC: National Academies Press, 2004.

[80] Institute of Medicine. Adverse effects of vaccines: Evidence and causality. URL: http://www.iom.edu/vaccineadverseeffects.

[81] Sugarman SD. Cases in vaccine court—legal battles over vaccines and autism. N Engl J Med 2007;357:1275-9.

[82] Goodman NW. MMR scare stories: Some things are just too attractive to the media. BMJ 2007;335:222.

[83] Chatterjee A, O'Keefe C. Current controversies in the USA regarding vaccine safety. Expert Rev Vaccines 2010;9:497-502.

[84] Gerber JS, Offit PA. Vaccines and autism: A tale of shifting hypotheses. Clin Inf Dis (CID) 2009;48:456-61.

[85] Tafuri S, Martinelli D, Prato R, Germinario C. From the struggle for freedom to the denial of scientific evidence: history of antivaccinationists in Europe. Ann Ig 2011; 23:93-9. [Italian].

[86] Measles epidemiology. URL: http://enwikipedia.org/wiki/measles#epidemiology.

[87] Gardner P. Prevention of meningococcal disease. N Engl J Med 2006;355(14):1466-72.

[88] Middleman AB. Immunization update: Pertussis, meningococcus, and human papillomavirus. Adolesc Med 2006;17:233-40.

[89] Ellenberg SS, Foulkes, MA, Midthun K. Evaluating the safety of new vaccines: Summary of a workshop. Am J Publ Health 2005;95:800-7.

[90] Harrison CH, Dwyer DM, Maples CT. Risk of meningococcal infection in college students. JAMA 1999;281:1906-10.

[91] Updated recommendations for meningococcal conjugate vaccines. ACIP. Centers for Disease Prevention and Control. MMWR 2011;60:72-6.

[92] Kumar A, Murray DL, Havlicheck DH. Immunizations for the college student: A campus perspective of an outbreak and national and international considerations. Pediatr Clin 2005;52:229-41.

[93] Bruce MG, Rosenstein NE, Capparella JM. Risk factors for meningococcal disease in college students. JAMA 2001;286:688-93.

[94] Meningococcal disease and college students. Recommendations of Advisory Committee on Immunizations Practices (ACIP). MMWR 2000:49(RR07):1-20.

[95] Prevention and control of meningococcal disease. recommendations of the Advisory Committee on Immunization Practices (ACIP). MMWR Recomm Rep 2005;54 (RR-7):1-21.

[96] Offit PA, Peter G. The meningococcal vaccine—public policy and individual choices. N Engl J Med 2003;349:2353-6.

[97] No authors. Meningococcal disease control in countries of the African meningitis belt. Wkly Epidemiol Rec 2014;89(20):206-14.

[98] Goodman AL, Masuet-Aumatell C, Halbert J, Zuckerman JN. Awareness of meningococcal diseases among travelers from the United Kingdom to the meningitis belt in Africa. Am J Trop Med Hyg 2014 Jun 2. pii:13-0763.

[99] Meningococcal vaccination: What every should know. URL: https://www.cdc.gov/vaccines/vpd/mening/public/index.html.

[100] Cohn AC, MacNeil JR, Clark TA, Ortega-Sanchez IR, Briere EZ, Meissner HC, et al. Prevention and control of meningococcal disease: recommendations of the Advisory Committee on Immunization Practices (ACIP). MMWR Recomm Rep 2013;66(RR-2):1-28.

[101] Hale SF, Camaione L, Lomaestro BM. MenHibrix: A new combination meningococcal vaccine for infants and toddlers. Ann Pharmacother 2014;48(3):404-11.

[102] Use of MenACWY-CRM vaccine in children aged 2 through 23 months at increased risk for meningococcal disease. MMWR 2014;63(24):527-30.

[103] Holst J, Oster P, Arnold R, Tatley MV, Naess LM, Aaberge IS, et al. Vaccines against meningococcal serogroup B disease containing outer membrane vesicles (OMV): Lesions from past programs andimplications for the future. Hum Vaccin Immunother 2013;9(6):1241-53.

[104] Galano A. Vacuna contra el virus del Papiloma Humano (VPH). Argentina. Buenos Aires, Argentina: Ministerio de Salud Presidencia de la Nacion, 2011. URL: www.msal.gov.ar.

[105] Van Limbergen EJ, Dok R, Laenen A, Hauben E, van den Weyngaert D, et al. HPV-related oropharyngeal cancers in Flanders (Belgium): A multicenter study. B-ENT 2014;19(1):7-14.

[106] Henley SJ, Singh S, King J, Wilson R, Ryerson B. Centers for Disease Control and Prevention (CDC). Invasive cancer incidence: United States, 2010. MMWR 2014;63(12):253-9.

[107] Machalek DA, Poynten M, Jin F, Fairley CK, Farnsworth A, Garland SM, et al. Anal human papillomavirus infection and associated neoplastic lesions in men who have sex with men: A systemic review and meta-analysis. Lancet Oncol 2012;13(5):487-500.

[108] Brotherton JM. Human papillomavirus vaccination: Where are we now? J Paediatr Child Health 2014. doi:10.1111/jpc.12627.

[109] Human Papillomavirus (HPV) Vaccination: What every should know. URL: https://www.cdc.gov/vaccines/vpd/hpv/public/index.html

[110] Markowitz LE, Hariri S, Lin C, Dunne EF, Steinau M, McQuillan G, et al. Reduction in human papillomavirus (HPV) prevalence among young women following HPV vaccine introduction in the United States. National Health and Nutrition Examination Surveys 2003-2010. J Infec Dis 2013;208(3):385-93.

[111] Franco EL, Mayrand M-H, Ratnam S. HPV DNA versus Papanicolaou screening tests for cervical cancer. N Engl J Med 2008;358:643-4.

[112] Meites E, Szilagyi PG, Cheson HW, Inger ER, Romero JR, Markowitz LE. MMWR 2019;86(32):698-702.

[113] American College of Obstetricians and Gynecologists. ACOG Committee opinion no. 558: Integrating immunizations into practice. Obstet Gynecol 2013;121(4):897-903.

[114] Mullins TL, Griffioen AM, Glynn S, Zimet GD, Rosenthal SL, Fortenberry JD, et al. Human papillomarvirus vaccine communication: perspectives of 11-12 year-old-girls, mothers, and clinicians. Vaccine 2013;31(42):4894-901.

[115] Lefkowitz ES, Kelly KMBS, Vasilenko SA, Maggs JL. Correlates of human papillomavirus vaccination among female university students. Women Health 2014 Jun 25.

[116] Centers for Disease Control and Prevention (CDC). Human papillomavirus vaccination coverage among adolescent girls, 2007-2012, and postlicensure vaccine safety monitoring, 2006-2013-United States. MMWR 2013;62(29):591-5.

[117] Christensen ND, Budgeon LR. Vaccines and immunization against human papillomavirus. Curr Probl Dermatol 2014;45:252-64.

[118] Johnston MI, Fauci AS. An HIV vaccine---evolving concepts. N Engl J Med 2007; 356: 2073-81.

[119] Hepatitis A Questions and answers for the public. URL: https://www.cdc.gov/hepatitis/hav/afaq.htm

[120] CDC Pink Book: Epidemiology and prevention of vaccine preventable diseases, 9th edition. Atlanta, GA: Centers for Disease Control and Prevention, 2006:182-3,194,263-4.

[121] Srivastava A, Mathias A, Yachha SK, Agarwal J, Aggarwal R. Need for immunization against hepatotropic viruses in children with chronic liver disease: A serological study. J Pediatr Gastroenterol Nutr 2014 May 16.

[122] Incidence of acute hepatitis B—United States, 1990-2002. MMWR 2004;52(51):1252-4.

[123] Sugunan AP, Bhattacharya H, Bhattacharya D, Mandal A, Ghosal SR, Rao RC, et al. Impact of hepatitis B immunization among the Nicobarese tribe - antibody titres and seroprotection five years after vaccination. Indian J Med Res 2014;139(3):427-30.

[124] Qureshi H, Javaid N, Alam SE, Bile KM. The evidence of mother to child transmission of hepatitis B virus infection in Pakistan and the need for hepatitis B immunization policy change. J Pak Med Assoc 2014;64(4):403-8.

[125] Asherio A, Zhang SM. Hepatitis B vaccination and the risk of multiple sclerosis. N Engl J Med 2001;344:327-32.

[126] Chicken pox vaccination: What everyone should know. URL: https://www.cdc.gov/vaccines/vpd/varicella/public/index.html.

[127] CDC Pink Book. Epidemiology and prevention of vaccine preventable diseases, 11th edition. Atlanta, GA: Centers for Disease Control and Prevention, 2011:292.

[128] Marin M, Zhang JX, Seward JF. Near elimination of varicella deaths in the US after Implementation of the vaccination program. Pediatrics 2011;128:214-20.

[129] Huang SS, Johnson KM, Ray GT et al. Healthcare utilization and cost of pneumococcal disease in the United States. Vaccine 2011;29:3398-412.

[130] Kyaw MH, Lynfield R, Schaffner W et al. Effect of introduction of the pneumococcal conjugate vaccine on drug-resistant Streptococcus pneumoniae. N Engl J Med 2006; 354:1455-63.

[131] Rivera-Olivero IA, Del Nogal B, Fuentes M, Cortez R, Bogaert D, Hermans PW, et al. Immunogenicity of a 7-valent pneumococcal conjugate vaccine (PCV7) and impact on carriage in Venezuelan children at risk of invasive pneumococcal diseases. Vaccine 2014 May 14. pii: S0264-410X(14)00553-2.

[132] Salvadori MI, Price VE, Canadian Paediatric Socity, Infectious Diseases and Immunization Committee. Preventing and treating infections in children with aspenia or hyposplenia. Paediatr Child Health 2014;19(5):271-8.

[133] Pneumococcal vaccination: What everyone should know. URL: https://www.cdc.gov/vaccines/vpd/pneumo/public/index.html.

[134] Use of PCV13 and PPVS23 for adults with immunocompromising conditions, Recommendations of the ACIP. MMWR 2012;61(40):816-9.

[135] Pekka NJ, Whitney CG. Updated recommendations for prevention of invasive pneumococcal disease among adults using PPSV23. MMWR 2010;59(34):1102-6.

[136] Use of 13-valent pneumococcal conjugate vaccine and 23-valent pneumococcal polysaccharide vaccine for adults with immunocompromising conditions: Recommendations of the Advisory Committee on Immunization Practices (ACIP). MMWR 2012;61(40):816-9.

[137] Madhi SA, Bamford L, Ngcobo N. Effectiveness of pneumococcal conjugate vaccine and rotavirus vaccine introduction into the South African public immunisation programme. S Afr Med J 2014;104(3 Suppl 1):228-34.

[138] Shakoor S, Kabir F, Khowaja AR, Qureshi SM, Jehan F, Qamar F, et al. Pneumococcal serotypes and serogroups causing invasive disease in Pakistan, 2005-2013. PLoS One 2014;9(6):e98796.

[139] Key facts about seasonal flu vaccine. URL: https://www.cdc.gov/flu/prvent/keyfacts.htm

[140] Kelso JM. Administering influenza vaccine to egg-allergic persons. Expert Rev Vaccines 2014;June 25:1-9.

[141] Nelson EA, Ip M, Tam JS, Mounts AW, Chau SL, Law SK, et al. Burden of influenza infection in hospitalized children below 6 months of age and above in Honk Kong from 2005 to 2011. Vaccine 2014 May 14. pii: S0264-410X(14)00601-X.

[142] Centers for Disease Control and Prevention. Prevention and control of influenza with vaccines. Recommendations of the Advisory Committee on Immunization Practices (ACIP). MMWR 2010;59(RR-8).

[143] Atkinson W, Wolfe S, Hamborsky J, eds. Epidemiology and prevention of vaccine-preventable diseases,11th edition. Washington, DC: Public Health Foundation 2011:142-3.

[144] Zerr DM, Englund JA, Robertson AS. Hospital-based influenza vaccination of children: An opportunity to prevent subsequent hospitalization. Pediatrics 2008; 121:345-8.

[145] Influenza vaccination coverage among pregnant women—U.S. 2011-2012 influenza season. MMWR 2012;61(38):758-64.

[146] Writing Committee of the Second WHO consultation on Clinical Aspects of human infection with Avian influenza (H5N1) virus. Update on Avian Influenza (H5N1) virus infection in humans. N Engl J Med 2008;358:261-73.

[147] Johnson LE, Clará W, Gambhir M, Fuentes RC, Marin-Correa C, Jara J, et al. Improvements in pandemic preparedness in 8 Central American countries, 2008-2012. BMC Health Serv Res 2014;14(1):209-12.

[148] Siston AM, Rasmussen SA, Honein MA, Fry AM, Seib K, Callaghan WM, et al. Pandemic 2009 influenza A (H1N1) virus illness among pregnant women in the United States. JAMA 2010;303(15):1517-25.

[149] Håberg SE, Trogstad L, Gunnes N, Wilcox AJ, Gjessing HK, Samuelsen SO et al. Risk of fetal death after pandemic influenza virus infection or vaccination. N Engl J Med 2013;368(4):333-40.

[150] Epperson S, Blanton L, Kniss K, Mustaquim D, Steffens C, Wallis T, et al. Influenza activity-United States, 2013-14 season and composition of the 2014-15 influenza vaccines. MMWR 2014;63(22):483-90.

[151] Atkinson W, Wolfe S, Hamborsky J, eds. Epidemiology and prevention of vaccine-preventable diseases,11th edition. Washington, DC: Public Health Foundation 2011:263-74.

[152] Yen C, Tate JE, Hyde TB, Cortese MM, Lopman BA, Jiang B, et al. Rotavirus vaccines: Current status and future considerations. Hum Vaccin Immunother 2014 Apr 22;10(6).

[153] Rotavirus vaccination: What everyone should know. URL: https://www.cdc.gov/vaccines/vpd/rotavirus/public/inde.html

[154] Seheri LM, Mwenda JM, Page N. Report of the 7th African Rotavirus Symposium, Cape Town, South Africa, 8th November 2012. Vaccine 2014 May 13. pii:S0264-410X(14)00657-4.

[155] Becker-Dreps S, Bucardo F, Vilchez S, Zambrana LE, Liu L, Weber DJ, et al. Etiology of childhood diarrhea following rotavirus vaccine introduction: A prospective, population-based study in Nicaragua. Pediatr Infect Dis J 2014 May 29.

[156] Monk HM, Motsney AJ, Wade KC. Safety of rotavirus vaccine in the NICU. Pediatrics 2014; May 19. pii: peds.2013-3504.

[157] Centers for Disease Control and Prevention. Prevention of rotavirus gastroenteritis among infants and children. MMWR 2009;58(RR-2):1-25.

[158] Provider information: Rotavirus VIS. URL: www.cdc.gov/vaccines.

[159] Anderson EJ. Time to begin a new chapter and expand rotavirus immunization. Clin Infect Dis 2014 June 18. pii:ciu475.

[160] Typhoid fever and paratyphoid fever: Vaccination. URL: https://www.cdc.gov/typhoid-fever/typhoid-vaccination.html.

[161] Garske T, Van Kerkhove MD, Yactayo S, Ronveaux O, Lewis, RF, Staples JE, et al. Yellow fever in Africa: estimating the burden of disease and impact of mass vaccination from outbreak and serological data. PLoS Med 2014;11(5):e1001638.

[162] Staples JE, Diallo M, Janusz ZB, Manengu C, Perea W, Yactayo S, et al. Yellow fever risk assessment in the Central African Republic. Trans R Soc Trop Med Hyg 2014 Jun 19 pii:tru086.

[163] WHO. Vaccines and vaccination against yellow fever: WHO Position Paper, June, 2013- Recommendations. Vaccine 2014 May 20. pii: S0264-410X(14)00707-5.

[164] Martins RD, Pavão AL, de Oliveira PM, Dos Santos PR, Carvalho SM, Mohrdieck R, et al. Adverse events following yellow fever immunization: Report and analysis of 67 neurological cases in Brazil. Vaccine 2014 May 14. pii: S0264-410X(14)00658-6.

[165] Wilder-Smith A, Halstead SB. Japanese encephalitis: Update on vaccines and vaccine recommendations. Curr Opin Infect Dis 2010;23(5):426-31.

[166] Japanese encephalitis vaccine. URL: https://www.cdc.gov/japaneseencephalitis/vaccine/index/html?

[167] Glezen WP, Alpers M. Maternal immunizations. Clin Infect Dis 1999;28:219-24.

[168] General recommendations on immunizations. Recommendations of ACIP. MMWR 2011;60(2):1-64.

[169] Heinonen OP, Shapiro S, Monson RR, Hartz SC, Rosenberg L, Slone D. Immunization during pregnancy against poliomyelitis and influenza in relation to childhood malignancy. Int J Epidemiol 1973;2(3):229-35.

[170] Chu HY, Englund JA. Maternal Immunization. Clin Infect Dis 2014 May 5. pii:ciu327.

[171] Zaman K, Roy E, Arifeen SE, Rahman M, Raqib R, Wilson E, et al. Effectiveness of maternal influenza immunization in mothers and infants. N Engl J Med 2008;359(15):1555-64.

[172] Moniz MH, Beigi RH. Maternal immunization: clinical experiences, challenges, and opportunities in vaccine acceptance. Hum Vaccin Immunother 2014;10(9):2562-70.

[173] Englund JA, Mbawuike IN, Hammill H, Holleman MC, Baxter BD, Glezen WP. Maternal immunization with influenza or tetanus toxoid vaccine for passive antibody protection in young infants. J Infect Dis 1993;168(3):647-56.

[174] Updated recommendations for the use of tetanus toxoid, reduced diphtheria toxoid, and acellular pertussis vaccine (Tdap) in pregnant women. Advisory Committee on Immunization Practice (ACIP) 2012. MMWR 2013;62(07):131-5.

[175] Gall SA, Myers J, Pichichero M. Maternal immunization with tetanus-diphtheria-pertussis vaccine: effect of maternal and neonatal serum antibody levels. Am J Obstet Gynecol 2011;204(4):334.e1-5.

[176] Healy CM, Rench MA, Baker CJ. Importance of timing of maternal combined tetanus, diphtheria, and acellular pertussis (Tdap) immunization and protection of young infants. Clin Infect Dis 2013;56(4):539-44.

[177] Service NH. Whooping cough vaccination in pregnancy. URL: http://www.nhs.uk/conditions/pregnancy-and-baby/pages/whooping-cough-vaccination-pregnant.aspx-safe.

[178] Munoz FM, Bond NH, Maccato M, Pinell P, Hammill HA, Swamy GK, et al. Safety and immunogenicity of tetanus diphtheria and acellular pertussis (Tdap) immunization during pregnancy in mothers and infants: a randomized clinical trial. JAMA 2014;311(17):1760-9.

[179] Jiménez-Truque N, Edwards KM. Maternal pertussis immunization: Can it help infants? JAMA 2014;311(17):1736-7.

[180] deMoraes-Pinto MI, Verhoeff F, Chimsuku L, Milligan PJ, Wesumperuma L, Broadhead RL et al. Placental antibody transfer: influence of maternal HIV infection and placental malaria. Arch Dis Child Fetal Neonatal Ed 1998;79(3):F202-5.

[181] Atkinson W, Wolfe C, Hamborsky J. Centers for Disease Control and Prevention. Epidemiology and prevention of vaccine-preventable diseases. The Pink Book, 12th ed. Washington DC: Public Health Foundation, 2011:287.

[182] Grosheide PM, Schalm SW, van Os HC, Fetter WP, Heijtink RA. Immune response to hepatitis B vaccine in pregnant women receiving post-exposure prophylaxis. Eur J Obstet Gynecol Reprod Biol 1993;50(1):5-8.

[183] Baker CJ, Rench MA, Edwards MS, Carpenter RJ, Hays BM, Kasper DL. Immunization of pregnant women with a polysaccharide vaccine of group B streptococcus. N Engl J Med 1988;319(18):1180-5.

[184] Baker CJ, Rench MA, McInnes P. Immunization of pregnant women with group B streptococcal type III capsular polysaccharide-tetanus toxoid conjugate vaccine. Vaccine 2003;21(24):3468-72.

[185] Munoz FM, Ferrieri P. Group B Streptococcus vaccination in pregnancy: moving toward a global maternal immunization program. Vaccine 2013;31(Suppl 4):D46-51.

[186] Madhi SA, Dangor Z, Heath PT, Schrag S, Izu A, Sobanjo-Ter Meulen A: Considerations for a phase-III trial to evaluate a group B streptococcal polysaccharide-protein conjugate vaccine in pregnant women for the prevention of early-and late-onset invasive disease in young infants. Vaccine 2013;31(Suppl 4);D52-7

[187] Mulholland K, Suara RO, Siber G, Roberton D, Jaffar S, N'Jie J, et al. Maternal immunization with Haemophilus influenzae type b polysaccharide-tetanus protein conjugate vaccine in the Gambia. JAMA 1996;275(15):1182-8.

[188] Englund JA, Glezen WP. Maternal immunization with Haemophilus influenze type b vaccines in different populations. Vaccine 2003;21(24):3455-9.

[189] Englund JA, Glezen WP, Thompson C, Anwaruddin R, Turner CS, Siber GR. Haemophilus influenza type b-specific antibody in infants after maternal immunization. Pediatr Infect Dis J 1997;16(12):1120-30.

[190] Shahid NS, Steinhoff MC, Hoque SS, Begum T, Thompson C, Silber GR. Serum, breast milk, and infant antibody after maternal immunisation with peumococcal vaccine. Lancet 1995;346(8985):1252-7.

[191] Munoz FM, Englund JA, Cheesman CC, Maccato ML, Pinell PM, Nahm MH, et al. Maternal immunization with pneumococcal polysaccharide vaccine in the third trimester of gestation. Vaccine 2001;20(5-6):826-7.

[192] Chaithongwongwatthana S, Yamasmit W, Limpongsanurak S, Lumbiganon P, DeSimone JA, Baxter JK et al. Pneumococcal vaccination during pregnancy for preventing infant infection. Cochrane Database Syst Rev 2012;7:CD004903.

[193] Shahid NS, Steinhoff MC, Begum T, Thompson CM, Siber GR. Placental and breast transfer of antibodies after maternal immunization with polysaccharide meningococcal vaccine: a randomized, controlled evaluation. Vaccine 2002;20(17-18):2404-9.

[194] Zheteyeva Y, Moro PL, Yue X, Broder K. Safety of meningococcal polysaccharaide-protein conjugate vaccine in pregnancy: A review of the Vaccine Adverse Event Reporting System. Am J Obstet Gynecol 2013;208(6):478.e-1-6.

[195] Brown GC, Carroll CJ. Antibody response of pregnant women to poliomyelitis vaccine and passive transfer to infants. J Immunol 1958;81(5):389-95.

[196] Harjulehto T, Aro T, Hovi T, Saxen L. Congenital malformations and oral poliovirus vaccination during pregnancy. Lancet 1989;1(8641):771-2.

[197] Belshe RB, Leone PA, Bernstein DI, Wald A, Levin MJ, Stapleton JT, et al. Efficacy of a trial of a herpes simplex vaccine. N Engl J Med 2012;366(1):34-44.

[198] Roth K, Ferreira VH, Kaushie C. HSV-2 vaccine: current state and insights into development of a vaccine that targets genital mucosal protection. Microb Pathog 2013;58:45-54.

[199] Pass RF, Zhang C, Evans A, Simpson T, Andrews W, Huang ML, et al. Vaccine prevention of maternal cytomegalovirus infection. N Engl J Med 2009;360(12):1191-9.

[200] Anderson LJ, Dormitzer PR, Nokes DJ, Rappuoli R, Roca A, Graham BS. Strategic priorities for respiratory syncytial virus (RSV) vaccine development. Vaccine 2013;31(Suppl 2):B209-15.

[201] Karron RA, Buchholz UJ, Collins PL. Live-attenuated respiratory syncytial virus vaccines. Curr Top Microbiol Immunol 2013;372:259-84.

[202] Haley DR. Improving immunization rates of underserved children: a historical study of 10 health departments. Int J Health Policy Manag 2014;2(4):193-7.

[203] Tapia-Conyer R, Betancourt-Cravioto M, Saucedo-Martinez R, Motta-Murguía L, Gallardo-Rincón H. Strengthening vaccination policies in Latin America: An evidence-based approach. Vaccine 2013;31(37):3826-33.

[204] Scheifele DW, Halperin SA, Bettinger JA. Childhood ition rates in Canada are too low: UNICEF. Paediatr Child Health 2014;19(5):237-8.

[205] Plotkin SA, Robinson JM. How and why vaccines are made. In: Kaufmann HE, Lambert PH, eds. The great challenge for the future. Basel, Switzerland: Birkhauser Verlag, 2005:23-36.

[206] Orenstein WA, Douglas RG, Rodewald LE, Hinman AR. Immunization in the United States: Success, structure, and stress. Health Aff (Millwood) 2005;24:599-610.

[207] Hinman AR. Control of communicable diseases. In: Wallace HM, Patrick K, Parcel GS, Igoe JB, eds. Principles and practices of student health. Volume One. Oakland, CA: Third Party Publishing Company, 1992:53-62.

[208] Centers for Disease Control and Prevention (CDC). Ten great public achievements: United States 1900-1999. MMWR 1999;48:241-3.

[209] Centers for Disease Control and Prevention (CDC). Vaccine preventable diseases. Improving vaccination coverage in children, adolescents and adults. A report on recommendations from the Task Force on Community Preventable services. MMWR 1999;48(RR-8):1-5.

[210] Centers for Disease Control and Prevention (CDC). Ten great public health achievements—United States, 2001-2010. MMWR 2011;60:619-23.

[211] Centers for Disease Control and Prevention (CDC). Ten great public health achievements—worldwide, 2001-2010. MMWR 2011;60:814-8.

[212] Delany I, Rappuoli R, De Gregorio E. Vaccines for the 21st century. EMBO Mol Med 2014;6(6):708-20.

[213] Verma R, Khanna P, Chawla S. Recommended vaccines for international travelers to India. Hum Vaccin Immunother 2015;11(10):2455-7.

[214] Maitezou H. Immunization of healthcare providers: a critical step toward patient safety. Vaccine 2014 May 23. pii:S0264-410X(14)00713-0.

[215] Lernout T, Theeten H, Leuridan E, Van Damme P. Do vaccines save lives? Yes they do! Acta Med Port 2014;27(2):160-2.

[216] Steffens MS, Dunn AG, Wiley KE, Leask J. How organisations promoting vaccination respond to misinformation on social medica: a qualitative investigation. BMC Public Health 2019;19(1):1348. doi: 10.1186/s12889-019-7659-3.

[217] Koutsaftiki C, Mammas IN, Papatheodoropoulou A, Koutsounaki E Theodoridou M, Spandidos DA. Paediatric virology and the indisputable value of prevention. Exp Ther Med 2019;18(4):3257-9.

[218] Nour R. A systematic review of methods to improve attitudes towards childhood vaccinations. Cureus 2019;11(7):e5067. doi: 10.7759/cureus.5067.

[219] Poland GA, Tiburt JC, Marcuse EK. Preserving civility in vaccine policy discourse: A way forward. JAMA 2019;322(3):209-10.

[220] Greydanus DE: Historical perspectives on the current anti-vaccine hysteria in the 21st entury. J Clin Trials 2013;S5:001. doi:10.4172/2167-0870.S5-001.

[221] Musa S, Skrijelj V, Kulo A, Habersaat KB, Smjecanin M, Primorac E, et al. Identifying barriers and drivers to vaccination: A qualitative interview study with health workers in the Federation of Bosnia and Herzegovina. Vaccine 2020; 38(8):1906-14.

[222] Tremouillaux-Guiller J, Moustafa K, Hefferon K, Gaobotse G, Makhzoum A. Plant-made HIV vaccines and potential candidates. Curr Opin Biotechnol 2020;61:209-16.

[223] Wei CJ, Crank MC, Shiver J, Graham BS, Mascola JR, Nabel GJ. Next- generation influenza vaccines: opportunities and challenges. Nat Rev Drug Discov 2020 Feb 14. doi: 10.1038/s41573-019-0056-x.

[224] Santoni M, Zampieri R, Avesani L. Plant virus nanoparticles for vaccine application. Curr Protein Pept Sci 2020 Feb 11. doi: 10.2174/1389203721666200212100255.

[225] Zhang L, Liu Y. Potential interventions for novel coronavirus in China: A systematic review J Med Viol 2020 Feb 13. doi: 10.1002/jmv.25707.

In: Child and Adolescent Health
Editors: A Tenenbaum and J Merrick
ISBN: 978-1-53617-825-8

Chapter 5

INGESTION OF A HICKORY TUSSOCK CATERPILLAR: A CASE REPORT

Anna Jain[1], MD, Patrick Jones[2], MD and Dilip R Patel[1,*], MD, MBA, MPH

[1]Department of Pediatric and Adolescent Medicine,
Western Michigan University Homer Stryker MD School of Medicine,
Kalamazoo, Michigan, United States of America
[2]Pediatric Gastroenterology, Bronson Children's Hospital,
Kalamazoo, Michigan, United States of America

ABSTRACT

Foreign body ingestion is a common childhood problem. The most common objects are coins and food, however, as young children explore their world by placing objects in their mouths, there is no limit to what can be ingested. The following case outlines identification and

[*] Correspondence: Professor Dilip R Patel, MD, MBA, MPH, Chair, Department of Pediatric and Adolescent Medicine, Western Michigan University Homer Stryker MD School of Medicine, 1000 Oakland Drive, Kalamazoo MI 49008, United States.
Email: dilip.patel@med.wmich.edu.

management of unusual and uncommon foreign body ingestion and highlights the importance of clinical suspicion and in-depth history.

INTRODUCTION

American Association of Poison Control National Poison Data System has estimated that in 2011, over 90,000 children presented to emergency departments (ED) with foreign body ingestion (1). This can be attributed to normal childhood development, wherein very young children explore and learn about their environment by placing objects in their mouth. In order to do so, they must achieve certain developmental milestones. Specifically, development of pincer grasp and ability of an infant to rake their hand along a surface, typically attained between 6-7 months of age, contribute to the etiology of foreign body ingestion in infancy. Typically developing 10 month old infant is able to cruise around and able to pull to stand and walk with both hands held up. Infants at this age can grasp, pick up, and release an object. Given the developmental capacity, infants at this age can put small objects in mouth and swallow. There may or may not be any complications depending up on the nature of the ingested foreign body or object.

CASE STORY

A 10 month old previously healthy male presented to ED with drooling and refusal to swallow. Symptoms began suddenly. He was playing in a corner of his grandmother's day care, located in a barn, when he began to cry and scream. Grandmother reported that patient began to drool excessively and refused to swallow anything, including saliva. Mother reported mild rash around his mouth with mucosal irritation of his lips that had resolved on arrival to ED. Parents were concerned for foreign body ingestion, but reported that when symptoms began, patient had been playing in an empty corner with a walker. He was taken to ED where X-ray of chest and abdomen was performed for suspicion of foreign object ingestion. X-ray was negative for radio-opaque object. He was observed over 10 minutes, during which he made no effort to swallow. As symptoms persisted, pediatric gastroenterology was consulted. Esophagogastroduodenocopy (EGD) was performed for concern for radiolucent foreign object. During the procedure, multiple small white filaments were found embedded in esophageal mucosa (see Figures 1-3).

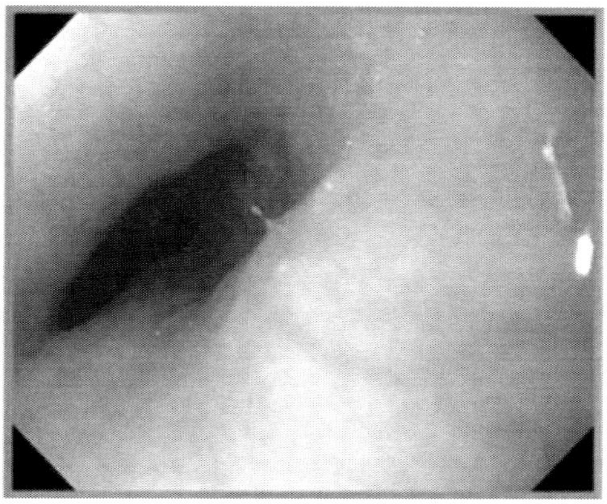

Figure 1. Courtesy of Patrick Jones, MD.

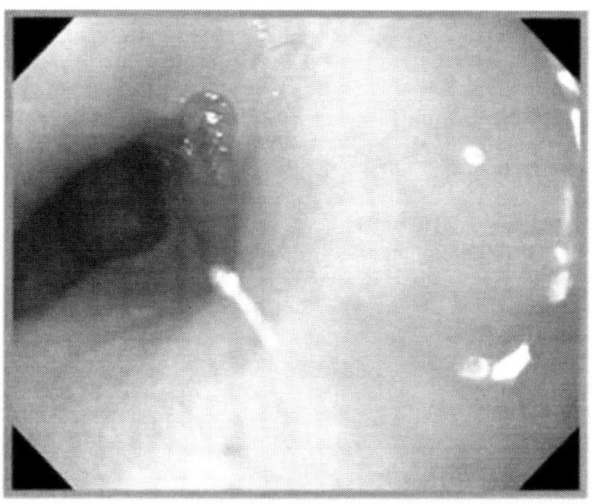

Figure 2. Courtesy of Patrick Jones, MD.

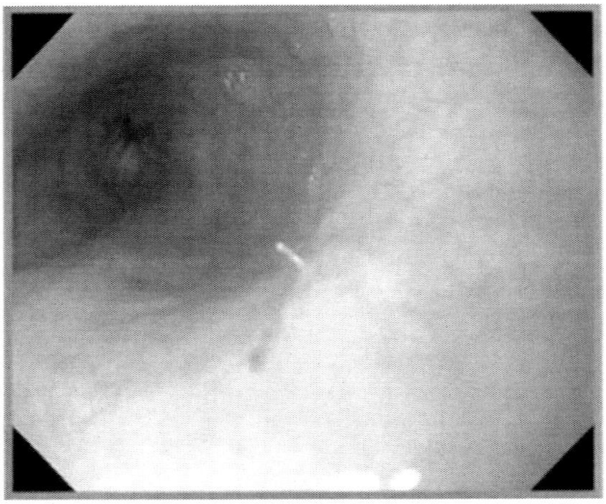

Figure 3. Courtesy of Patrick Jones, MD.

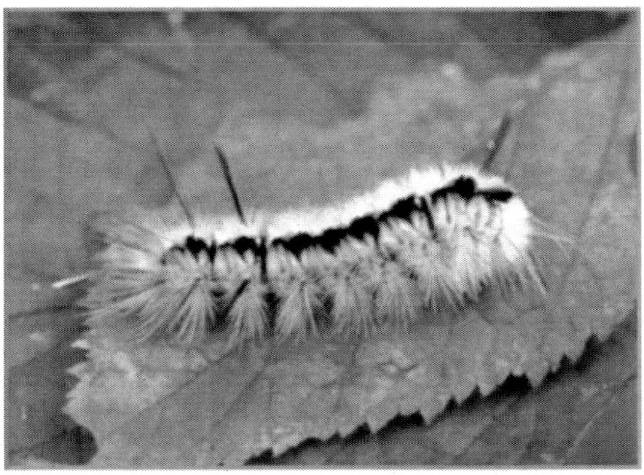

Figure 4. Hickory tussock caterpillar.

These filaments were difficult to remove as they broke apart when pulled. Ultimately, small biopsies were done to remove these filaments. Pathologic exam revealed scattered eosinophils and filaments were described as white-pink soft tissue up to 0.2-0.3 cm.

At the same time, grandmother thoroughly searched patient's play area and reported that "the only thing [she] could find was a half a caterpillar". Based on the EGD findings, filaments could be consistent with caterpillar hairs. The half-caterpillar was examined and filaments appeared to match hairs covering the body of the caterpillar. Furthermore, caterpillar has been preliminarily identified as a hickory tussock caterpillar, known to cause contact dermatitis (see Figure 5). Contact dermatitis was treated with antihistamine and corticosteroid orally. Patient improved, was discharged in subsequent two days.

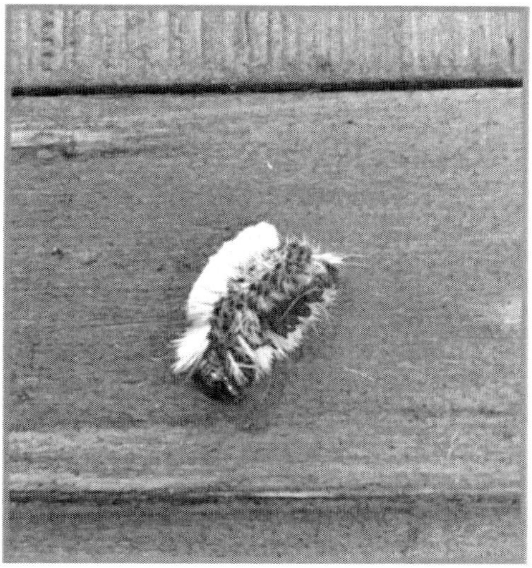

Figure 5. Specimen recovered from scene of incident.

DISCUSSION

The hickory tussock or lophocampa caryae caterpillar is native to the eastern United States (see Figure 4) (2). When provoked, these insects will extend hairs that barb into predators and cause contact dermatitis (3,4). There are many reports of skin contact with these insects, but few reports of ingestion (4). One report identified a few cases in Pennsylvania where children presented with drooling, refusal to drink, and diffuse urticaria, similar to this patient (5). A review of literature suggests that this may be the first documented case of hickory tussock ingestion in Michigan.

REFERENCES

[1] Kay M, Wyllie R. Pediatric foreign bodies and their management. Curr Gastroenterol Rep 2005;7(3):212-18.

[2] Pitetti RD, Kuspis D, Krenzelok EP. Caterpillars: An unusual source of ingestion. Pediatr Emerg Care 1999;15(1):33-6.

[3] Lee D, Pitetti RD, Casselbrant ML. Oropharyngeal manifestations of lepidopterism. Arch Otolaryngol Head Neck Surg 1999;125(1):50-2.

[4] Hossler EW. Caterpillars and moths: Part II. Dermatologic manifestations of encounters with lepidoptera. J Am Acad Dermatol 2010;62(1):13-28.

[5] Tripi PA, Lee R, Keiper JB, Jones AW, Arnold JE. An unusual case of ingestion of a moth cocoon in a 14-month-old girl. Am J Otolaryngol 2010;31(2):123-6.

In: Child and Adolescent Health
Editors: A Tenenbaum and J Merrick
ISBN: 978-1-53617-825-8

Chapter 6

A MULTILEVEL MODELING ANALYSIS OF PREDICTORS OF NEONATAL HYPOGLYCEMIA AMONG DIABETIC AND NON-DIABETIC MOTHERS

Brook T Alemu[1,*], PhD, MPH, Matthew Hoch[2], PhD, Bonnie Van Lunen[3], PhD, ATC, FNATA and Muge Akpinar-Elci[3], MD, MPH

[1]Western Carolina University, School of Health Sciences, Cullowhee, North Carolina, [2]University of Kentucky, College of Health Sciences, Lexington, Kentucky and [3]Old Dominion University, College of Health Sciences, Norfolk, Virginia, United States of America

ABSTRACT

Neonatal hypoglycemia (NH) is the most frequently encountered metabolic disorder of newborn infants and has been linked to various

[*] Corresponding Author's Email: balemu@wcu.edu.

adverse health outcomes. The risk of developing hypoglycemia among infants of diabetic mothers (IDMs) is even higher. The purpose of this chapter is to construct multilevel models that include individual-level and contextual-level characteristics to predict NH in diabetic and non-diabetic mothers. We analyzed a stratified probability sampling of 3.7 million pediatric hospital discharges using the 2012 Kids' Inpatient Database. Neonates (first 28 days after birth) with a diagnosis of hypoglycemia were included in the study. Groups were compared using the Rao-Scott Chi-Square test for categorical variables. Hierarchical models were constructed to simultaneously examine individual and contextual predictors of NH. As 20% of the variability in the rate of NH is accounted by hospitals, our specification of hierarchical modeling was appropriate to account for the variability among hospitals. We estimated that 67,124 pediatric discharges were associated with NH. Among hypoglycemic neonates, 30% were IDMs. Race, morbidity, small for gestational age, large for gestational age, prematurity, delivery by caesarian section, diabetes status, history of substance/alcohol abuse, elective admission, emergency service use, teaching hospitals, large hospitals, Medicaid insurance, privately owned hospitals, and rural hospitals were significantly associated with NH. IDMs had more than a 5-fold increased risk of developing NH compared to infants of non-diabetic mothers. The Hispanic health paradox was also observed in our study. Future research should focus on the long term clinical significance of NH by including more robust individual and environmental risk factors.

Introduction

Neonatal hypoglycemia (NH) is the most common metabolic abnormality in infants and it is associated with numerous negative health outcomes (1). Estimates for NH are between 3% and 29% of all pregnancies in the United States (US) (2). As glucose is an essential primary substrate for the brain, neurons and glial cells are susceptible to hypoglycemia (3). Therefore, neonates with hypoglycemia are prone to various acute (4) and chronic health problems (5). In the short run, newborns may experience jitteriness, hypotonia, lethargy, irritability, apnea, tachypnea, poor feeding, hypothermia, and seizures (6). Later in their life, they may experience a neurodevelopmental delay or even death (7).

The risk of developing hypoglycemia among infants of diabetic mothers (IDMs) is even higher (8). Hypoglycemia occurs in approximately

3-20% of neonates born to mothers with diabetes (6-8), with an estimated incidence rate of approximately 27% among IDMs compared to 3% among full-term healthy infants of non-diabetic women (9). Previous research on NH mainly focused on individual-level risk factors such as poor maternal glycemic control, neonatal weight at birth, and gestational age at delivery as predisposing risk factors for the development of NH in diabetic pregnancies (10). However, contextual risk factors such as household income, type of insurance, hospital characteristics, and regional variations were not considered in these studies.

NH is a highly preventable medical condition (11) and yet it poses a significant threat to the health of newborns. Due to a lack of adequate knowledge about the potential individual and contextual risk factors, the prevention of NH has been difficult (12). Therefore, considering these multilevel characteristics in assessing the determinants of NH is necessary to understand the complex relationship among various influencing factors. In addition, since NH is strongly associated with poor maternal health (13), the identification of the risk factors is important to improve the mothers' health through effective prevention measures that can reduce high-risk pregnancies.

The purpose of the current study is to construct multilevel models that include individual-level and contextual-level characteristics in order to predict NH in diabetic and non-diabetic mothers. Addressing this topic using a large nationally representative database is necessary to guide the prevention and control of adverse health outcomes associated with hypoglycemia.

OUR STUDY

We used the 2012 Kid's Inpatient Database (KID) developed by the Healthcare Cost and Utilization Project (HCUP). The KID is the largest publicly available all-payer pediatric (=20 years of age) inpatient care database in the US. The 2012 KID database includes 4,179 hospitals and 3,195,782 pediatric discharges. HCUP categorizes hospital regions as northeast, midwest, south, and west. In addition to demographic and clinical measures, hospital ownership, teaching status, location, bed size, and other important hospital characteristics were also included in the database. In total, 70 children's hospitals (400,835 pediatric discharges) and 4,109 hospitals that admit all patients (2,794,947 pediatric discharges) were included in the 2012 database. As we are interested only in neonates, this analysis is limited to uncomplicated and complicated in-hospital births. Hospital discharges with missing, invalid, or inconsistent ages were excluded from the HCUP KID.

Inclusion/exclusion criteria

Subjects were eligible to be included in the study if they were neonates (first 28 days after birth), had a diagnosis of hypoglycemia (ICD-9-CM = 775.6), and were born in the 44 HCUP participating hospitals in the year 2012. All other pediatric cases occurred in the US community, non-rehabilitation hospitals were excluded.

Variables

The current study included both individual and contextual level characteristics of NH. International classification of diseases, 9th version (ICD-9-CM codes), Diagnostic Related Groups (DRGs), Clinical Classifications Software Category (DXCCS1-DXCCS25), and Clinical classification software category for all procedures (PRCCS1- PRCCS15) was used to extract the independent variables. The dependent variable, NH, was extracted as a dichotomous variable using the ICD-9-CM code 775.6. The complete list of codes used to identify variables are listed in appendix A.

The individual characteristics included in the analysis were gender, race, prematurity, small-for-gestational-age (birth weight <10th percentile), large-for-gestational-age (birth weight >90th percentile), mortality, admission type (elective, non-elective), admission day (weekend, weekday), indicator of emergency service use, comorbidities including jitteriness, hypotonia, lethargy, irritability, apnea, tachypnea, poor feeding, hypothermia, sepsis, seizures, neurodevelopmental deficits were included. Indicator of maternal diabetes status (type 1, type2, gestational), history of substance/alcohol abuse, and delivery mode (caesarian, normal).

Contextual variables such as region (Northeast, Midwest, South, West), insurance type (Medicare, Medicaid, Private insurance, Self-pay, No charge), median household income for patient's zip code, admission season (January-March, April-June, July-September, October-December), hospital bed size (1-99, 100-399, = 400), ownership (public, private), teaching status, and location (rural, urban) were included in the analysis.

Statistical analysis

KID's inpatient core file and the hospital file were used. All analyses were weighted to account for the complex probability sampling of the dataset and permit inferences regarding the risk factors for NH. Descriptive and inferential statistics were performed taking complex survey design into consideration. Groups were compared using the Rao-Scott Chi-Square test for categorical variables. Values were presented as numbers (n), percentages (%), and odds ratios (OR).

Hierarchical logistic models were constructed to simultaneously examine individual and contextual predictors of NH. The proposed statistical analysis is appropriate because of 1) the nested structure of the data and 2) unlike Ordinary Least Squares models (OLS), hierarchical models enable us to investigate and explain the sources of both the within and between variations of higher-level factors. Random-intercept models were applied to identify key factors that can independently predict NH among diabetic and non-diabetic mothers. A p-value < 0.05 was considered statistically significant for all tests. SAS® version 9.3 was used for data analysis (Institute Inc., Cary, NC, USA).

Table 1. Individual-level characteristics of neonatal Hypoglycemia

Variables	Hypoglycemic	Non-Hypoglycemich	Total	P Value
Unweighted sample n	51,880	1,055,693	1,107,573	
Weighted population size n	67,124	3,666,636	3,733,760	
Gender n, (%)				
Male	38,495 (57.38)	1,868,004 (50.97)	1,906,499 (51.09)	<.0001
Female	28598 (43.62)	1796628 (49.03)	1,825,227 (48.91)	
Race n, (%)				
White	33,575 (55.35)	1,757,304 (52.34)	1,790,879 (52.39)	<.0001
Black	10,129 (16.70)	479,259 (14.27)	489,388 (14.32)	
Hispanic	9,459 (15.59)	675,793 (20.13)	685,252 (20.05)	
Other$	7,493 (12.35)	445,429 (13.27)	452,922 (13.25)	
SGA n, %				
SGA£	33,808 (50.37)	348,156 (0.09)	381,964 (10.23)	<.0001
Non-SGA	33,316 (49.63)	3,318,480 (99.91)	3,351,796 (89.77)	
LGA n, (%)				
LGA¥	9,723 (14.49)	204,808 (6.00)	214,532 (5.75)	<.0001
Non- LGA	57,401 (85.51)	3,461,828 (94.00)	3,519,228 (94.25)	
Morbidity n, (%)				
With Comorbidities	7,902 (11.77)	64,541 (1.76)	72,443 (7.97)	<.0001
Without Comorbidities	59,222 (88.23)	3,602,094 (98.24)	3,661,316 (92.03)	
Mortality n, (%)				
Died	515 (0.77)	10,408 (0.28)	10,923 (0.29)	<.0001
Alive	66,599 (99.23)	3,656,010 (99.72)	3,722,609 (99.71)	
Prematurity n, (%)				
Premature	27,064 (40.32)	270,550 (7.38)	297,614 (7.97)	<.0001
Non-Premature	40,060 (59.68)	3,396,086 (92.62)	3,436,146 (92.03)	
Delivery Mode n, (%)				
Cesarean Section	29,903 (44.55)	114,2704 (31.16)	117,2607 (31.41)	<.0001
Normal Delivery	37,221 (55.45)	2,523,931 (68.84)	2,561,152 (68.59)	
Mothers' Diabetic Status n, (%)				
Diabetic	20,674 (30.80)	259,243 (7.07)	279,917 (7.50)	<.0001
Non-Diabetic	46,450 (69.20)	3,407,393 (92.93)	3,453,843 (92.50)	
Admission Day n, (%)				
Weekday	53,029 (79.00)	2,929,102 (79.89)	2,982,131 (79.87)	<.0001
Weekend	14,095 (21.00)	737,532 (20.11)	751,627 (20.13)	
Elective Admission Status n, %				
Elective	164 (0.24)	8,391 (0.23)	8,555 (0.23)	<.0001
Non-Elective	6,6874 (99.76)	3,654,687 (99.77)	3,721,561 (99.77)	
Emergency Dept. Service n, (%)*				
Serviced	88 (0.001)	2,214 (0.001)	2,302 (0.06)	<.0001
Not Serviced	67,037 (99.9)	3,664,422 (99.9)	3,731,459 (99.94)	
History of Sub/alc. Abuse n, (%)				
Indicated	1,566 (2.33)	27,584 (0.75)	29,150 (0.78)	<.0001
Not-Indicated	65,558 (97.67)	3,639,052 (99.25)	3,704,610 (99.22)	

KID, Kid's Inpatient Database 2012. All analyses were weighted to account for the complex probability sampling of the dataset. $Other Race, Asian/Pacific Islander; Native American; unspecified; £SGA, small for gestational age; ¥LGA, large for gestational age.

FINDINGS

A weighted total of 3,733,760 in-hospital births were included in the 2012 KID's inpatient database (see Table 1). A total of 67,124 (5%) neonates were hypoglycemic. Among neonates included in the study 51% were

Table 2. Contextual level characteristics of neonatal hypoglycemia

Variables	Hypoglycemic	Non-Hypoglycemic	Total	P Value
Unweighted sample n	51,880	1,055,693	1,107,573	
Weighted population size n	67,124	3,666,636	3,733,760	
Type of Insurance				
Medicaid	30,843 (46.04)	169,5905 (46.38)	1,726,748 (46.37)	<.0001
Medicare	276 (0.41)	12,991 (0.36)	1,326,7 (0.36)	
Private insurance	31,799 (47.46)	1,687,688 (46.15)	1,719,487 (46.18)	
Other [%]	4,081 (6.09)	259,998 (7.1)	264,079 (7.09)	
Teaching status n, (%)				
Teaching	38,050 (56.69)	1,813,077 (49.6)	1,851,127 (49.58)	<.0001
Non-Teaching	29,074 (43.31)	1,853,559 (50.55)	1,882,633 (50.42)	
Bed Size n, (%)				
Small (1-99)	6,187 (9.22)	406,305 (11.08)	412,492 (11.05)	<.0001
Medium (100-399)	16,811 (25.04)	935,351 (25.51)	952,162 (25.50)	
Large (≥ 400)	44,126 (65.74)	2,324,980 (63.41)	2,369,106 (63.45)	
Ownership n, (%)				
Private	49,286 (73.43)	2,651,655 (72.32)	2,700,941 (72.34)	<.0001
Public	17,838(26.57)	1,014,981 (27.68)	1,032,819 (27.66)	
Neighborhood Income[#]				
1st Quartile (1 - 38,999)	18,405 (27.92)	1,023,540 (28.41)	1,041,945 (28.40)	<.0001
2nd Quartile (39,000 - 47,999)	15,945 (24.19)	886,723 (24.61)	902,668 (24.61)	
3rd Quartile (48,000 - 62,999)	16,086 (24.40)	886,738 (24.61)	902,824 (24.61)	
4th Quartile (63,000+)	15,489 (23.49)	805,520 (22.36)	821,009 (22.38)	
Admission Season				
January-March	15,388 (22.93)	880,221 (24.01)	895,609 (23.99)	<.0001
April-June	16,034 (23.89)	889,119 (24.25)	905,153 (24.25)	
July-September	18,080 (26.94)	975,669 (26.61)	993,749 (26.62)	
October-December	17,605 (26.23)	920,905 (25.12)	938,510 (25.14)	
Hospital Location				
Rural	5,576 (8.31)	441,988 (12.05)	447,564 (11.99)	<.0001
Urban	61,548 (91.69)	3,224,647 (87.95)	3,286,195 (88.01)	
Hospital Region				
Northeast	11,645 (17.35)	603,344 (16.45)	614,988 (16.47)	<.0001
Midwest	14,847 (22.12)	779,609 (21.26)	794,456 (21.28)	
South	25,813 (38.46)	1,395,779 (38.07)	1,421,592 (38.07)	
West	14,820 (22.08)	887,905 (24.22)	902,725 (24.18)	

KID, Kid's Inpatient Database 2012. All analyses were weighted to account for the complex probability sampling of the dataset. [+]NH, neonatal hypoglycemia; [%]Other Insurance = Self-pay, No charge, Other; [#]Income = Median Household Income for patient's Zip code divided into 4 quartiles; Emergency = HCUP Emergency Department service indicator.

male, while 52% were White, 14% Black, 20% Hispanic, 13% other (Asian/Pacific and Native Americans). Among neonates with hypoglycemia 50% were small for gestational age, 15% were large for gestational age, 12% had comorbidities, 40% were premature, 44% were delivered by cesarean section, 30% were born from mothers with diabetes, and 2% of the births were associated with mothers with a history of substance/alcohol abuse. Almost all mothers were admitted through non-elective admission (99%) and close to 80% of births occurred during weekdays.

The majority of newborns had some form of insurance coverage including 46% with Medicaid, 46% with private insurance and 7% with other types of coverages (self-pay and no charge) (see Table 2). The median household income in the zip code of patient's residence were proportionately distributed into 28% ($1-$38,999), 25% ($39,000-$47,999), 25% ($48,000 - $62,999), and 22% ($63,000 and above). The majority of births occurred in urban hospitals (88%), in hospitals with bed size greater than or equal to 400 (36%) between July and September (27%). Furthermore, the majority of hospitals were large (63%), privately owned (72%) and well distributed geographically among the four hospital regions including Northeast (17%), Midwest (21%), South (38%), and West (24%). Fifty-seven percent of neonates with hypoglycemia were born in teaching hospitals.

Table 3 reports the results from the random intercept model that shows the bivariate relationship between the specified variables and NH. In this analysis male sex (OR 1.3, 95% CI 1.27-1.31), Black (OR 1.1, 95% CI 1.05-1.11), Hispanic (OR 0.8, 95% CI 0.77-0.81) and Other race (Asian/Pacific and Native Americans, OR 0.8, 95% CI 0.82-0.87), morbidity (OR 2.7, 95% CI 2.57-2.73), small for gestational age (OR 9.6, 95% CI 9.41-9.72), large for gestational age (OR 2.9, 95% CI 2.81-2.95), prematurity (OR 7.0, 95% CI 6.78-7.15), delivery by caesarian section (OR 1.9, 95% CI 1.79-1.85), diabetes status (OR 5.6, 95% CI 5.46-5.65), history of substance/alcohol abuse (OR 1.2, 95% CI 1.08-1.22), elective admission (OR 0.8, 95% CI 0.64-0.92), emergency service use (OR 1.5, 95% CI 1.17-2.00), admission between July and September (OR 1.1, 95%

CI 1.03-1.08), admission between October and December (OR 1.1, 95% CI 1.06-1.11), neighborhood income above $63,000 (OR 0.9, 95% CI 0.94 - 0.99), teaching hospitals (OR 1.7, 95% CI 1.58-1.87), medium hospital bed size (OR 1.2, 95% CI 1.04 - 1.29), large hospital bed size (OR 1.4, 95% CI 1.26-1.55), privately owned hospitals (OR 1.1, 95% CI 1.05-1.24), urban hospitals (OR 2.0, 95% CI 1.84-2.24), and Medicaid insurance (OR 1.2, 95% CI 1.01-1.35) were significantly associated with NH.

Table 3. OR, 95% CIs, and P from bivariate random intercept models for individual-level and contextual-level risk factors

Variables	ORs	95% CI	P value
Male	1.3	1.273 - 1.313	<.0001
Black	1.1	1.052 - 1.107	<.0001
Hispanic	0.8	0.769 - 0.812	0.0002
Other	0.8	0.820 - 0.869	<.0001
Morbidity	2.7	2.573 - 2.734	<.0001
SGA	9.6	9.409 - 9.718	<.0001
LGA	2.9	2.812 - 2.945	<.0001
Premature	7.0	6.782 - 7.150	<.0001
Cesarean Section	1.9	1.795 - 1.852	<.0001
Diabetic	5.6	5.455 - 5.648	<.0001
Substance	3.2	2.971 - 3.343	<.0001
Elective	0.8	0.635 - 0.920	0.0046
Weekend	1.0	1.022 - 1.062	<.0001
Emergency#	2.2	1.646 - 2.833	0.0018
2nd Quartile (39,000 - 47,999)	0.9	0.970 - 1.017	0.0833
3rd Quartile (48,000 - 62,999)	0.9	0.931 - 0.978	0.1898
4th Quartile (63,000+)	0.9	0.944 - 0.997	0.0008
Lower Income	1.0	1.018 - 1.058	0.0001
Midwest€	1.2	1.123 - 1.190	<.0001
South	1.1	1.111 - 1.172	<.0001
West	1.1	1.081 - 1.135	<.0001
2nd Quarter Admission	1.0	0.999 - 1.045	<.0001
3rd Quarter Admission	1.1	1.033 - 1.079	0.0291
4th Quarter Admission	1.1	1.057 - 1.105	<.0001
Teaching Status	1.7	1.579 - 1.865	<.0001
Medium Bed Size (100-399) Ω	1.2	1.035 - 1.290	<.0001
Large Bed Size (≥ 400)	1.4	1.263 - 1.549	<.0001
Privately Owned	1.1	1.053 - 1.244	0.0016
Urban Hospitals	2.0	1.838 - 2.242	<.0001
Medicaid∞	1.2	1.008 - 1.352	0.0389
Private insurance	1.0	1.017 - 1.056	0.0002
Other%	0.9	0.830 - 0.898	<.0001

OR, unadjusted odds ratio; SGA, small for gestational age; LGA, large for gestational age; CI, confidence interval; #Emergency, HCUP Emergency Department service indicator; €Northeast region used as a reference; Ω Small (1-99) used as a reference; ∞Medicare used as a reference; %Other Insurance = Self-pay, No charge.

Table 4. OR, 95% CI, and P values from model 3 that indicate the relationship between individual and contextual level predictors and neonatal hypoglycemia

Variables	ORs	95% CI	P value
Male	1.2	1.18-1.23	<.0001
Black	1.0	0.90-1.06	0.5739
Hispanic	0.7	0.61-0.80	<.0001
Other	0.8	0.78-0.91	<.0001
Morbidity	5.0	4.63-5.40	<.0001
SGA	9.7	9.25-10.27	<.0001
LGA	3.1	2.86-3.34	<.0001
Premature	3.8	3.44-4.15	<.0001
Cesarean Section	1.5	1.50-1.59	<.0001
Diabetic	5.1	4.81-5.41	<.0001
Substance	2.1	1.92-2.29	<.0001
Elective	1.0	0.79-1.57	0.5470
Weekend	1.1	1.03-1.08	<.0001
Emergency#	1.5	1.10-2.00	0.0106
2nd Quartile (39,000 - 47,999)	1.0	0.94-1.05	0.7809
3rd Quartile (48,000 - 62,999)	0.9	0.90-1.04	0.4293
4th Quartile (63,000+)	1.0	0.93-1.10	0.8046
Midwest€	0.9	0.85-1.10	0.8046
South	0.9	0.87-1.10	0.4293
West	0.9	0.87-1.09	0.7809
2nd Quarter Admission	1.0	1.00-1.06	0.0002
3rd Quarter Admission	1.1	1.02-1.13	0.0040
4th Quarter Admission	1.1	1.05-1.15	0.0747
Teaching Status	1.2	1.10-1.34	0.0001
Medium Bed Size (100-399) Ω	1.1	0.92-1.24	0.2939
Large Bed Size (≥ 400)	1.1	0.94-1.23	0.4090
Privately Owned	1.0	0.90-1.14	0.8254
Urban Hospitals	1.4	1.21-1.52	<.0001
Medicaid∞	0.9	0.67-1.09	0.2124
Private insurance	0.9	0.68-1.13	0.3010
Other%	0.8	0.60-1.04	0.2124

*OR, unadjusted odds ratio; SGA, small for gestational age; LGA, large for gestational age; CI, confidence interval; #Emergency, HCUP Emergency Department service indicator; €Northeast region used as a reference; Ω Small (1-99) used as a reference; ∞Medicare used as a reference; %Other Insurance = Self-pay, No charge.

Using the estimate obtained from the empty model, the intra-class correlation coefficient (ICC) which indicates how much of the total variation in the probability of NH is accounted for by the hospitals were calculated. Hierarchical model assumes that the dichotomous outcome from the hierarchical model comes from an unknown latent continuous variable with a level-1 residual that follows a logistic distribution with a mean of 0 and a variance of 3 (14). As a result, 3.29 were used as the level-

1 variance (V_P) while the hospital variance ($V_H = 0.8381$) were obtained from the model.

$$ICC = V_H / [(V_H + V_P)] * 100$$
$$ICC = [0.8381 / (0.8381 + 3.29)] * 100 = 20\%$$

The above calculation indicates that 20% of the variability in the rate of NH is accounted by hospitals, leaving 80% of the variability to be accounted by patients. The result also indicates that there is a statistically significant amount of variability ($V_H = 0.8381$; $Z = 26.74$; $p < .0001$) in the odds of developing hypoglycemia between the hospitals.

In the model that was constructed to observe the relationship between individual level predictors and NH (table not presented), female sex (OR 0.8, 95% CI 0.81-0.85), Hispanic (OR 0.8, 95% CI 0.78-0.83), Other race (Asian/Pacific and Native Americans, OR 0.9, 95% CI 0.84-0.90), morbidity (OR 2.6, 95% CI 2.49-2.66), small for gestational age (OR 3.9, 95% CI 3.82-3.98), large for gestational age (OR 2.8, 95% CI 2.76-2.92), prematurity (OR 1.9, 95% CI 1.87-1.99), delivery by caesarian section (OR 1.4, 95% CI 1.38-1.44), diabetes status (OR 2.0, 95% CI 1.95-2.04), history of substance/alcohol abuse (OR 1.2, 95% CI 1.10-1.25), elective admission (OR 0.8, 95% CI 0.64 - 0.92), and emergency service use (OR 1.4, 95% CI 1.02-1.82) were significantly associated with NH.

The final model that combines both the individual and contextual level predictors is presented in Table 4. In this analysis male sex (OR 1.2, 95% CI 1.18-1.23), Hispanic (OR 0.7, 95% CI 0.61-0.80) and other race (Asian/Pacific and Native Americans, OR 0.8, 95% CI 0.78-0.91), morbidity (OR 5.0, 95% CI 4.63-5.40), small for gestational age (OR 9.7, 95% CI 9.25-10.27), large for gestational age (OR 3.1, 95% CI 2.86-3.34), prematurity (OR 3.8, 95% CI 3.44-4.15), delivery by caesarian section (OR 1.5, 95% CI 1.50-1.59), diabetes status (OR 5.1, 95% CI 4.81-5.41), history of substance/alcohol abuse (OR 2.1, 95% CI 1.92-2.29), weekend admission (OR 1.1, 95% CI 1.03-1.08), emergency service use (OR 1.5, 95% CI 1.10-2.00), teaching hospitals (OR 1.2, 95% CI 1.10-1.34), and rural hospitals (OR 1.4, 95% CI 1.21-1.52) were significantly associated with NH.

DISCUSSION

In our analysis of the 2012 HCUP KID database, which included more than 3.7 million patient discharges, indicated a 5% (67,124) prevalence of NH. Our main hypothesis was confirmed by the strong association found between NH and diabetic mothers. Statistically significant associations were found both in the bivariate random intercept model (OR 5.6) and multivariate model (OR 5.1). Most studies of NH used small databases from single medical facilities, mainly focused on clinical factors without having proper comparison groups. Our study used a large nationally validated database to determine the individual and contextual risk factors of NH both in diabetic and non-diabetic mothers. The results of the current study highlight the increased risk (5 fold) of NH among diabetic mothers compared to non-diabetic mothers at the national level. As NH is associated with acute and potentially permanent neurological damage (5, 11), hospitals across the US should develop a more effective method and devise management strategies to identify fetuses from diabetic mothers so that intervention during the neonatal period can be made.

Pertaining to the association between the other individual-level risk factors and NH, our results were consistent with data from the literature. For example, Bollepalli et al. (10) found that large for gestational age/macrosomic infants had 3.5-fold higher odds of developing hypoglycemia compared to non-macrosomic infants. Higher frequencies of maternal diabetes and large for gestational age infants were also observed by Flores-le Roux et al. (15). Similar to our findings, Ramos et al. (16) indicated that the frequency of hypoglycemia was statistically associated with prematurity, macrosomia and Ponderal index. Furthermore, Hispanic health paradox was also observed in our study. The paradox states that despite lower socioeconomic status Hispanics have comparable or better health outcomes than whites (17). Similar to what the paradox states, we found that Hispanic neonates are 30% less likely to develop NH compared to whites. Better breastfeeding habits, lower birth trauma, protective dietary practices, and strong social networks and support are thought to be the main factors explaining these paradoxical health outcomes (18). Overall, the findings related to the individual risk factors examined by the current study were consistent with the literature.

Regarding the contextual characteristics, the most robust association, as evidenced by the statistical significance in the multivariate analysis, were found in rural and teaching hospitals. Infants born in these hospitals appear to have a significantly higher chance of developing NH compared to urban and non-teaching hospitals. It is well supported that disparity of overall health and health outcomes of rural populations are significantly different than urban populations. In general, people who live in rural areas tend to have poorer health outcomes due to multiple factors including but not limited to a sedentary lifestyle, higher alcohol consumption, higher smoking rates, shortage of resources for clinical care, and lower socioeconomic status (19). It appears that these poorer health outcomes in the general rural population are also reflected in the health outcomes of neonates born in rural hospitals. These may be due to the fact that rural mothers tend to be less educated, younger, single (20), more likely to deliver by caesarian section, more likely to deliver low birthweight and premature infants, travel longer distance to access medical care, and receive less prenatal care (21, 22). In order to balance neonatal outcomes between rural and urban hospitals, targeted intervention efforts that incorporate the particular healthcare needs of rural communities should be introduced across hospitals in the US.

Regarding neonatal outcomes in teaching hospitals, our findings were also consistent with data on the literature. Sloan et al. (23) found that teaching hospitals had higher postoperative complications in four of six surgical procedures. In a study that included 16.9 million Medicare patients, Yuan et al. (24) found that teaching hospitals had the highest mortality rates. Using the Veteran Affairs hospital data Khuri et al. (25) also found that complication rates were higher in teaching hospitals in six of seven specialties and four of eight operations.

We recognize that there are limitations associated with this study. Because of the structure of the KID database, we were not able to track patients over time to determine the long-term health impact of NH on, for example, neurological and cognitive developments. Therefore, interpretation of the results should consider the retrospective cross-sectional nature of the study design. Our analyses were also limited to the variables that were provided by the data. Although the variables included in the study are sufficient to understand the overall risk factors of NH, variables such as educational background, employment status, and individual income could have provided more insightful results. Furthermore, as the data include only community, non-rehabilitation hospitals, other types of hospitals such as Veterans' Administration and Indian Health System facilities were not included. Our findings may have been underestimated by the exclusion of states and hospitals. Despite these limitations, however, the KID database is the only nationally validated database that is available to conduct outcomes research on the pediatric population and the use of such validated databases should be encouraged in other areas of public health research.

We found that IDMs have more than 5-fold increased risk of developing NH compared to infants of non-diabetic mothers. In addition, the increased risk of NH in male, premature, macrosomic, small for gestational age, large for gestational age, and neonates born from mothers with a history of substance or alcohol abuse were also the most relevant results associated with the individual risk factors. Increased awareness of NH in these subgroups should be encouraged to improve and changes clinical practices across hospitals in the US. Future research should focus on the long term clinical significance of NH by including a more robust individual and environmental risk factors.

ACKNOWLEDGMENTS

This research project was not funded. The authors have no financial disclosures to declare and no conflicts of interest to report. As this work did not involve human subject participants, informed consent was not obtained. Nonetheless, the study was conducted in accordance with the 1964 Declaration of Helsinki and we received IRB approval for our circumscribed analysis. The current study does not involve animals.

APPENDIX A: CODES FOR THE IDENTIFICATION OF VARIABLES IN THE KID'S INPATIENT DATABASE

Variables	ICD-9-CM/ PRCCS/ DXCCS/ DRG24
NH	775.6 (ICD-9-CM)
Large for Gestational Age	766.1 (ICD-9-CM)
Small for Gestational Age	764.0, V21.30- V21.35 (ICD-9-CM)
Prematurity	386, 387, 388, 375 (DRG24)
History of Alcohol/Substance Abuse	660, 661 (DXCCS); 52,433,521,523 (DRG24)
Complicated Pregnancy	219 (DXCCS)
Delivery by Cesarean Section	669.7; V3001(ICD-9-CM)/ 134, 134,740,741,742,743,744,745,746,747,748,749 (PRCCS)/ 370, 371 (DRG24)
Indicator of Diabetic Status (Type I, Type II, Gestational)	250.01-250.93, 775.0, 648.03, 648.83 (ICD-9-CM)/ 49, 50, 186 (DXCCS)/295 (DRG24)
Comorbidities	
Jitteriness	796.9 (ICD-9-CM)
Hypotonia	781.3 (ICD-9-CM)
Lethargy	780.7 (ICD-9-CM)
Irritability	799.22 (ICD-9-CM)
Apnea	786.03 (ICD-9-CM)
Tachypnea	786.06 (ICD-9-CM)
Poor feeding	783.3 (ICD-9-CM)
Hypothermia	991.6 (ICD-9-CM)
Sepsis	995.91, 771.81 (ICD-9-CM)
Seizures	345.0-345.9 (ICD-9-CM)
Neurodevelopmental Delay	315.0-315.9 (ICD-9-CM)

ICD-9-CM = International classification of diseases, 9th version; PRCCS = Clinical classification software category for all procedures; DRG24 = Diagnostic related groups, version 24; DXCCS = Clinical classifications software category for all diagnosis.

REFERENCES

[1] Najati N, Saboktakin L. Prevalence and underlying etiologies of neonatal hypoglycemia. Pakistan J Biol Sci 2010;13(15):753.

[2] DePuy AM, Coassolo KM, Som DA, Smulian JC. Neonatal hypoglycemia in term, nondiabetic pregnancies. Am J Obstet Gynecol 2009;200(5):e45-51.

[3] De AK, Biswas R, Samanta M, Kundu CK. Study of blood glucose level in normal and low birth weight newborns and impact of early breast feeding in a tertiary care centre. Ann Nigerian Med 2011;5(2):53.

[4] Alkalay AL, Flores-Sarnat L, Sarnat HB, Farber SJ, Simmons CF. Plasma glucose concentrations in profound neonatal hypoglycemia. Clin Pediatrics 2006;45(6):550-8.

[5] Boluyt N, van Kempen A, Offringa M. Neurodevelopment after neonatal hypoglycemia: A systematic review and design of an optimal future study. Pediatrics 2006;117(6):2231-43.

[6] Hay WW, Rozance PJ. Continuous glucose monitoring for diagnosis and treatment of neonatal hypoglycemia. J Pediatrics 2010;157(2):180-2.

[7] Osier FH, Berkley JA, Ross A, Sanderson F, Mohammed S, Newton CR. Abnormal blood glucose concentrations on admission to a rural Kenyan district hospital: prevalence and outcome. Arch Dis Child 20031;88(7):621-5.

[8] Rozance PJ, Hay WW. Hypoglycemia in newborn infants: features associated with adverse outcomes. Neonatology 2006;90(2):74-86.

[9] Cordero L, Treuer SH, Landon MB, Gabbe SG. Management of infants of diabetic mothers. Arch Pediatr Adolesc Med 1998;152(3):249-54.

[10] Agrawal RK, Lui K, Gupta JM. Neonatal hypoglycaemia in infants of diabetic mothers. J Paediatr Child Health 2000;36(4):354-6.

[11] Burns CM, Rutherford MA, Boardman JP, Cowan FM. Patterns of cerebral injury and neurodevelopmental outcomes after symptomatic neonatal hypoglycemia. Pediatrics 2008;122(1):65-74.

[12] Mehta A. Prevention and management of neonatal hypoglycaemia. Arch Dis Child Fetal Neonatal Ed 1994;70(1):F54.

[13] García-Patterson A, Aulinas A, María MÁ, Úbeda J, Orellana I, Ginovart G, et al. Maternal body mass index is a predictor of neonatal hypoglycemia in gestational diabetes mellitus. J Clin Endocrinol 2012;97(5):1623-8.

[14] Pedersen J. Weight and length at birth of infants of diabetic mothers. Eur J Endocrinol 1954;16(4):330-42.

[15] Flores-le Roux JA, Sagarra E, Benaiges D, Hernandez-Rivas E, Chillaron JJ, de Dou JP, et al. A prospective evaluation of neonatal hypoglycaemia in infants of women with gestational diabetes mellitus. Diab Res Clin Pract 2012;97(2):217-22.

[16] Ramos GA, Hanley AA, Aguayo J, Warshak CR, Kim JH, Moore TR. Neonatal chemical hypoglycemia in newborns from pregnancies complicated by type 2 and gestational diabetes mellitus–the importance of neonatal ponderal index. J Matern Fetal Neonatal Med 2012;25(3):267-71.

[17] Ruiz JM, Hamann HA, Mehl MR, O'Connor MF. The Hispanic health paradox: From epidemiological phenomenon to contribution opportunities for psychological science. Group Processes Intergr Relat 2016l;19(4):462-76.

[18] Ruiz JM, Steffen P, Smith TB. Hispanic mortality paradox: a systematic review and meta-analysis of the longitudinal literature. Am J Public Health 2013;103(3):e52-60.

[19] Coburn AF, Wakefield M, Casey M, Moscovice I, Payne S, Loux S. Assuring rural hospital patient safety: what should be the priorities? J Rural Health 2004;20(4):314-26.

[20] Vartak S, Ward MM, Vaughn TE. Patient safety outcomes in small urban and small rural hospitals. J Rural Health 2010;26(1):58-66.

[21] Moscovice I, Wholey DR, Klingner J, Knott A. Measuring rural hospital quality. J Rural Health 2004;20(4):383-93.

[22] Kozhimannil K. Rural-urban differences in childbirth care, 2002-2010, and implications for the future. Med Care 2014;52(1):4.

[23] Sloan FA, Conover CJ, Provenzale D. Hospital credentialing and quality of care. Soc Sci Med 2000;50(1):77-88.

[24] Yuan Z, Cooper GS, Einstadter D, Cebul RD, Rimm AA. The association between hospital type and mortality and length of stay: a study of 16.9 million hospitalized Medicare beneficiaries. Med Care 2000;38(2):231-45.

[25] Khuri SF, Najjar SF, Daley J, Krasnicka B, Hossain M, Henderson WG, et al. Comparison of surgical outcomes between teaching and nonteaching hospitals in the Department of Veterans Affairs. Ann Surgery 2001;234(3):370.

In: Child and Adolescent Health
Editors: A Tenenbaum and J Merrick
ISBN: 978-1-53617-825-8

Chapter 7

IDENTIFYING FACTORS ASSOCIATED WITH AUTISM SPECTRUM DISORDER BASED ON A COMPREHENSIVE NATIONAL SURVEY

Kotwoallama R Zerbo, Chen Mo, DrPH, Jingjing Yin*, PhD and Hani M Samawi, PhD
Department of Biostatistics, Epidemeology and Environmental Sciences, Jiann-Ping Hsu College Public Health, Georgia Southern University, Statesboro, Georgia, United States of America

ABSTRACT

In this chapter we aim to identify factors associated with childhood autism spectrum disorders (ASD) based on the National Survey of Children's Health. Methods: The National Survey of Children's Health is a cross-sectional survey of parents' report of their child health conditions. We performed a secondary analysis of this survey data to determine the association between parent-reported autism spectrum disorder diagnosis and possible risk factors. The logistic regression model for complex survey data was applied. Results: Child health, health insurance, and

* Corresponding Author's Email: Jingjing Yin, Email: jyin@georgiasouthern.edu.

family health and activities were significantly associated with ASD diagnosis. Specifically, the odds of reporting autism spectrum disorder for children with history of anxiety disorder is seven times higher than that of those without; the odds of autism spectrum disorder diagnosis is 45% and 36% less in children uninsured and those privately-insured compared to those publicly insured. Additionally, children whose primary language was Spanish have reduced odds of 50%. Conclusions: Our study highlights associated factors of childhood ASD and as such it can be used as a stepping stone for future studies, especially cohort studies to validate the direction of important associations.

INTRODUCTION

Autism spectrum disorders (ASD) are neurodevelopmental disorders that can cause significant social, communication and behavioral challenges (1). Children affected by ASD often demonstrate unusual interests and behaviors, such as not responding to name, avoiding eye contact and preferring to be alone, experiencing delayed speech and language skills, repeating words or phrases over, and demonstrating flat or inappropriate facial expressions (1). The prevalence of ASD has gradually increased in the last few years (2-4). During 1997 to 2014, the prevalence of ASD had increased from 0.47% to 17.1% (5). According to a 2014 surveillance report from the Centers for Disease Control and Prevention's (CDC) Autism and Developmental Disability Monitoring (ADDM) Network, about 1 in 68 children has been identified with ASD (1, 6). The emotional and economic burden of childhood ASD is vast and in many cases leads to reduced family earnings (7). Summary studies from the United States of America, the United Kingdom, and Ireland revealed that the cost of lifetime care for children with ASD is over $1.4 million (8).

Many studies have investigated associated with ASD in an effort to clarify etiologies. However, it is also importance to identify associated factors in order to properly manage the treatment of ASD. The United Kingdom National Health Service identifies five main categories of risk factors for ASD: genetic, environmental, psychological, neurological factors and other health conditions (9). In the past, ASD was thought to be largely genetic in nature and many studies have focused on genetic, neurological factors, perinatal and neonatal factors (10-12). Our study assesses the epidemiological factors associated with parent-reported childhood ASD in the United States based on a secondary analysis of the National Survey of Children's Health (NSCH 2011-2012). The survey categories the variables into five categories: child's health, neighborhood safety, family health and activities, demographical attributes, and health insurance coverage.

OUR STUDY

The National Survey of Children's Health (2011-2012) is a nationally representative telephone survey. This survey is a cross-sectional, complex, probability sample (i.e., survey was conducted within each of the geographic State individually with different sampling weights) of parents' report of their child health status including ASD diagnosis. The survey reported ASD as three categories (current diagnosis, ever told but not currently diagnosed and never diagnosed with the disease). For the purpose of our study, ASD has been converted into two categories (never diagnosed versus ever or currently diagnosed). Due to the confounding effect of early intervention of ASD which could reduce the symptoms of ASD, we combined "ever had diagnosed" and "currently being diagnosed" groups into "ever diagnosed with ASD." In such way, the confounding effect of "early intervention" is lessened since no intervention done for the "never diagnosed" group. Furthermore, as ASD is a chronic life-long condition, it would not expect to resolve. Although symptoms can subside substantially with intervention, ASD symptoms would be present and have an influence on someone throughout his/her life. Therefore, the two categories of ASD diagnosis (never versus ever diagnosed) were considered sufficient. We recognize a limitation of the study is that the ASD diagnosis record in the NSCH survey is based on parent self-reports instead of the validated diagnosis obtained from physicians.

We performed univariate analysis on all variables that were surveyed in NSCH. The variables recorded as part of the National Survey are 1) child's health condition: child's overall health status, condition of child's teeth, oral health status, BMI status, premature birth and chronic health conditions such as diabetes, asthma, joint, muscle and bone problem, brain injury and anxiety; 2) neighborhood safety: supportive neighborhood, safe communities, safe school; 3) family health and activities: physical, mental health status of parents, exposure to secondhand smoking, time spent watching TV, childcare-induced parental stress, and some adverse childhood experience such as divorce, domestic violence, insufficient income, exposure to drug abuse; 4) demographics: child age, gender, family structure, race, poverty level and health insurance coverage.

Statistical analysis

Since the NSCH data is from a complex survey with stratification by geographical State with unequal sampling weights, we obtained the descriptive summary results, such as frequencies and sample means by using PROC SURVEYFREQ and PROC SURVEYMEANS in SAS 9.4. These procedures are common statistical procedures in SAS for handling complex survey sample designs (13, 14). The categories of the following covariates: anxiety, brain injury, joint, muscle and bone condition, and Spanish language with initially three levels (similar as ASD), were combined "ever had" and "currently having" corresponding conditions into a single level and resulting in binary variables with "ever and currently have" versus "never had" corresponding conditions. The significance level was set to be 0.05.

Table 1. Multivariate table for the factors significantly associated with ASD diagnosis in the final model

Effects	Multivariate analysis OR	Multivariate analysis 95% CI		P-value	Univariate Analysis OR	Univariate Analysis 95% CI		P-value
Demographics								
Child age	0.93	0.89	0.96	<.0001	0.94	0.91	0.97	0.0004
Gender								
Male vs. Female	4.38	3.54	5.41	<.0001	4.09	3.34	5.02	<.0001
Spanish language[1]								
Yes vs. No	0.50	0.35	0.71	<.0001	0.69	0.51	0.94	0.0175
Child health								
Anxiety								
Yes vs. No	8.69	7.22	10.47	<.0001	13.75	11.66	16.21	<.0001
Child overall health[2]								
Fair/poor	1.45	0.96	2.19	0.0557	5.12	3.71	7.07	<.0001
Good	1.93	1.53	2.44	<.0001	3.63	2.98	4.43	<.0001
Joint muscle & bone								
Yes vs. No	1.74	1.29	2.34	0.00	3.43	2.72	4.34	<.0001
Premature								
Yes vs. No	1.50	1.18	1.89	0.00	1.87	1.51	2.30	<.0001
Health Insurance								
Insurance type [3]								
Uninsured	0.55	0.32	0.93	0.0364	0.31	0.19	0.52	<.0001
Private	0.64	0.52	0.79	0.00	0.39	0.32	0.46	<.0001
Family Health and activities								
Parental stress[4]								
Yes vs. No	4.45	3.64	5.44	<.0001	8.65	7.32	10.22	<.0001

[1] Coded "Yes" if he primary language spoken at home is Spanish.

[2] Excellent/very good as reference level.

[3] Public insurance as reference level.

[4] Coded "Yes" if their parents responded "Usually" or "Always" to one or more of three questions: - child was much harder to care for than other children; - often bothered a lot by their child's behavior; - angry with child.

In order to assess factors associated with childhood ASD (ever diagnosed versus never diagnosed), logistic regression models for complex survey were fitted using PROC SURVEYLOGISTIC in SAS 9.4. First, univariate logistic regression model of each of the independent variables versus ASD diagnosis were fitted and those significantly associated variables were considered as candidate variables to be fitted into the multivariate logistic model. The stepwise model selection is applied for determining the multivariate regression model. Note all significant associations identified by the logistic regression models cannot directly concluded as risk factors and causalities since the findings are based on data from a cross-sectional survey. We recognized the survey design as cross-sectional study to be another limitation to our study. Table 1 presents the results of the final multivariable logistic regression model after stepwise selection.

FINDINGS

Among the 95,677 survey participants, 1967 (2.06%) children have ever been diagnosed with ASD, and 83,515 (87.29%) children have never been diagnosed with the condition; ASD information of 10,195 (10.66%) children was missing, and the majority of the missing data was due to unstable diagnosis of ASD before the age of two (3, 15). Therefore, the survey did not include the ASD diagnosis for children less than two years old. Note that the prevalence of ASD is low (2%); thus, for certain associated factors, we approximate the relative risk by the odds ratio calculated from the logistic regression models.

The information about ASD is missing among 10,195 children. In order to evaluate if the distributions of the covariates are significantly different for the samples with Autism data compared to the samples without, frequencies of the factors of interest are calculated for the two groups, respectively. Table 2 presents the corresponding frequencies, from which, we see that the distributions of most covariates in non-missing and missing groups are similar. The only exception is the mean age, as in the sample with missing ASD information, age is significantly smaller (<1 year old) based on the fact that the survey recorded ASD data on children aged two or older (since the diagnosis of ASD is less accurate at earlier ages). Therefore, we conclude that the part of missing data does not affect the associations between the covariates of interest and the diagnosis of childhood ASD.

Table 2. Descriptive statistics and univariate analysis results

Parameter	Sample with Autism data		Sample without Autism data		Univariate Analysis Results				
	N	**Mean**	**N**	**Mean**	**OR**	**LCL**	**UCL**	**Estimate**	**P**
Demographics									
Age									
Child age	85482	9.83	10195	0.64	0.94	0.91	0.97	-0.06	0.0004
	N	%	**N**	%					
Gender									
Male	44055	51.61	5151	50.57	4.09	3.34	5.02	1.41	<.0001
Female	41309	48.39	5035	49.43	-	-	-	-	-
Spanish Language									
Yes	11100	13.31	1555	15.67	0.69	0.51	0.94	-0.37	0.0175
No	72291	86.69	8367	84.33	-	-	-	-	-
Federal Poverty level									
≥400% FPL	31172	36.47	3459	33.94	0.65	0.49	0.88	-0.43	0.0046
200-399% FPL	26117	30.56	2804	27.51	0.81	0.6	1.09	-0.21	0.1661
100-199% FPL	15325	17.93	1856	18.21	0.87	0.62	1.22	-0.14	0.4159
0-99% FPL	12852	15.04	2074	20.35	-	-	-	-	-
Income [1]									
Very Often	4675	5.58	542	5.41	2.34	1.67	3.28	0.85	<.0001
Somewhat Often	13150	15.70	1474	14.72	1.68	1.34	2.1	0.52	<.0001
Rarely	25666	30.64	2458	24.54	1.16	0.96	1.39	0.15	0.1247
Never	40286	48.09	5541	55.33	-	-	-	-	-
Child Health									
BMI									
Overweight/ obese	12754	29.14	32	36.78	1.57	1.32	1.86	0.45	<.0001
Underweight	2494	5.70	7	8.05	1.49	1.09	2.03	0.4	0.01
Normal weight	28522	65.16	48	55.17	-	-	-	-	-
Overall health									
Fair/poor	2226	2.61	166	1.63	5.12	3.71	7.07	1.63	<.0001
Good	8525	9.98	741	7.27	3.63	2.98	4.43	1.29	<.0001
Excellent/ very good	74687	87.42	9283	91.10	-	-	-	-	-
Premature									
Yes	9556	11.29	1194	11.75	1.87	1.51	2.3	0.62	<.0001
No	75065	88.71	8966	88.25	-	-	-	-	-
Low birthweight									
Yes	Yes	Yes	Yes	Yes	Yes	Yes	Yes	Yes	Yes
No	No	No	No	No	No	No	No	No	No

Table 2. (Continued)

Parameter	Sample with Autism data		Sample without Autism data		Univariate Analysis Results				
	N	Mean	N	Mean	OR	LCL	UCL	Estimate	P
Diabetes [2]									
Ever not current	93	0.11	7	0.07	3.5	0.83	14.75	1.25	0.088
Current	364	0.43	6	0.06	1.67	0.74	3.79	0.51	0.219
No	84987	99.47	10165	99.87	-	-	-	-	-
Anxiety									
Yes	5017	5.88	47	37.01	13.75	11.66	16.21	2.62	<.0001
No	80349	94.12	80	62.99	-	-	-	-	-
Asthma [2]									
Ever not current	5075	5.95	116	1.14	1.16	0.86	1.55	0.14	0.338
Current	8007	9.39	220	2.17	1.38	1.08	1.77	0.32	0.0093
No	72209	84.66	9823	96.69	-	-	-	-	-
Brain									
Yes	2783	3.26	70	0.69	1.52	1.13	2.06	0.42	0.0063
No	82645	96.74	10105	99.31	-	-	-	-	-
Joint muscle & bone									
Yes	3039	3.56	163	1.60	3.43	2.72	4.34	1.23	<.0001
No	82348	96.44	10007	98.40	-	-	-	-	-
Teeth									
Fair/poor	4771	5.58	82	1.63	2.84	2.14	3.77	1.04	<.0001
Good	15366	17.99	525	10.42	1.58	1.3	1.93	0.46	<.0001
Excellent/ very good	65289	76.43	4432	87.95	-	-	-	-	-
Oral health									
Yes	14597	17.13	133	2.63	1.28	1.05	1.57	0.25	0.0175
No	70628	82.87	4921	97.37	-	-	-	-	-
Family Health and activities									
Mother physical health									
Fair/Poor	7995	10.17	599	6.10	2.12	1.68	2.67	0.75	<.0001
Good	17680	22.49	1691	17.21	1.43	1.19	1.73	0.36	0.0002
Excellent/ Very good	52942	67.34	7536	76.69	-	-	-	-	-
Father physical health									
Fair/poor	5191	7.68	370	4.41	1.54	1.19	2.01	0.43	0.0012
Good	14665	21.70	1405	16.76	1.32	1.1	1.59	0.28	0.003
Excellent/ very good	47737	70.62	6607	78.82	-	-	-	-	-
Mother mental health									
Fair/Poor	4990	6.35	448	4.57	3.09	2.39	3.99	1.13	<.0001
Good	14975	19.07	1496	15.25	1.72	1.42	2.08	0.54	<.0001
Excellent/	58556	74.57	7868	80.19	-	-	-	-	-

Parameter	Sample with Autism data		Sample without Autism data		Univariate Analysis Results				
	N	Mean	N	Mean	OR	LCL	UCL	Estimate	P
Very good									
Father mental health									
Fair/Poor	2908	4.31	209	2.50	3.12	2.4	4.05	1.14	<.0001
Good	11069	16.40	1042	12.44	1.43	1.17	1.76	0.36	0.0006
Excellent/ Very good	53531	79.30	7123	85.06	-	-	-	-	-
Smoker in household									
Yes	19871	23.47	2261	22.41	1.09	0.9	1.32	0.0885	0.3611
No	64778	76.53	7826	77.59	-	-	-	-	-
In house tobacco exposure [4]									
Some and inside	4425	5.23	197	1.95	1.25	0.89	1.75	0.22	0.2018
Some but not inside	15442	18.24	2062	20.45	1.05	0.85	1.3	0.05	0.6778
None	64778	76.53	7826	77.60	-	-	-	-	-
TV watching									
0 hour	4619	5.43	1184	23.56	0.79	0.53	1.17	-0.24	0.2291
1 hour or less	36025	42.34	2505	49.84	0.71	0.55	0.91	-0.34	0.0077
1 to 4 hours	35230	41.41	1046	20.81	0.75	0.58	0.96	-0.29	0.0209
4 or more hours	9209	10.82	291	5.79	-	-	-	-	-
Adverse family experiences [5]									
None	46135	54.64	7382	73.31	1.34	1.11	1.63	0.3	0.0027
One	19839	23.50	2034	20.20	1.72	1.4	2.1	0.54	<.0001
Two or more	18458	21.86	654	6.49	-	-	-	-	-
Parental stress [6]									
Yes	8058	9.45	522	5.14	8.65	7.32	10.22	2.16	<.0001
No	77203	90.55	9643	94.86	-	-	-	-	-
Family mental health [7]									
Yes	8176	9.76	373	3.72	1.69	1.33	2.14	0.52	<.0001
No	75629	90.24	9643	96.28	-	-	-	-	-
Divorce									
Yes	16650	19.83	426	4.24	1.39	1.12	1.73	0.33	0.0028
No	67317	80.17	9610	95.76	-	-	-	-	-
Alcohol or Drug [8]									
Yes	9691	11.54	368	3.67	1.22	0.94	1.59	0.2	0.1286
No	74289	88.46	9664	96.33	-	-	-	-	-
Domestic violence [9]									
Yes	5718	6.84	193	1.93	1.38	0.98	1.96	0.32	0.066
No	77852	93.16	9831	98.07	-	-	-	-	-
Parent in Jail [10]									
Yes	5406	6.43	236	2.35	1.41	0.96	2.07	0.34	0.0807
No	78634	93.57	9801	97.65	-	-	-	-	-

Table 2. (Continued)

Parameter	Sample with Autism data		Sample without Autism data		Univariate Analysis Results				
	N	Mean	N	Mean	OR	LCL	UCL	Estimate	P
Neighborhood safety									
Neighborhood violence									
Yes	7140	8.52	114	1.14	1.38	1.06	1.79	0.32	0.0154
No	76632	91.48	9922	98.86	-	-	-	-	-
Supportive neighborhood									
No	11298	13.52	1836	18.55	1.82	1.45	2.27	0.6	<.0001
Yes	72257	86.48	8060	81.45	-	-	-	-	-
Safe neighborhood									
Never/ Sometimes	7953	9.48	912	9.14	1.55	1.18	2.05	0.44	0.0019
Usually/ always	75949	90.52	9069	90.86	-	-	-	-	-
Safe school									
Never/ Sometimes	3442	5.49	17	15.32	1.71	1.25	2.33	0.54	0.0007
Usually/ always	59212	94.51	94	84.68	-	-	-	-	-
Health insurance coverage									
Insurance type									
Private	56988	67.48	6078	60.60	0.39	0.32	0.46	-0.95	<.0001
Uninsured	3735	4.42	304	3.03	0.31	0.19	0.52	-1.17	<.0001
Public	23730	36.32	3647	36.36	-	-	-	-	-

[1] The question was "How often do you feel the family income is not enough to support the child?"

[2] Categories: Does not have the condition, Ever told but does not currently, Currently has condition

[3] Overall healthy contains both mental and physical health status

[4] Categories: no smoker, some smoker but no smoking inside, some smoker and smoking inside the house

[5] Considered the following: (1) socioeconomic hardship, (2) divorce/separation of parent, (3) death of parent, (4) parent served time in jail, (5) witness to domestic violence, (6) victim of neighborhood violence, (7) lived with someone who was mentally ill or suicidal, (8) lived with someone with alcohol/drug problem, (9) treated or judged unfairly due to race/ethnicity

[6] Coded "Yes" if their parents responded "Usually" or "Always" to one or more of three questions: - child was much harder to care for than other children; - often bothered a lot by their child's behavior; - angry with child.

[7] Child lived with anyone who was mentally ill or suicidal, or severity depressed for more than a couple weeks

[8] Child lived with anyone who had a problem with alcohol or drugs

[9] Child saw parents hit, kip, slap, punch or beat each other up

[10] Child lived with a parent who served time in jail after he/she was born.

Descriptive analysis of all covariates

In the complete data set with information of ASD diagnosis, the mean age of children when the survey was taken was 9.83 ranging from 2 to 17 years and the percentages of male and female were 51.61% and 48.39% respectively. There are 87.42% of the children were reported to be in excellent or very good overall health, 9.98% in good overall health and 2.61% in fair or poor overall health. In addition, 11.29% were reported to have had premature birth, 5.88% had anxiety disorder, 3.56% had joint, muscle or bone problems. Furthermore, 43.45% of parents reported parental stress associated with caregiving and 9.64% of survey participants spoke Spanish in their home. The majority of participants reported to have private insurance (52.56%), and the rest to have public insurance (45.18%) and very few to have no insurance (2.26%). The left half of Table 2 lists all frequencies of each of the candidate variables that were studied in this paper.

Univariate analysis of individual covariate and ASD

The right half of Table 2 give results of univariate logistic regression models, i.e., estimated odds ratio and corresponding 95% confidence intervals and p-values. Variables found to be significantly (at level 0.05) associated with Childhood ASD without controlling for other confounders are:

- *Demographic factors*: age (one year increase, OR=0.94, p-value=0.0004), gender (male versus female, OR=4.09, p<.0001), Spanish as primary household language (yes versus no, OR=0.69, p=0.0175), How often do you feel income is not enough (very often, OR=2.34, p<.0001; sometimes, OR=1.68, p<.0001; rarely, OR=1.16, p=0.1247 versus never).
- *Child health*: weight (overweight, OR=1.57, p<.0001; underweight, OR=1.49,p=0.01 versus normal weight), child

overall health (poor, OR=5.12, p<.0001; good, OR=3.63, p<.0001 versus excellent), premature (yes versus no, OR=1.87, p<.0001), low birth weight (yes versus no, OR=1.68, p<.0001), anxiety (yes versus no, OR=13.75, p<.0001), history of brain injury (yes versus no, OR=1.52, p=0.0063), history of joint muscle & bone problems (yes versus no, OR=3.43, p<.0001), condition of child's teeth (poor, OR=2.84, p<.0001; good, OR=1.58, p<.0001 versus excellent) and history of oral health problem (yes versus no, OR=1.28, p=0.0175).

- *Family health and activities*: mother (poor, OR=2.12, p<.0001; good, OR=1.43, p=0.0002 versus excellent) and father's (poor, OR=1.54, p=0.0012; good, OR=1.32, p=0.003 versus excellent) physical health; mother (poor, OR=3.09, p<.0001; good, OR=1.72, p<.0001 versus excellent) and father's (poor, OR=3.12, p<.0001; good, OR=1.43, p=0.0006 versus excellent) mental health; smoker in the household (yes versus no, OR=1.09, p=0.3611); the in-house tobacco exposure (in-house, OR=1.25, p=0.2018; outside house OR=1.05, p=0.6778 versus none); TV watching (none, OR=0.79, p=0.2291; =1 hour, OR=0.71, p=0.0077; 1-4 hours, OR=0.75, p=0.0209 versus =4 hours); adverse family experiences (none, OR=1.34, p=0.0027; one, OR=1.72, p<.0001 versus = two); parental stress due to caring for the child (yes versus no, OR=8.65, p<.0001), lived with anyone with mental health issue (yes versus no, OR=1.69, p<.0001); divorce (yes versus no, OR=1.39, p=0.0028).
- *Neighborhood safety*: neighborhood violence (yes versus no, OR=1.38, p=0.0154), supportive neighborhood (yes versus no, OR=1.82, p<.0001), safe neighborhood (never/sometimes versus usually/always, OR=1.55, p=0.0019) and safe school (never/sometimes versus usually/always, OR=1.71, p=0.0007).
- *Health insurance type* (private, OR=0.39, p<.0001; uninsured, OR=0.31, p<.0001 versus public).

Multivariate analysis controlling for potential confounders

All of the significant variables (i.e., univariate p-value<0.05) listed in Table 2 were included as candidate variables to be fitted into the multivariable logistic regression model and the fitness of the model was evaluated by stepwise model selection. However, some of these variables were removed due to their statistical insignificance (i.e., adjusted p-value>0.05) in the multivariable model.

Table 1 presents the results of the final multivariable logistic regression model after stepwise selection. In general, the factors of children themselves such as demographic and child health were found to be significantly associated with ASD diagnosis after controlling for potential confounders. Also health insurance type was found to significantly affect the ASD diagnosis in the multivariate analysis. More specifically, the conditional odds of parent reported ASD diagnosis for males is 3.38 (with 95% C.I. as (2.54, 4.41)) times higher than that of females, so that the risk of ASD in male children are three times more than that of female children; for children with a history of anxiety, the odds is 7.69 (6.22, 9.47) times higher than those without; also children whose care induces stress on the parents (as defined in the NSCH survey, parental stress refers to "parents experiencing more stress in caring for their child"), the conditional odds of ASD diagnosis is 3.45 (2.64, 4.44) times higher than those whose parents did not report care-induced stress.

A history of joint, muscle and bone condition increases the conditional odds of ASD by 74% (29%, 134%). Premature birth increases the risk of ASD by 50% (18%, 89%). Child with poor and good overall health are 1.45 (0.96, 2.19) and 1.93 (1.53, 2.44) times more likely to be diagnosed as ASD compared to child with excellent overall health. For one-year increase in age, the conditional odds of ASD diagnosis decreases by 7% (4%, 11%); the conditional odds of ASD diagnosis is 45% (7%, 68%), and 36% (21%,48%) less in children uninsured, and those privately insured compared to those publicly insured. Additionally, children whose primary language is Spanish had a reduced odds of ASD diagnosis by 50% (29%, 65%).

In summary, a child with the following conditions has higher conditional odds of ASD diagnosis: male, younger age, non-Spanish primary language, with anxiety, with poorer overall health, with history of joint, muscle or bone problems, born premature and with parents experiencing childcare-induced stress. The results also suggest that children with public health insurance have significantly increased conditional odds of being diagnosed with ASD compared with those uninsured and those with private health insurance.

Comparison of prevalence of factors in ASD versus non-ASD groups

Table 3 shows the prevalence data for the associated factors in the final model and factors that were significant univariately and/or were believed to be related to ASD diagnosis in previous studies. The prevalence results are consistent with the results from univariate and multivariable analysis which have been discussed above. Among all variables in the final model, the prevalence difference of male (28.45%), anxiety (37.24%), poorer child overall health (21.86%) and parental stress (34.80%) in the group of ASD diagnosis versus without ASD diagnosis are more than 20%. In detail, among the ASD diagnosis, the prevalence of male (79.40%) is 28.45% higher than that in the non-ASD diagnosis group (50.95%). Therefore, more male children were diagnosed with ASD and we conclude male children have higher risk of ASD. Similarly, children with premature birth have higher risk of ASD (7.05% higher in ASD versus non-ASD).

However, not all associations with ASD can be interpreted as risk directly. For example, the prevalence of anxiety and parental stress is 42.26% and 43.45% in the group with ASD diagnosis and 5.02% and 8.65% in the group without ASD diagnosis, respectively. In other words, children with ASD diagnosis can be considered as more likely to suffer from anxiety and parental stress; in the other way, anxiety and parental stress can potentially increase the risk of childhood ASD.

The independent variables, that were not included in the final model but with a prevalence difference ranging from 10-20% are income (11.25%), obesity (11.74%), child's teeth (14.02%), mother's physical (12.86%) and mental (15.10%) health, father mental health (13.29%) and adverse family experiences (15.13%). In addition, the prevalence difference of father's physical health (8.79%) and family mental health (9.21%) are close to 10%. The rest of the factors not in the final model have prevalence difference below 10%.

Table 3. Prevalence data of associated factors of ASD in the final model and other interested factors

Parameter	**ASD**				
	Yes		**No**		
	N	**%**	**N**	**%**	**% Difference**
Factors in the final model					
Demographics					
Child age [1]	-	-	-	-	-
Gender					
Male	1561	79.40	42494	50.95	**28.45
Female	405	20.60	40904	49.05	-28.45
Spanish language					
Yes	186	9.64	10914	13.40	-3.76
No	1744	90.36	70547	86.60	3.76
Child health					
Anxiety					
Yes	827	42.26	4190	5.02	37.24
No	1130	57.74	79219	94.98	***-37.24
Child overall health					
Fair/poor	208	10.59	2018	2.42	8.17
Good	459	23.36	8066	9.66	13.70
Excellent/very good	1298	66.06	73389	87.92	**-21.86
Joint muscle & bone					
Yes	257	13.13	2782	3.33	9.80
No	1700	86.87	80648	96.67	-9.80
Premature					
Yes	351	18.18	9205	11.13	7.05
No	1580	81.82	73485	88.87	-7.05
Health Insurance					
Insurance type					
Uninsured	44	2.26	3691	4.47	-2.22

Parameter	ASD				
	Yes		No		
	N	%	N	%	% Difference
Private	1025	52.56	55963	67.83	-15.27
Public	881	45.18	22849	27.69	*17.48
Family health and activity					
Parental stress					
Yes	852	43.45	7206	8.65	34.80
No	1109	56.55	76094	91.35	***-34.80
Factors not in the final model but was significant in the univariate model					
Demographics					
Income 2					
Very Often	217	11.24	4458	5.45	5.80
Somewhat Often	431	22.33	12719	15.54	6.79
Rarely	566	29.33	25100	30.67	-1.34
Never	716	37.10	39570	48.35	*-11.25
Child Health					
BMI					
Overweight/obese	431	38.65	12323	28.89	9.76
Underweight	85	7.62	2409	5.65	1.98
Normal weight	599	53.72	27923	65.46	*-11.74
Low birthweight					
Yes	254	13.75	7125	9.01	4.75
No	1593	86.25	71991	90.99	-4.75
Brain					
Yes	134	6.83	2649	3.17	3.65
No	1829	93.17	80816	96.83	-3.65
Teeth					
Fair/poor	242	12.30	4529	5.43	6.88
Good	491	24.96	14875	17.82	7.14
Excellent/very good	1234	62.74	64055	76.75	*-14.02
Oral health					
Yes	410	20.92	14187	17.04	3.88
No	1550	79.08	69078	82.96	-3.88
Family Health and activities					
Mother physical health					
Fair/Poor	323	18.03	7672	9.99	8.05
Good	487	27.19	17193	22.38	4.81
Excellent/Very good	981	54.77	51961	67.63	*-12.86
Father physical health					
Fair/poor	157	11.17	5034	7.61	3.56
Good	377	26.81	14288	21.59	5.23
Excellent/very good	872	62.02	46865	70.81	-8.79

Parameter	**ASD**				
	Yes		**No**		
	N	**%**	**N**	**%**	**% Difference**
Mother mental health					
Fair/Poor	244	13.62	4746	6.19	7.43
Good	476	26.56	14499	18.90	7.67
Excellent/Very good	1072	59.82	57484	74.92	*-15.10
Father mental health					
Fair/Poor	131	9.32	2777	4.20	5.12
Good	343	24.40	10726	16.23	8.17
Excellent/Very good	932	66.29	52599	79.57	*-13.29
Adverse family experiences [3]					
None	776	39.86	45359	54.99	*-15.13
One	501	25.73	19338	23.44	2.29
Two or more	670	34.41	17788	21.57	12.85
Family mental health [4]					
Yes	361	18.75	7815	9.54	9.21
No	1564	81.25	74065	90.46	-9.21
Divorce					
Yes	528	27.33	16122	19.65	7.68
No	1404	72.67	65913	80.35	-7.68
Neighborhood safety					
Neighborhood violence					
Yes	284	14.72	6856	8.38	6.35
No	1645	85.28	74987	91.62	-6.35
Supportive neighborhood					
No	1497	77.73	70760	86.68	-8.96
Yes	429	22.27	10869	13.32	8.96
Safe neighborhood					
Never/Sometimes	270	13.95	7683	9.37	4.58
Usually/always	1665	86.05	74284	90.63	-4.58
Safe school					
Never/Sometimes	137	8.61	3305	5.41	3.20
Usually/always	1454	91.39	57758	94.59	-3.20

[1] Child age is a continuous variable.

[2] The question was "How often do you feel the family income is not enough to support the child?"

[3] Considered the following: (1) socioeconomic hardship, (2) divorce/separation of parent, (3) death of parent, (4) parent served time in jail, (5) witness to domestic violence, (6) victim of neighborhood violence, (7) lived with someone who was mentally ill or suicidal, (8) lived with someone with alcohol/drug problem, (9) treated or judged unfairly due to race/ethnicity

[4] Child lived with anyone who was mentally ill or suicidal, or severity depressed for more than a couple weeks

[*] Difference >10%; ** difference > 20%; *** difference > 30%.

Discussion

This study identifies factors that are significantly associated with parent-reported childhood ASD through a secondary analysis of a national survey data. Of the five categories investigated, demographics, child health, health insurance, and family health and activities were significantly associated with ASD diagnosis after controlling for potential confounders. Specifically, a child's age and gender were found to be significant in the final multivariate model. Overall health status and certain health conditions such as premature birth, history of anxiety disorder and of joint, muscle or bone conditions are associated with ASD diagnosis; additionally, parental stress, Spanish as a primary household language and type of insurance were found to be associated with ASD diagnosis. Some of the variables (such as income, BMI, parents physical and mental health) which were not included in the final multivariate model possess potential importance for ASD even they were not significant.

Our study concluded that parent reported childhood ASD is significantly associated with premature birth as found in previous studies. Both the prevalence data of premature and low birthweight supports the results from our multivariable analysis. The prevalences are higher in the group of childhood ASD diagnosis compared to non-ASD diagnosis. Lampi et al. concluded that the risk of childhood autism increased if the child's birth weight is very low (<1500 g) and moderately low (<2500 g), very low gestational age (less than 32 weeks), and small for gestational age (birth weight < 10th percentile of same birth aged children) [16]. Shcendel and Bhasin concluded that the birth weight of <2500 g and preterm birth at <33 weeks' gestation were associated with an approximately twofold-increased risk of autism according to multivariable analyses (17). Our results' consistency with the previous findings reinforce that perinatal and neonatal factors are important in childhood ASD (12).

Age is a significant factor in predicting the likelihood of parent reported childhood ASD. Our results suggest that the odds of ASD diagnosis decreases as age increases. This result may be due to the timing of identifying ASD (1, 3, 15). The detection of childhood ASD can be detected at 18 months or younger; however, the diagnosis of ASD is not stable at the early ages and the diagnosis needs to be verified as the children grow older (1, 3, 18-20). A study of Stenberg et al. (18) discussed that the detection of ASD among 18 months old children might not be possible in the general population. Among the siblings of children with ASD, Zwaigenbaum et al. (20) found that the percentage of confirmation of ASD diagnosis was higher among children who have been diagnosed at 24 months than those at 18 months. Another study from Ozonoff et al. (19) concluded that, although the stability of ASD diagnosis was high at both 18 and 24 months among siblings of children with ASD, almost half of the ASD outcomes were not identified at 24 months and ASD diagnosis was not confirmed until 36 months. They suggested screening of ASD should be repeated multiple times during the first years of life among high risk children (19). Furthermore, since the symptoms of ASD can often subside substantially with early intervention, so the current trend for ASD screening is as early as possible and repeated when the child is older.

Our study concluded that gender is significantly associated with childhood ASD. The odds of parent reported ASD diagnosis in girls is lower than that of boys. According to the prevalence data in our study, the percent difference of male versus female in ASD diagnosis group and non-ASD diagnosis group is large. Findings from previous studies vary. Some studies found that boys have higher odds of developing ASD than girls (21-24). In addition, the prevalence of childhood ASD diagnosis is clearly higher in boys than in girls by the latest CDC surveillance report of 2014. On the other hand, Reinhardt et al. did not find significant effects of gender or a diagnostic group by sex interaction and suggested that the phenotype in males and females early in development were similar (25). Some research suggested that girls with ASD were diagnosed later than boys (26).

Additionally, in both univariate and multivariate logistic models, parental stress is significantly associated with childhood ASD and the prevalence of parental stress is much higher in the group with parent-reported positive diagnosis compared to group without. Many studies have corroborated the correlation between parental stress and childhood ASD. In fact, parental stress due to caring a child affected by ASD is widely discussed in the literature (27-30). In a study on the impact of childhood ASD on parental stress, Rao determined that parents of children with ASD experienced more parental stress than parents of children without the disease (30). It can be argued such association is due to the fact that children with ASD diagnosis require more care so parent is likely to experience more stress. Alternatively, since both mother and father's mental health was found to be significantly associated with ASD in the univariate analysis, parent mental health may affecting their ability to handle stress. In such case, parent stress is possibly a mediator for the effect of parent mental health on childhood ASD.

The type of insurance coverage was found to be significantly associated with the diagnosis of childhood ASD in our study. Publicly-insured children (such as Medicaid or SHIP) had more ASD diagnosis than privately-insured and non-insured children. A study on disparities in ASD diagnosis is in agreement with our results (31). Liptack et al. concluded that children with Medicaid and State Children's Health Insurance Program (SHIP) had better access to health services than uninsured children (31). Furthermore, Wang et al. (32) determined that the total cost associated with childhood ASD in public insurance, notably Medicaid, was higher than private insurance. The study argued that the limited coverage of childhood ASD from private insurance may be the cause for the disparities. It is not uncommon for families with a child of ASD, even if fairly well off, to seek additional coverage from public insurance due to large expense of ASD treatments. On the other hand, it is also generally believed that parents with private insurance have higher income and education, living in safer neighborhoods and perhaps are more likely to be aware of ASD; hence, their children may be exposed to less environmental factors rendering this population less prone to childhood ASD. Therefore, less diagnostic and less healthcare cost in the privately insured population is due to less prevalence of ASD for children with private insurance. Since this is a secondary analysis of a cross-sectional survey reported by parent, further study is needed to warrant the causes of the health insurance disparities.

Income was significant in the univariate model. The survey asked "How often do you feel the family income is not enough to support the child," and parent answered "more often" are more likely to have a child with ASD than those answered "never." And many factors are related to income, such as parent stress and insurance type and neighborhood safety. On the other hand, supporting an ASD child is large economic burden due to high cost of ASD treatment and usually requiring parents spend more time from their work to be with the child.

The analysis yielded that non-Hispanic children have higher odds of ASD diagnosis compared to Hispanic children. This finding is in accordance with previous findings which concluded that the prevalence of ASD is low in Hispanic children. Another study concluded that the disparity in primary care services may contribute to the disparity in ASD diagnosis among Hispanic and non-Hispanic children (33). The study found that over 80% primary care physicians have developmental screening protocol but only about 30% had Spanish language versions (33). In addition, since the survey data is based on parent reported data, among Latino parents there may be less awareness of symptoms of childhood ASD; or parent may not report related symptoms due to cultural stigma. The lower odds of ASD diagnosis in Hispanic children does not mean that the actual prevalence of childhood ASD is less among this population. Some of the factors, such as income, teeth and oral health and neighborhood safety were found to be significantly associated with ASD diagnosis in the univariate analysis; however, they became insignificant when fitted into multivariable model. Hispanic families usually have lower income and the neighborhoods that they live in are less safe and supportive than that of non-Hispanic families. And the access of dental healthcare is less among the Hispanic family. It is possible that those factors are related to disparities for Hispanic children so that their effects were confounded due to muticolinearity with Hispanic in the multivariate analysis. It would be interesting to explore in more detail based on the prospective study.

Bone, joint or muscle condition was found to be significantly correlated with the diagnosis of childhood ASD and prevalence of experience with bone, joint or muscle problems is larger in the group with

ASD diagnosis in our study. Our finding supports a recent study by Barnabe et al. which concluded that children with ASD also experience worse conditions of bones, joints, muscles and teeth (34). The mechanistic research from Barnabe et al. demonstrated that cellular calcium homeostasis or the concentration of calcium in extracellular fluid plays an essential role in susceptibility from ASD, and therefore, suggested that pre-natal or peri-natal calcium levels may be correlated with development of ASD (34). The condition of child's teeth is also related to the concentration of calcium. In our study, there is considerable difference between the proportion of child with excellent/good teeth condition in the group with ASD diagnosis (62.74%) and without (76.75%). On the other hand, Lee et al. concluded that children with ASD were at increased risk of injury, thus potentially inducing more bone, joint or muscle problems (35). Additionally, studies have linked autism to inflammation; inflammation is known to be associated with bone, joint and muscle problems; hence such association between bone, joint and muscle problems with ASD can be mediated by inflammation (36, 37). Further potential reasons for Bone, joint, muscle and teeth issues would be nutrition, access to well child and dental care as well as whether enforcing the healthy habits such as brushing teeth. However, these potential confounders are not surveyed in the NSCH study.

BMI was not found to be a significant factor associated with childhood ASD and it does not have a large prevalence difference in children diagnosed with ASD and without. However, it was found to be a significant factor in the univariate analysis: child with overweight or obese is 57% (32%, 86%) more likely to have ASD. The univariate result agrees with current literature which suggests that obese is correlated with childhood ASD. Two recently published studies suggested that overweight and obese were associated with ASD (38, 39). Other potential factors which associated with both ASD and obesity are sedentary life style, unhealthy diet and medications. However, these potential confounders are not surveyed in the NSCH study.

On the basis of our prevalence data, the factors that are not in the final model generally have lower prevalence difference between children with

ASD diagnosis and without. Some of the factors that were expected to be significantly associated do not have considerable prevalence differences (from 10% to 20%). The percent difference of mother's physical and mental health is higher than father's. Mothers are usually the primary care provider and the health of a pregnant mother affects that of the fetus and later child. Prevalence of poorer father's mental health has a higher percent difference than that of the physical health. While taking care of a child, father's mental health might be an important environmental factor to influence the child's mental health. Furthermore, genetics/heredity of mental health issues such as anxiety and depression are believed to be significantly associated with child's mental health. Similar to adverse family experiences, a child that lives with parents who have poorer health, particularly poorer mental health, have more adverse family experiences compare to the others.

The National Survey of Children Health (NSCH) data is obtained through a population complex survey method so that the resulting sample is representative of the US children population. Results from analysis of the NSCH data are s generalizable. However, this is a cross-sectional survey so the results points to possible association but not causation. Additionally, the survey data collected provides insight on parent-reported childhood ASD diagnosis, and no physician verification of the diagnosis was provided. Without external validation of ASD diagnosis, we cannot rule out the inclusion of bias in the secondary data analysis.

In summary, our study identified associated factors of childhood ASD based on the secondary analysis of the NSCH data. Our results indicated that younger children, boys, children with a history of anxiety, joint, bone and muscle condition, children born prematurely and those who have poorer overall health are more likely to be reported to have a diagnosis of childhood ASD. Additionally, children living in non-Hispanic household, those that are publicly insured and those who's care cause more parental stress were more likely to have childhood ASD than their counterparts. The study results are significant to the literature of childhood ASD. Our study highlights associated factors of childhood ASD and as such it can be used as a stepping stone for future studies, especially cohort studies to validate the direction of important associations. Furthermore, we recommend future studies to use validated physician diagnostic data.

ACKNOWLEDGMENTS

We are grateful to the Center of Child and Adolescent Health for providing us with the data set of 2011 National Survey of Children's Health. Conflict of interest: There is no conflict of interest. JY and HMS conceived and designed the project. CM performed the preliminary data analysis and KRZ performed the final data analysis, and both were under the guidance of JY. KRZ and CM co-wrote the early drafts of this manuscript under the guidance of JY. All co-authors edited the manuscript and approved its final version.

REFERENCES

[1] National Institute of Mental Health. Autism spectrum disorders 2016. URL: http://www.nimh.nih.gov/health/topics/autism-spectrum-disorders-asd/index.shtml.

[2] Blumberg SJ, Bramlett MD, Kogan MD, Schieve LA, Jones JR, Lu MC. Changes in prevalence of parent-reported autism spectrum disorder in school-aged US children: 2007 to 2011–2012. Natl Health Stat Rep 2013;65(20):1-7.

[3] Centers for Disease Control and Prevention. Autism spectrum disorder (ASD) URL: http://www.cdc.gov/ncbddd/autism/index.html.

[4] Johnson CP. Early clinical characteristics of children with autism. Autism spectrum disorders in children New York. New York: Marcell Dekker, 2004:85-123.

[5] Boyle CA, Boulet S, Schieve LA, Cohen RA, Blumberg SJ, Yeargin-Allsopp M, et al. Trends in the prevalence of developmental disabilities in US children, 1997–2008. Pediatrics 2011;127(6):1034-42.

[6] Baio J. Prevalence of autism spectrum disorder among children aged 8 years: Autism and Developmental Disabilities Monitoring Network, 11 Sites, United States, 2010. MMWR 2014;63(SS02):1-21.

[7] Shimabukuro TT, Grosse SD, Rice C. Medical expenditures for children with an autism spectrum disorder in a privately insured population. J Autism Dev Disord 2008;38(3):546-52.

[8] World Health Organization. Comprehensive and coordinated efforts for the management of autism spectrum disorders 2013. URL: http://apps.who.int/gb/ebwha/pdf_files/EB133/B133_4-en.pdf.

[9] National Health Service Choices. Autism spectrum disorder: Causes 2016. URL: http://www.nhs.uk/Conditions/Autistic-spectrum-disorder/Pages/Causes.aspx.

[10] Bilder D, Pinborough-Zimmerman J, Miller J, McMahon W. Prenatal, perinatal, and neonatal factors associated with autism spectrum disorders. Pediatrics 2009;123(5):1293-300.

[11] Chaste P, Leboyer M. Autism risk factors: genes, environment, and gene-environment interactions. Dialogues Clin Neurosci 2012;14(3):281-92.

[12] Gardener H, Spiegelman D, Buka SL. Perinatal and neonatal risk factors for autism: a comprehensive meta-analysis. Pediatrics 2011:128(2):344-55.

[13] SAS Institution Inc. Base SAS® 9.4 procedures guide: Statistical procedures, second edition. Cary, NC: SAS Institute, 2013.

[14] SAS Institution Inc. SAS/STAT® 9.22 user's guide: PROC SURVEYREG statement, first edition. Cary, NC: SAS Institute, 2010.

[15] Lord C, Risi S, DiLavore PS, Shulman C, Thurm A, Pickles A. Autism from 2 to 9 years of age. Arch Gen Psychiatry 2006;63(6):694-701.

[16] Lampi KM, Lehtonen L, Tran PL, Suominen A, Lehti V, Banerjee PN, et al. Risk of autism spectrum disorders in low birth weight and small for gestational age infants. J Pediatrics 2012;161(5):830-6.

[17] Schendel D, Bhasin TK. Birth weight and gestational age characteristics of children with autism, including a comparison with other developmental disabilities. Pediatrics 2008;121(6):1155-64.

[18] Stenberg N, Bresnahan M, Gunnes N, Hirtz D, Hornig M, Lie KK, et al. Identifying children with autism spectrum disorder at 18 months in a general population sample. Paediatr Perinat Epidemiol 2014;28(3):255-62.

[19] Ozonoff S, Young GS, Landa RJ, Brian J, Bryson S, Charman T, et al. Diagnostic stability in young children at risk for autism spectrum disorder: a baby siblings research consortium study. J Child Psychol Psychiatry 2015;56(9):988-98.

[20] Zwaigenbaum L, Bryson SE, Brian J, Smith IM, Roberts W, Szatmari P, et al. Stability of diagnostic assessment for autism spectrum disorder between 18 and 36 months in a high-risk cohort. Autism Res 2016;9(7):790-800.

[21] Giarelli E, Wiggins LD, Rice CE, Levy SE, Kirby RS, Pinto-Martin J, et al. Sex differences in the evaluation and diagnosis of autism spectrum disorders among children. Disabil Health J 2010;3(2):107-16.

[22] Kumazaki H, Muramatsu T, Kosaka H, Fujisawa TX, Iwata K, Tokoda A, et al. Sex differences in cognitive and symptom profiles in children with high functioning autism spectrum disorders. Res Autism Spect Disord 2015;13:1-7.

[23] Sun X, Allison C, Auyeung B, Matthews FE, Sharp SJ, Baron-Cohen S, et al. The Mandarin Childhood Autism Spectrum Test (CAST): Sex differences. J Autism Dev Disord 2014;44(9):2137-46.

[24] Werling DM, Geschwind DH. Sex differences in autism spectrum disorders. Curr Opin Neurology 2013;26(2):146.

[25] Reinhardt VP, Wetherby AM, Schatschneider C, Lord C. Examination of sex differences in a large sample of young children with autism spectrum disorder and typical development. J Autism Dev Disord 2015;45(3):697-706.

[26] Begeer S, Mandell D, Wijnker-Holmes B, Venderbosch S, Rem D, Stekelenburg F, et al. Sex differences in the timing of identification among children and adults with autism spectrum disorders. J Autism Dev Disord 2013;43(5):1151-6.

[27] Bebko JM, Konstantareas MM, Springer J. Parent and professional evaluations of family stress associated with characteristics of autism. J Autism Dev Disord 1987;17(4):565-76.

[28] Estes A, Munson J, Dawson G, Koehler E, Zhou X-H, Abbott R. Parenting stress and psychological functioning among mothers of preschool children with autism and developmental delay. Autism 2009;13(4):375-87.

[29] Hastings RP. Child behaviour problems and partner mental health as correlates of stress in mothers and fathers of children with autism. J Intellect Disabil Res 2003;47(4-5):231-7.

[30] Rao PA, Beidel DC. The impact of children with high-functioning autism on parental stress, sibling adjustment, and family functioning. Behav Modification 2009;33(4):437-51.

[31] Liptak GS, Benzoni LB, Mruzek DW, Nolan KW, Thingvoll MA, Wade CM, et al. Disparities in diagnosis and access to health services for children with autism: data from the National Survey of Children's Health. J Dev Behav Pediatrics 2008;29(3):152-60.

[32] Wang L, Mandell DS, Lawer L, Cidav Z, Leslie DL. Healthcare service use and costs for autism spectrum disorder: A comparison between medicaid and private insurance. J Autism Dev Disord 2013;43(5):1057-64.

[33] Zuckerman KE, Mattox K, Donelan K, Batbayar O, Baghaee A, Bethell C. Pediatrician identification of Latino children at risk for autism spectrum disorder. Pediatrics 2013;132(3):445-53.

[34] Barnabei VM, Rasmusson RL, Bett G. Autism and induced labor: Is calcium a potential mechanistic link? Am J Obstet Gynecol 2014;210(5):494.

[35] Lee L-C, Harrington RA, Chang JJ, Connors SL. Increased risk of injury in children with developmental disabilities. Res Dev Disabil 2008;29(3):247-55.

[36] Medicine JH. Brain inflammation a hallmark of autism, large-scale analysis shows. ScienceDaily 2014 Dec 10. URL: https://www.sciencedaily.com/releases/2014/12/141210073857.htm.

[37] Doshi-Velez F, Avillach P, Palmer N, Bousvaros A, Ge Y, Fox K, et al. Prevalence of inflammatory bowel disease among patients with autism spectrum disorders. Inflamm Bowel Dis 2015;21(10):2281-8.

[38] Broder-Fingert S, Brazauskas K, Lindgren K, Iannuzzi D, Van Cleave J. Prevalence of overweight and obesity in a large clinical sample of children with autism. Acad Pediatrics 2014;14(4):408-14.

[39] Zuckerman KE, Hill AP, Guion K, Voltolina L, Fombonne E. Overweight and obesity: Prevalence and correlates in a large clinical sample of children with autism spectrum disorder. J Autism Dev Disord 2014;44(7):1708-19.

SECTION TWO: FROM CANNABIS TO FOOD

In: Child and Adolescent Health
Editors: A Tenenbaum and J Merrick
ISBN: 978-1-53617-825-8

Chapter 8

MEDICAL CANNABINOIDS IN TREATMENT RESISTANT EPILEPSY DISORDERS

Yasmeen Razvi[1], BSc(C), Stephanie Chan[1], BSc(C), Angelo Fefekos[2], MBA, Henry Lam[1], MLS, Carlo DeAngelis[1], PharmD and Edward Chow[1,*], MBBS
[1]Sunnybrook Health Sciences Centre, University of Toronto, Toronto and [2]MedReleaf, Markham, Ontario, Canada

Cumulating evidence suggests that cannabinoid-based products provide therapeutic benefits to individuals with childhood-onset, treatment-resistant epilepsy (TRE) disorders. The most recent literature review on the topic was published in 2017 by O'Connell et al, which included 18 studies. A greater number of studies have been conducted on pediatric patients than adults, which have shown a general trend towards decreased seizure frequency following the use of cannabinoids. There is however, a unified recommendation to increase the number of randomized control trials (RCTs) investigating the safety and efficacy of this drug, particularly in adult TRE populations where high quality data is currently lacking. Since the release of this review, two additional RCTs assessing the effectiveness of cannabidiol (CBD) for childhood-onset TRE have been published and found cannabidiol to be effective in decreasing the

[*] Corresponding Author's Email: Edward.Chow@sunnybrook.ca.

incidence of seizures. Future studies should assess drug-drug interactions resulting from the use of cannabinoids in conjunction with standard antiepileptic regimens, as well as further assess other relevant safety measures. Furthermore, vulnerable subsets of these populations, including individuals with severe cognitive impairments should be included in future studies due to their present exclusion from the literature, along with patients of diverse ethnic backgrounds. Finally, the varying chemical profiles of cannabinoids should be compared to determine the most effective and ideal methods for optimization of their effects.

INTRODUCTION

The use of cannabinoids for a wide variety of therapeutic purposes dates as far back as 400 AD (1). Emerging literature suggests that drugs containing active ingredients derived from cannabinoids may significantly decrease the incidence of seizures experienced by patients with treatment-resistant epilepsy (TRE) disorders. TRE is defined as a distressing affliction arising from an inability to reach prolonged remission of seizures even after receiving a minimum of two standard treatment regimens, which significantly impacts patient quality of life (2).

Despite the long history of use and documented therapeutic effects of medical cannabinoids, an overwhelming need still exists to conduct robust and high quality clinical trials to validate the safety and efficacy of cannabinoid-based treatment regimens in epileptic patient populations.

CURRENT EVIDENCE

The current literature on the use of cannabis for TRE is summarized in table 1. A comprehensive, literature review of 18 studies on the use of cannabinoids for TRE in both pediatric and adult patients was published in 2017 by O'Connell et al. (3). Studies on adult patients were mainly case reports and surveys focusing on the use of smoked cannabinoids (4–9). Three case reports on adult patients aged 24, 29, and 45 years found reductions in seizure frequency following the use of smoked cannabinoids, with only the 29-year old experiencing worsening of seizures following cessation of cannabinoid use (5-7). Two other studies on adult patients reported increased seizure frequency following the administration of cannabinoids in some cases (4, 9). The first study was a case report from 1967 on a 20-year old with tonic-clonic seizures who had previously achieved seizure remission, but experienced a series of seizures following an extended period of marijuana use (4). The second study consisted of a survey of patients at a tertiary epilepsy center (n = 310) who were both ex-cannabinoid (n = 297) and active cannabinoid users (n = 13) (9). Of the active cannabinoids users, 2 reported improvements in the incidence and severity of seizures. However, 7 ex-cannabinoid users reported a worsening of seizure incidence and severity following cannabinoid consumption, in contrast with the results of other studies.

Two older RCTs on adult patients did not find any significant difference between the cannabidiol (CBD) and placebo group (10-11). The first of these studies, published in 1986 by Ames and Cridland, was a RCT conducted on institutionalized, epileptic adults with cognitive disabilities (n = 12) who were randomized to receive either 200-300 mg of CBD (n = 6) or a placebo (n = 6) over a 3-week period (10). There was no significant difference observed in the incidence and severity of seizures between both groups and no AEs were reported. The second study, presented as an unpublished abstract by Trembly and Sherman at the 1990 International Conference on Cannabis and Cannabinoids, was a 6-month, double-blind crossover study in a sample of adult patients with TRE (n = 12) (11). Similar to the previous study, there was no significant difference in the incidence and severity of seizures between the treatment and placebo groups and no AEs were reported. In both cases, results were limited by small sample sizes ($n \leq 12$) and may be considered somewhat outdated, demonstrating the need for further research in this population(10–12).

Studies on pediatric patients focused largely on orally administered CBD extracts and were mainly case series, case reports, and surveys (13-17). Most of these studies concluded that cannabinoids produced

Table 1. Summary of available literature on cannabis use for epilepsy

Reference	Year	Study Design	Sample Size	Patient Age (Years)	TRE Disorder	Cannabinoid Compound	Efficacy	Adverse Events
Consroe et al. (5)	1975	Case report	1	24	• Generalized	Smoked cannabis	Near complete remission	• None
Ellison et al. (6)	1990	Case report	1	29	• Focal	Smoked cannabis	Decreased seizure frequency	• Increased frequency of seizures following cessation
Mortati et al. (7)	2007	Case report	1	45	• Focal	Smoked cannabis	Greater than 90% reduction in seizure frequency	• None
Keeler & Reifler (4)	1967	Case report	1	20	• Not specified	Smoked cannabis	Increased seizure frequency	• Increased frequency of seizures following marijuana use
Hamerle et al. (9)	2014	Survey	310	18+	• Not specified	Smoked cannabis	Decreased seizure frequency in 2 patients; increased seizure frequency in 7	• Increased frequency of seizures following marijuana use
Ames & Cridland (10)	1986	RCT	12 (treatment n = 6, placebo n = 6)	18+	• Not specified	200-300 mg CBD per day (n = 6)	No significant difference between treatment & placebo	• None
Trembly & Sherman (11)	1990	RCT	12	18+	• Not specified	300 mg CBD per day	No significant difference between treatment & placebo	• None

Reference	Year	Study Design	Sample Size	Patient Age (Years)	• TRE Disorder	Cannabinoid Compound	Efficacy	• Adverse Events
Porter & Jacobson (13)	2013	Survey	19	2-16	• Dravet syndrome (n = 13) • Doose syndrome (n = 4) • Lennox-Gastaut syndrome (n = 1) • Idiopathic epilepsy (n = 1)	CBD	Decreased seizure frequency in 16 (84%) patients; complete remission in 2 (11%)	• Somnolence • Decreased appetite
Maa & Figi (14)	2014	Case report	1	5	• Dravet syndrome	Tincture of CBD and THC	Decrease from 50 seizures per day to 2-3 per month	• Somnolence
Gedde & Maa (15)	2013	Survey	11	<18	• Doose syndrome (n = 4) • Dravet syndrome (n = 2) • Idiopathic epilepsy (n = 2) • Lennox-Gastaut syndrome (n = 1) • Metachromatic leukodystrophy (n = 1) • Cortical dysplasia (n = 1)	CBD	Decreased seizure frequency in all; complete remission in 8	• Somnolence
Cunha et al. (18)	1980	RCT	15 (treatment n = 8, placebo n = 7)	22-35	• Not specified	200-300 mg CBD per day (n = 8)	Decreased seizure frequency in 3 and complete remission in 4 (treatment); decreased seizure frequency in 1 (placebo)	• Somnolence • Gastric discomfort

Table 1. (Continued).

Reference	Year	Study Design	Sample Size		Patient Age (Years)	TRE Disorder	Cannabinoid Compound	Efficacy	Adverse Events
Devinsky et al. (19)	2016	Multicenter, open-label trial		214	1-30	• Generalized	CBD	Decreased frequency of seizures per month from 30.0 (IQR 11.0–96.0) to 15.8 (IQR 5.6–57.6) (n = 137) from baseline to end of treatment	• Somnolence • Diarrhea • Decreased appetite
Tzadok et al. (17)	2016	Retrospective, multicenter cohort study		74	1-18	• Generalized	CBD-enriched cannabinoids	Decreased seizure frequency in 89% of patients	• Somnolence • Increased frequency of seizures • GI irritability
Press et al. (16)	2015	Open-label, retrospective chart review		75	0.08-18	• Generalized	Oral cannabinoid extracts	Decreased seizure frequency in 57% of patients	• Somnolence • Increased frequency of seizures
Devinsky et al. (20)	2017	RCT		120 (treatment n = 61, placebo n = 59)	2-18	• Dravet syndrome	20 mg/kg oral solution of CBD per day (n = 61)	38.9% (treatment) & 13.3% (placebo) reduction in seizures ($p = 0.01$) from baseline to end of treatment	• Somnolence • Diarrhea • Decreased appetite
Thiele et al. (21)	2018	RCT		171 (treatment n = 86, placebo n = 85)	2-55	• Lennox-Gastaut syndrome	20 mg/kg oral CBD per day (n = 86)	43.9% (treatment) & 21.8% (placebo) reduction in seizures from baseline to end of treatment	• Somnolence • Diarrhea • Pyrexi • Decreased appetite • Vomiting

significant therapeutic benefits, and have potential use in the clinical setting. A 2013 survey on the use of CBD-enriched cannabis was administered to parents of children with TRE (n = 19) through a Facebook group that facilitated the exchange of information related to CBD in the treatment of TRE (13). Most patients included in the study had Dravet syndrome (n = 13) and had tried an average of 12 different antiepileptic drugs prior to using CBD. Most parents (84%) reported a reduction in the incidence of seizures in their children when using CBD-enriched cannabis, of which 11% (n = 2) reported complete remission of seizures. A case report on a 5-year old female with Dravet syndrome named Charlotte reported highly favourable results following cannabinoid therapy, which has since garnered significant media attention (14). Charlotte was administered a tincture of CBD and tetrahydrocannabinol (THC), a formulation which has come to be known as Charlotte's Web amongst the community, alongside her standard antiepileptic regimen. Charlotte's seizures decreased significantly from approximately 50 convulsive seizures per day at baseline to approximately 2-3 nocturnal convulsions per month, with sustained symptom relief for 20 months following the study. Another survey administered to parents of children with TRE disorders who used CBD extracts (n = 11) found a decrease in motor seizures in all patients, with 8 patients reportedly experiencing near or complete seizure remission (15).

Four higher quality studies included in the review showed significant improvements in childhood-onset TRE following the administration of cannabinoids. The first, published in 1980 by Cunha et al. (18), randomized patients to receive a 200-300 mg daily dose of CBD (n = 8) or placebo (n = 7) for up to 4.5 months. It was found that amongst the CBD group, 4 patients were nearly seizure-free and 3 had mild improvements throughout the trial, with 1 patient experiencing no improvements. Only 1 patient in the placebo group demonstrated improvements in their condition. A later multicenter, open-label trial conducted by Devinsky et al. (19) on pediatric patients with TRE (n = 214) found a reduction in the median frequency of motor seizures per month from 30.0 at baseline (IQR 11.0–96.0) to 15.8 (IQR 5.6–57.6) in the efficacy analysis group (n = 137) over

12 weeks. A retrospective, multicenter study by Tzadok et al. (17) assessed seizure frequency in pediatric patients (n = 74) with TRE on regimens of CBD-enriched cannabinoids and found that 89% of patients (n = 66) reported an overall decrease in seizure frequency. Finally, an open-labeled, single-centre retrospective chart review of a population of pediatric patients with TRE using oral cannabinoid extracts found that 57% of patients (n = 43) experienced improvements in seizure control and 33% (n = 25) experienced a greater than 50% reduction in seizures (16).

Since the publication of this review, a double-blind, RCT was conducted by Devinsky et al. (20) and subsequently published in the New England Journal of Medicine. Pediatric patients with treatment-resistant Dravet syndrome (n = 120), aged 2 to 18 years, were randomized to receive a 20 mg/kg oral solution of CBD per day (n = 61) or placebo twice per day (n = 59) in a double-blind fashion. The primary endpoint was the difference in the incidence of motor seizures between the baseline and treatment period. There was found to be a statistically significant difference in the change of seizure incidence between treatment and placebo groups, with changes of -38.9% and -13.3% respectively (p = 0.01) from baseline to end of treatment.

An additional placebo controlled double-blind RCT by Thiele et al. (21) recently published in Lancet was conducted as a multicenter assessment of the effectiveness of cannabidiol as adjunct treatment for patients aged 2 to 55 (n = 171) suffering from Lennox-Gastaut syndrome, a rare form of TRE. Patients were randomized to receive either 20 mg/kg of oral CBD per day (n = 86) or a placebo (n = 85). The percent change in incidence of seizures per month between the baseline and treatment period was used as the primary endpoint. The treatment group experienced a change of -43.9% (IQR −69.6 to −1.9) in the incidence of seizures, compared to -21.8% (IQR −45.7 to 1.7) in the placebo group from baseline to end of treatment. Additionally, there was a median difference of −17.21 (p = 0.0135) and −19.45 (p = 0.0096) in seizure frequency during the 14-week treatment and 12-week maintenance period respectively between the treatment groups.

An RCT on the use of cannabis in tuberous sclerosis complex (TSC), a childhood-onset disorder in which most patients experience epileptic seizures, is currently being conducted and is expected to be published within the following year.

FUTURE DIRECTIONS

Overall, the available literature suggests that the use of cannabinoids to manage TRE may result in a significant decrease in seizure frequency when compared to placebo. There is also a clear shift in the literature towards the conduct of robust, high quality clinical trials validating these effects, as compared to earlier anecdotal, case reports, and survey-based studies. That said, there are still several limitations to the data that currently exists. Cannabinoids have been administered in previous studies, predominently as an adjunct therapy alongside standard antiepileptic regimens however, potential drug-drug interactions have not yet been thoroughly studied or understood. Specifically, interactions of cannabis with valproate and clobazam should undergo further investigation as several studies have found that patients experience increased sedation when these drugs are administered concurrently, likely due to increased plasma concentrations of epileptic drugs caused by a change in liver enzyme activity (19, 22). Furthermore, dose-response studies are required to better establish best-practice applications of cannabis. Current literature focuses largely on doses of around 20 mg/kg of oral CBD but does not report on effects of titration up or down. Individuals with severe cognitive impairments have been excluded from many previous studies, however make up a considerable proportion of the population of TRE patients. Further research should be conducted into the use of cannabinoids for TRE in this sub-population, as they too may be able to benefit from this treatment, however, its safety and tolerability should be carefully considered. Future trials should also aim to have representative ethnic diversity in their study populations as most available studies have been made up largely of Caucasian patients, with the most recent RCT consisting of a 90% Caucasian population (21). Once implemented into common practice, real-world data should be obtained to validate the longer-term safety and efficacy of cannabinoids for treating of TRE. Finally, due to the varying chemical profiles of cannabinoids, an important future consideration is comparing different cannabinoid products to determine the most effective and ideal methods for optimization of their effects.

Overall, the quality of information available around the use of cannabinoid-based therapies for childhood-onset TRE disorders is improving, and will continue to grow. Limitations and gaps in the literature should be taken into consideration moving forward, and with the eventual growth of knowledge, clinicians may be able to begin considering administering cannabinoids more regularly in clinical practice, especially when other treatments have failed.

ACKNOWLEDGMENT

We thank the generous support of Bratty Family Fund, Michael and Karyn Goldstein Cancer Research Fund, Joey and Mary Furfari Cancer Research Fund, Pulenzas Cancer Research Fund, Joseph and Silvana Melara Cancer Research Fund, and Ofelia Cancer Research Fund

REFERENCES

[1] Zlas J, Stark H, Seligman J, Levy R, Werker E, Breuer A, et al. Early medical use of cannabis. Nature 1993;363(6426):215.

[2] Kwan P, Arzimanoglou A, Berg AT, Brodie MJ, Allen Hauser W, Mathern G, et al. Definition of drug resistant epilepsy: Consensus proposal by the ad hoc Task Force of the ILAE Commission on Therapeutic Strategies. Epilepsia 2009;51(6):1069-77.

[3] O'Connell BK, Gloss D, Devinsky O. Cannabinoids in treatment-resistant epilepsy: A review. Epilepsy Behav 2017;70:341-8.

[4] Keeler MH, Reifler CB. Grand mal convulsions subsequent to marijuana use. Case report. Dis Nerv Syst 1967;28(7 Pt 1):474-5.

[5] Consroe PF, Wood GC, Buchsbaum H. Anticonvulsant nature of marihuana smoking. JAMA 1975;234(3):306-7.

[6] Ellison JM, Gelwan E, Ogletree J. Complex partial seizure symptoms affected by marijuana abuse. J Clin Psychiatry 1990;51(10):439-40.

[7] Mortati K, Dworetzky B, Devinsky O. Marijuana: An effective antiepileptic treatment in partial epilepsy? A case report and review of the literature. Rev Neurol Dis 2007;4(2):103-6.

[8] Gross DW, Hamm J, Ashworth NL, Quigley D. Marijuana use and epilepsy: prevalence in patients of a tertiary care epilepsy center. Neurology 2004;62(11):2095-7.

[9] Hamerle M, Ghaeni L, Kowski A, Weissinger F, Holtkamp M. Cannabis and other illicit drug use in epilepsy patients. Eur J Neurol 2014;21(1):167-170.

[10] Ames FR, Cridland S. Anticonvulsant effect of cannabidiol. S Afr Med J 1986;69(1):14.

[11] Trembly B, Sherman M. Double-blind clinical study of cannabidiol as a secondary anticonvulsant. Marijuana '90 international conference on cannabis and cannabinoids, 1990.

[12] Mechoulam R, Carlini EA. Toward drugs derived from cannabis. Naturwissenschaften 1978;65(4):174-9.

[13] Porter BE, Jacobson C. Report of a parent survey of cannabidiol-enriched cannabis use in pediatric treatment-resistant epilepsy. Epilepsy Behav 2013;29(3):574-7.

[14] Maa E, Figi P. The case for medical marijuana in epilepsy. Epilepsia 2014;55(6):783-6.

[15] Gedde M, Maa E. Whole cannabis extract of high concentration cannabidiol may calm seizures in highly refractory pediatric epilepsies. In press at the 67th annual meeting of the American Epilepsy Society; December 6–10, 2013.

[16] Press CA, Knupp KG, Chapman KE. Parental reporting of response to oral cannabis extracts for treatment of refractory epilepsy. Epilepsy Behav 2015;45:49-52.

[17] Tzadok M, Uliel-Siboni S, Linder I, Kramer U, Epstein O, Menascu S, et al. CBD-enriched medical cannabis for intractable pediatric epilepsy: The current Israeli experience. Seizure 2016;35:41-4.

[18] Cunha JM, Carlini EA, Pereira AE, Ramos OL, Pimentel C, Gagliardi R, et al. Chronic administration of cannabidiol to healthy volunteers and epileptic patients. Pharmacology 1980;21(3):175-85.

[19] Devinsky O, Marsh E, Friedman D, Thiele E, Laux L, Sullivan J, et al. Cannabidiol in patients with treatment-resistant epilepsy: An open-label interventional trial. Lancet Neurol 2016;15(3):270-8.

[20] Devinsky O, Cross JH, Laux L, Marsh E, Miller I, Nabbout R, et al. Trial of cannabidiol for drug-resistant seizures in the dravet syndrome. N Engl J Med 2017;376(21):2011-20.

[21] Thiele EA, Marsh ED, French JA, Mazurkiewicz-Beldzinska M, Benbadis SR, Joshi C, et al. Cannabidiol in patients with seizures associated with Lennox-Gastaut

syndrome (GWPCARE4): a randomised, double-blind, placebo-controlled phase 3 trial. Lancet 2018;391(10125):1085-96.

[22] Geffrey AL, Pollack SF, Bruno PL, Thiele EA. Drug-drug interaction between clobazam and cannabidiol in children with refractory epilepsy. Epilepsia 2015;56(8):1246-51.

In: Child and Adolescent Health
Editors: A Tenenbaum and J Merrick
ISBN: 978-1-53617-825-8

Chapter 9

THE MECHANISTIC ROLE OF CYTOADHERENCE IN THALASSEMIA'S PROTECTION AGAINST MALARIA

Leena Elbedour*[*], *MHS, Salman Elbedour, PhD and Mohammed Hassan Almasudi, PhD
Department of Molecular Microbiology and Immunology, Johns Hopkins Bloomberg School of Public Health, Baltimore, Maryland, United States of America, Psychology and Special Education program, Al-Ahliyya Amman University, Amman, Jordan, Human Development and Psychoeducational Studies, Howard University, Washington, DC, United States of America and Department of Psychology, King AbdulAziz University, Faculty of Educational Graduate Studies, Jeddah, Saudi Arabia

ABSTRACT

Although the protective effect conferred against malaria by thalassemia was first recognized by Haldane in 1949, it has been sickle cell disease's

[*] Corresponding Author's Email: lelbedour@gmail.com.

protective role against malaria that has dominated the scientific literature. By recognizing mechanisms of this protective effect in sickle cell, the same mechanisms may possibly apply to thalassemia. Cytoadherence is the process employed by Plasmodium falciparum during the erythrocytic stages of infection in the human host. Infected erythrocytes attach to microcapillary endothelial tissues, enabling them to avoid splenic clearance, and thus continue the asexual reproductive cycle and the severe symptoms characteristic of malaria. Cytoadherence as a means of immune evasion will be discussed in regards to its efficiency in infected erythrocytes from sickle cell and thalassemic patients. Both intracellular and intercellular components of the infected erythrocyte and the endothelial cells will be of interest in testing the hypothesis that thalassemia confers protection against malaria through the mechanism of cytoadherence inhibition. As the human host and the pathogen have co-evolved in an effort to establish a symbiotic balance, it is essential to recognize patterns of human adaptation in order to gain insight into the evolution of the pathogen.

INTRODUCTION

Alterations in the structure and function of the human erythrocyte could be inferred to modify malarial infection. In regions of past or present endemic malaria, hemoglobinopathies appear to have been selected for, and include HbC, HbS, and thalassemic erythrocytes (1, 2). HbC is commonly referred to as hemoglobin C, and is caused by a single amino acid substitution mutation in ß-globin, in which glutamic acid at position 6 is replaced by lysine (2). Similarly, HbS, or sickle cell hemoglobin, also occurs due to a substitution mutation of glutamic acid at position 6; however, rather than a lysine, it is modified to a valine (2, 3). HbS is estimated to be found in frequencies of at least 18% in sub-Saharan Africa, the Middle East and parts of India (4). HbC is also a common variant, particularly in West Africa, however its distribution in malaria endemic regions is more limited than that of HbS (4, 5). The homozygous genotype CC is also less clinically severe than the homozygous SS genotype, which leads to severe sickle cell anemia (4). Homozygous genotype CC and heterozygous genotype AC have been shown to confer strong and mild protection against severe malaria, respectively (4). In contrast, while heterozygosity for the sickle trait has been shown to confer protection against severe malaria as well, the homozygous form of the trait frequently culminates in fatality due to severe sickle cell anemia (6). Research has also supported the clinical observations that HbAS protects against uncomplicated malaria and asymptomatic parasitemia (5). Therefore, as HbAS has been shown to offer a wider range of protection than either HbAC or HbCC, it will later be used as a model of comparison for the mechanistic protection of thalassemia against malaria (4).

Of the approximately 350,000 infants born with hemoglobin variants each year, 20% of these infants suffer from a thalassemia (7). In fact, hematologic disorders are the most common monogenic disorders in the world, affecting 5% of the human population, 1.7% of which are thalassemic (8). The thalassemic blood disorders can be distinguished as either a-thalassemia or ß-thalassemia (9). Both thalassemias are typically distributed equally among males and females (8). While a-thalassemia tends to occur in individuals of African and Southeast Asian descent, ß-thalassemia is more common in individuals of Mediterranean, African, and Southeast Asian descent (8).

a-thalassemia occurs as a result of deletions of the four genes controlling a-globin chain production on chromosome 16, thus creating fewer a-globin chains, unpaired ß-globin chains, and unstable tetramers differing from the a2ß2 configuration characteristic of normal hemoglobin (9, 10). The same process occurs in ß-thalassemia, but rather, deletions of the two genes controlling ß-globin chain production on chromosome 11 take place, ß-globin chains are reduced, and a-globin chains are left unpaired (8, 9).

The prototypical forms of a-thalassemia vary based on the number of deletions of the genes, while ß-thalassemia forms vary based on the degree of ß-globin chain production (8). An a-thalassemia silent carrier is distinguished by a single gene deletion, and is asymptomatic (8). Two deletions results in a variant known as a-thalassemia trait, which is similarly asymptomatic (8). a-thalassemia intermedia, or hemoglobin H (HbH) disease, is caused by deletions of three of the four genes, and leads to moderate to severe hemolytic anemia, hemolysis, and splenomegaly (8,

9). Deletions of all four of the a-globin genes is characterized by a lack of a-globin chain production and culminates in a-thalassemia major with hemoglobin Bart's (Hb Bart's), in which nonimmune hydropis fetalis occurs and typically kills the fetus (8, 9, 11). A defect of a single gene regulating ß-globin production leads to ß-thalassemia trait, an asymptomatic variant (8). When increased to two gene defects with a moderate to mild decline in ß-globin production, ß-thalassemia intermedia develops, with similar symptoms to ß-thalassemia major but to a lesser severity (8, 12, 13). In contrast, ß-thalassemia major results from a significant decrease in ß-globin, although it is still characterized by two gene defects (8, 12). Its signs and symptoms include jaundice, skeletal abnormalities, splenomegaly, and growth retardation (8, 12). This variant requires the patient to receive lifelong blood transfusions from an early age, in order to ensure hemoglobin levels remain higher than 9.5 g per dL (8, 12). Consequently, excess iron builds up as a result of transfusions, which the body is unable to remove, thus necessitating the use of an iron chelator (8).

It had previously been believed that perhaps the only external factor playing a role in the evolution of thalassemia was the social construct of consanguinity, in which the recessive trait was more likely to occur in children of intermarriages (8, 14). In 1949, however, John BS Haldane (1892-1964) added a fresh perspective on the issue by proposing that thalassemia had arisen out of evolutionary pressures to evade malaria and promote survival (8, 15). By 1954, these same pressures had been linked to sickle cell trait by Anthony C Allison (1925-2014), who collected evidence that had not yet been supported for thalassemia (8). Since then, research has remained fixated on locating the exact mechanisms by which these hematologic disorders may confer protection against malaria, oftentimes gaining insight from commonalities among these disorders. The aim of this essay is to build evidence for the hypothesis that thalassemia grants protection against malaria through the mechanism of cytoadherence inhibition, in a manner similar to that of sickle cell.

MALARIAL CYTOADHERENCE

The molecular mechanism of cytoadherence in the pathogenesis of malaria centers on the infected red blood cells' (IRBCs) evasion of splenic clearance, made feasible by their attachment to the capillary and post-capillary venular endothelium of critical tissues (16, 17). Knoblike protrusions on the surface of IRBCs composed of parasite-derived proteins play a fundamental role in the interaction between the IRBC and endothelial receptors (18). The major parasitic ligand that facilitates cytoadherence is the P falciparum erythrocyte membrane protein 1 (PfEMP1), which is located to the knoblike protrusions (18). The domain structure of PfEMP1consists of a variable number of Duffy binding-like (DBL) or cysteine-rich interdomain regions (CIDR) (19). The number of each domain in a particular PfEMP1 protein varies and the number and arrangement of the domains is contingent upon the homologous recombination events in the var gene, which encodes PfEMP1 (19). Variation in PfEMP1 dictates which receptors the IRBC bind to in host tissues, including endothelial cells, uninfected erythrocytes, monocytes, and platelets, creating a complex system of organ-specific targets (19, 20).

The conserved intracellular domain of PfEMP1, ATS, has been shown to bind with the knob-associated histidine-rich protein (KAHRP), which localizes in the erythrocyte membrane and serves to organize the knobs; this interaction thus anchors the PfEMP1 and contributes to the stability of the knoblike protrusions (20, 21). Stability is further heightened by the synergy of other proteins of parasitic origin, including sequestrin, PfHRP2, trypsin, PfEMP2, PfEMP3, ring-infected erythrocyte surface antigen (RESA), mature parasite-infected erythrocyte surface antigen (MESA), and VLA-4 (20-22). It has been inferred that their functions are in part to increase the rigidity and adhesiveness of the IRBC (21). These are just a few of the numerous protein families mobilized by the parasite.

All of these proteins are assembled intracellularly by the parasite through an intricate trafficking system of protein vesicles (24). As the erythrocytes have no nucleus, organelles, or protein synthesis to offer, plasmodium must utilize amino acids, such as cysteine, glutamate, methionine, proline, and tyrosine, from the breakdown of hemoglobin (23, 24). Within the IRBC, the parasite is separated from the host cytosol by its own plasma membrane and the parasitophorous vacuole membrane (PVM), through which it is able to export 10% of its own proteome to the erythrocyte cytosol or membrane (23, 24). This percentage was calculated based on the discovery of an amino acid motif, termed PEXEL, near the N-terminus of 463 parasitic proteins exported to the host cytosol (24). Other exported proteins do not contain the PEXEL motif, and thus have been classified as PEXEL-negative exported proteins (PNEPs); the transport mechanism of PNEPs has not been determined thus far (17).

Maurer's clefts serve as a compartment for the parasitic protein on route to the erythrocyte membrane, and connect to the PVM via a tubulovesicular network (TVN) (23, 24). Conflicting research has shown that Maurer's clefts may either serve as independent structures or form a continuous structure with the TVN (23). They have been described as unilamellar membrane profiles in the IRBC's cytoplasm, which connect to the trafficking system that includes vesicles and an actin filament network (24). Although the exact functions of the Maurer's clefts remain relatively ambiguous, knock-out experiments of membrane-associated histidine-rich protein-1 (MAHRP1) or skeleton binding protein-1 (SBP1), both of which are resident integral membrane proteins of Maurer's clefts, demonstrated the absence of PfEMP1 export to the IRBC surface (25, 26). Maurer's clefts have also been identified in the transport of KAHRP and PfEMP3 (23). Due to their probable role in protein packaging and transport, Maurer's clefts have been compared to the Golgi apparatus of host eukaryotic cells, although a possible relation between the two has not yet been traced (24).

Actin filaments of host origin have been implicated as acting as cables used by vesicles to transfer parasitic proteins from the Maurer's clefts to the erythrocyte membrane (5, 27). This interpretation was supported through the use of immune-labeling, in which human antibodies for actin reacted to the long filaments found in the IRBC, confirming its composition (5). It has been hypothesized that the actin structures are integral to the uninfected erythrocyte's membrane, and are then commandeered by the parasite as it develops intracellularly (5, 27). Prior to infection, it is believed that actin joins the proteins 4.1R, p55, and tropomodulin in crosslinking the heterodimer spectrin in the erythrocyte membrane; this ultimately allows for the hexagonal array that constitutes the membrane (5, 28). The exported parasitic protein PfEMP3 has been suspected as a possible mediator of the appropriation of host cell cytoskeleton, due to its role in destabilizing the erythrocyte membrane through its interface with a-spectrin in the membrane (5, 27). Moreover, MESA may also contribute through its disruption of the interactions between p55 and 4.1R (5). Interestingly, as the erythrocyte membrane seemingly deteriorates, the actin network created by the parasite simultaneously expands (5). Proteins that appear to link with actin include PfEMP1 and KAHRP (5). As KAHRP is the predominant protein in the construction of knobs, its interaction with actin may serve to anchor the filaments to the knob, while concurrently interacting with spectrin and the cytoplasmic region of PfEMP1 (5). PfEMP1 may also concurrently bind with spectrin (5). Controversy still exists over whether actin employs a myosin motor for movement or whether it uses a treadmilling mechanism (5). Functionality of the exporteome (exported proteome) and other structures, such as the vesicles, Maurer's clefts, and actin, require further research; currently, tangible measurements of the IRBC include parasite growth rate, parasite shape and structure, cytoadherence, knob presence, protein export, Maurer's clefts morphology, membrane rigidity, and nutrient uptake (24).

It has been supported however that PfEMP1 on the IRBC surface interacts with a wide range of host receptors. Endothelial receptors recognized for binding IRBCs include P-selectin, platelet glycoprotein IV (CD36), Inter-Cellular Adhesion Molecule-1 (ICAM-1), Vascular Cell Adhesion Molecule-1 (VCAM-1), thrombospondin, E-selectin, and chrondroitin-4-sulfate (CSA), although it is still unclear whether they play individual roles or whether they work together synergistically (22, 29).

CD36, in particular, is found throughout endothelial tissues, as well as on blood monocytes and platelets, reinforcing findings that suggest it is the major cytoadherent host receptor (16, 30). After binding PfEMP1 on the

IRBC, CD36 stimulates the aggregation of monocytes and platelets, promotes cytokine activation, fibrin deposition, and overall inflammation (16). CD36 also plays a role in activating macrophages and monocytes in the removal of obsolete cells (30).

In cerebral microcapillaries, however, the primary cytoadherent endothelial receptor is ICAM-1, whose interaction with the PfEMP1 ligand results in the severe cerebral symptoms characteristic of malaria (16, 30).

The endothelial receptor with the prime cytoadherent capacity in pregnant women is CSA, which is found throughout the placental tissues and is held in place by proteoglycans recognized as CSPG (31). The endothelium of the placenta functions very similarly to the endothelium surrounding organs, and its CSA receptors actively bind the parasite protein VAR2CSA (31, 32). A member of the extensive PfEMP1 protein family, VAR2CSA has been identified in all P. falciparum genomes, in which its variants' amino acids are 75-83% identical (31, 32). Interestingly, this genetic conservation contrasts with the antigenic variation recognized in PfEMP1. This cytoadherence has been shown to lead to severe maternal anemia, stillbirth, and low birth weight in pregnant women suffering from placental malaria (31, 33).

As the parasite initiates infection in the red blood cell, it first forms a ring stage parasite; IRBC with ring stage malaria can be detected in peripheral vascular circulation (34). Upon maturing into the trophozoite and schizont stages, however, the IRBCs initiate sequestration in microcapillary endothelial linings of vital organs, including the heart, gut, liver, lungs, kidney, adipose tissues, and brain (34). PfEMP1, with its variant arrangement, is also able to bind complement receptor 1 of other non-infected erythrocytes, creating rosettes which may successfully obstruct post-capillary venule flow (16, 35). This congestion culminates in changes to microcirculatory blood flow, and subsequently, to metabolic functions of critical tissues, which ultimately results in tissue hypoxia and the development of major symptoms of severe malaria (19, 22, 36). A direct result of cytoadherence may also include activation of intracellular signaling pathways in the endothelial cells, as well as changes in gene expression and immunoregulatory molecules (cytokines, nitric oxide synthase), (16, 22). One such example is the endothelial activation of leukocytes, which fosters coagulation, the cascade release of TNF, IL-1, and IL-6 from monocytes, and the activation of dendritic cells, all of which may promote inflammation that further damages tissues (16, 19). Nitric oxide synthesis also decreases in cases of severe malaria due to the consumption of L arginine, from which nitric oxide is produced (19, 37). Findings have suggested that L arginine concentrations increase due to increases in parasite biomass and hemolysis (19). In healthy individuals, nitric oxide is a vasodilator and also contributes to an anti-inflammatory response of the endothelia (19). The association between the activation of microvascular endothelial cells and the severity of disease has been strengthened through biopsy samples taken from live malaria patients (19). The more endothelial receptors present to bind the IRBC, the higher the rate of cytoadherence and the subsequent inflammation (19).

As this attack escalates, the parasite makes sure to further safeguard itself. As observed in a wide range of pathogenic mechanisms, PfEMP1's diversity also allows for the immune evasion of IgG responses, complement activation, opsonization, and antibody dependent cytotoxity (19). The Plasmodium has thus built up a vast array of dynamic machinery to combat human immunity.

SICKLE CELL AND ITS ALTERATION OF MALARIAL CYTOADHERENCE

In response to this parasitic threat, natural selection has advanced humans' means of defense in the malaria endemic regions of the world. As plasmodium's invasion of erythrocytes elicits the severe symptoms of malaria most readily associated with mortality, modifications of the erythrocytes' hemoglobin have evolved. One such divergence is the sickle cell trait common throughout the world (2). Data supports that HbAS decreases the escalation of mild malaria to severe malaria, and also decreases not only all-cause malaria mortality in children, but also mortality due to severe malarial anemia (19, 38). However, HbAS parasite densities have been measured to be approximately the same as those observed in HbAA cases (19).

Mechanistically, sickle trait's protective effect against malaria has also been linked to two primary roots of action: disruption of intracellular development and diminished cytoadherence (2). The disruption of the IRBC's intra-networking may be connected with the generation of methemoglobin and radical oxygen species from the sickle cell hemoglobin (2). The superoxide anion radicals (O2-) created can then be converted into hydrogen peroxide (H2O2) by the abundant hydrogen dismutase (39). In a healthy RBC, superoxides would be neutralized by catalase and glutathione peroxidase (39). Methemoglobin would be returned to its ferrous hemoglobin state through the work of met-Hb reductase (39). As witnessed in HbC and unpaired a- and ß-hemoglobin, HbS undergoes the oxidation of its iron from a ferrous state (Fe2+) state, to the ferric (Fe3+) and ferryl (Fe4+) states (5). Ferryl hemoglobin can substantially alter the actin filament networking through oxidation, creating shorter actin filaments than seen in infected HbAA erythrocytes, and which are unlikely to be attached to Maurer's clefts, vesicles, or knobs. Under conditions of excessive oxidative stress, such as in the case of sickle cell RBCs, the cycle of methemoglobin production increases to then produce hemichromes, which create a destabilizing effect on the erythrocyte membrane by decreasing spectrin-protein 4.1-actin interaction (5, 39). The parasite itself creates hemichrome upon transforming from the ring to the trophozoite stage, yet it appears that as the hemoglobinopathies also induce hemichrome production, its excess is thus destructive to the parasite (10).

Hemichrome formation can either be reversible, in which the sixth heme ligand in the electron spin resonance spectra is the distal histidine, or irreversible, in which it is an alternate amino acid residue from the hemoglobin (39). The more methemoglobin, superoxides, or hydrogen peroxide present to promote oxidative conditions, the more rapid the accumulation of hemichrome occurs (39). Hemichrome is able to form Heinz body-like aggregates, binding to several membrane proteins, one of which includes the band 3 protein (40). Co-clustering of the Heinz bodies, band 3 protein, and surface IgG has been documented to commonly occur in sickle erythrocytes (41). This co-clustering has also been noted to occur in thalassemic RBC (41). Interestingly, a certain degree of variability occurs in co-clustering, in that the Heinz bodies can also associate with other membrane proteins, such as glycophorin and ankyarin to varying extents (41). The rigid obstruction of the membrane created by Heinz bodies has been shown to contribute to the hemolysis common to hemoglobinopathic RBCs and this may ultimately play a hand in diminishing cytoadherence (42).

The destructive nature of the hemichrome can also be witnessed in its role as a reactant in the chemical formation of hydroxyl radicals, by way of the iron-catalyzed Haber-Weiss reaction (39). Hemichrome is further able to easily release heme, whose free, oxidized form is classified as hemin (39). The iron-protoporphyrin complex is ferroprotoporphyrin, or heme, when the iron is in the ferrous state (43). Once the iron is in the ferric state, ferriprotoporphyrin, or hemin, is created (43). Free heme in the plasma activates hematopoietic cells to release heme oxygenase I, which then degrades heme into carbon monoxide (5, 37). Carbon monoxide has been implicated in regulating malarial inflammation of the brain and other organs (5, 37).

Hematin is the hydroxide of heme that contains Fe (III) (44). Hematin has been shown to be present in higher concentrations in individuals suffering from malaria, sickle cell disease, and ischemia reperfusion (28, 45). Due to its hydrophobic qualities, hematin may also become membrane-bound (39. Simultaneously, membrane-bound hematin has been detected in higher concentrations in patients with sickle cell, thalassemia, and G6PD-deficiency (39). Besides inflammation and an increase in reactive oxygen species, hematin has also been implicated in causing cellular damage and lipid peroxidation (28). Lipid peroxidation can lead to increases in lipid hydroperoxides, secondary lipid products, conjugated diene hydroperoxides and volatile alkanes, all of which then lead to the increased permeability and disorder of the membrane (39, 43). Destabilization of the membrane is accompanied by a swelling of the RBC, potassium leak, alteration of membrane mechanisms of osmosis, and hematin cross-linkage of the membrane proteins band 4.1, spectrin, and actin (39). All of these events may either directly or indirectly contribute to the cytoadherent abilities of the IRBC.

The membrane is not the only structure of the sickle IRBC that is altered. Although the parasite still develops normally in HbS, the Maurer's clefts form abnormally, creating an amorphous shape distinct from the typical unilamellar arrangement (5, 46). Moreover, the majority of transport vehicles float in the cytoplasm, rather than connecting to actin (5, 46). Thus, the trafficking network is altered and cytoadherent ligand (such as PfEMP1) transport to the erythrocyte plasma membrane is impaired; this includes a reduced surface level and an abnormal cell-surface distribution (5, 46).

Additionally, in comparison to HbAA erythrocytes, HbAS and HbSS erythrocytes have abnormal knob morphology and distribution (5, 46). Consequences of this variation include a reduced adherence to human microvascular endothelial cells, reduced interaction with monocytes, and subsequently, less elevated levels of TNF and other cytokines typical of mild and severe malaria (5). There is evidence that many of the phenomena documented in sickle cell IRBCs also occur in thalassemic IRBCs.

THALASSEMIA

Research regarding the thalassemias and their relationship to malaria has varied in regards to a and ß thalassemia. Each has individually been compared to sickle cell in the literature, although the majority of data concerns a thalassemia. Both forms of thalassemia, however, have been shown to have no effect on uncomplicated malaria, which indicates that this particular blood disorder does not function through a mechanism of parasite replication inhibition (47). Like sickle cell, thalassemia has been shown to reduce the incidence of the manifestations of severe malaria (47).

Studies have shown that a thalassemia confers a similar form of protection against P falciparum as sickle cell, weakening the cytoadherent ability of the IRBCs to microcapillary endothelial cells (5). a-thalassemic IRBCs have abnormal PfEMP1/knob morphology, number, and function, as in the case of HbS IRBCs, leading to similar changes in interaction with microcapillary endothelial cells and monocytes (19). The mechanism behind these phenomena has not yet been identified. Fairhurst et al. (19) speculate that there are several mechanisms that may play a potential role. The first is that the hemichrome binding of band 3 proteins may obstruct Maurer's cleft networking of proteins to the membrane, whether that is to the cytoplasmic or to the extracellular surfaces of the IRBC (19). Another possibility cited was that ferric iron may oxidize membrane proteins and lipids, preventing the parasite from utilizing them in the remodeling of the host membrane (19).

a-thalassemic RBCs contain unpaired ß -globin chains, thus forming unstable ß4 tetramers, similar in instability to HbS, and leading to oxidative hemoglobin forms (48). The same pattern is witnessed in ß thalassemia, with unpaired a-globin chains and unstable a4 tetramers present (49). As with HbS, thalassemic hemoglobin may transition to the higher oxidative states of methemoglobin, reversible hemichromes, irreversible hemichromes, and Heinz bodies (48). Thus, under oxidative stress, membrane proteins, such as band 3, spectrin, and actin are cross-linked much in the same manner as those found in HbS (48). Moreover, lipid peroxidation of the membrane lipids once again alters membrane chemistry, resulting in a changed permeability (48).

Due to the oxidation-induced instability of the hemoglobin variants, as well as the parasite-mediated changes to the host's RBC cell membranes, increased numbers of membrane-bound autologous IgG and complement may form (50, 51). The autologous IgG is anti-band 3 specific, a site recognized for its hemichrome aggregates (51). This immune response thus marks the erythrocytes for destruction by macrophages and consequent removal by the spleen, a mechanism commonly used for erythrocyte senescence (51). In the case of ß thalassemia, as well as HbS and HbH, RBCs containing the ring form of the parasite were phagocytized by monocytes at a rate higher than that of normal RBCs (50). Phagocytosis was identified as being mediated by complement (50). The same process, however, was not recognized in cases of a thalassemia (50). The discrepancy has been traced to differing degrees of oxidative damage generated by the two thalassemias, with ß thalassemia predicted to create more damage (50). This conjecture was based on work involving HbH, in which higher oxidative damage resulted in higher ring phagocytosis (50). Furthermore, other studies have demonstrated the thalassemias' variation in pathophysiology, with a thalassemia characterized by more stable membrane mechanics than ß thalassemia, and a chains binding to the band 3 protein with a higher affinity (50, 52, 53).

The significance of the finding lies in that if enough rings are eliminated from the body, fewer trophozoites and schizonts will develop to then cytoadhere and sequester in the microvasculature, thus preventing the onset of severe malaria and lowering the mortality risk (50). Both methods would likely result in lower ring numbers. In comparison, no variation in phagocytosis was seen between trophozoites of normal and thalassemic (or any hemoglobinopathic) RBCs (50). Another advantage of ring phagocytosis is that it is less likely to damage monocyte function than trophozoite or schizont phagocytosis (50). The mature forms of the parasite harbor hemozoin, a remnant pigment of the oxidative damage of hemoglobin (50). Hemozoin diminishes the efficiency of the monocyte upon ingestion through several pathways: higher numbers of inflammatory cytokines are released, monocytes can no longer effectively dispose of ingested bacteria, repeated cycles of phagocytosis becomes difficult, upon interferon gamma stimulation monocytes can no longer express class II and other membrane antigens, and monocytes can no longer process antigens effectively (50). Finally, Ayi et al. (50) also showed that ring-parasitized RBCs are more likely than mature forms of the parasite to be killed by monocytes via oxidative burst. Due to the oxidative damage previously afflicted by the thalassemic hemoglobin, further oxidation may additionally contribute to impairing the parasite (50). For all these reasons, enhanced ring phagocytosis has attracted attention in the scientific community as a possible drug target for malaria.

In coordination with cytoadherence, microcytosis has also been shown to provide protection against severe malaria progression in homozygous a thalassemia cases (54, 55). However, as noted for all other forms of thalassemia, microcytic homozygous a thalassemia does not reduce parasite density (54, 55). Microcytosis occurs when erythrocyte counts are increased, and each erythrocyte contains a lower concentration of hemoglobin; thus, more erythrocytes must undergo hemolysis by the parasite to effectively destroy the cells and induce severe anemia (54). Remarkably, the microcytosis itself leads to mild anemia, yet natural selection may favor mild anemia in order to avoid the generally fatal severe malarial anemia (54). Williams et al. (56) support that that homozygous a thalassemia is more protective against malaria than the heterozygous form. Their work shows that homozygote patients' malarial mortality rates were 60% lower than those of healthy patients, while heterozygote patients' malarial mortality rates were 40% lower than those of healthy patients (56). This distinction may be due to the occurrence of microcytosis in homozygotes, which has not been detected in heterozygotes (56).

As microcytosis forces the parasite to exert extra energy, it may prove to be biologically beneficial to the human host, and should consequently be further researched as a possible mode of action in targeting malaria. For example, it may provide insight into other malarial Plasmodium species which also stimulate severe anemia (54). Researchers in the field may choose to investigate other mutations that result in microcytosis, as they may also play a role in protecting against malaria (54). Other hemoglobinopathies, including ß thalassemia and homozygous Hb E, similarly involve high microerythrocyte numbers, although less data is available to support these findings (54). It is unknown whether the same mechanism is employed in each of these disorders.

It is predicted that in thalassemia patients microcytosis and cytoadherence inhibition may not function independently, but rather, may work synergistically. As each microcytic erythrocyte contains less hemoglobin, parasitic hemolysis may result in less hemoglobin release, thus diminishing the level of inflammation that occurs as a result (54). Cytoadherence inhibition would also result in reduced inflammation of the endothelium, and thus both events could weaken the parasite's control of the immune system. Symptoms of severe malaria, including cerebral malaria, acidosis, and hyperlactaemia all manifest in both heterozygous and homozygous a thalassemia cases, and should be studied to assess the effect of microcytosis upon them (54). Moreover, homozygous a thalassemia patients have lower complement receptor 1 (CR1) expression, which is associated with the IRBC's rosetting on noninfected RBCs, as well as the removal of senescent RBCs (54). As rosetting is a common mechanism used in the development of severe malaria, how it functions alongside microcytosis in preventing severe malarial anemia should be examined (54). Due to the cytoadherent pathways established in rosetting, cytoadherence of the endothelial microvasculature and monocytes should also be considered.

a-thalassemic IRBCs have likewise shown impaired adherence to the human umbilical vein endothelial cells, in a process where cytoadherence is conferred by the parasite ligand VAR2CSA with chondroitin-4-sulfate (CSA) (33, 57, 58). CSA is described as being located on the proteoglycan matrix in both the intervillous space and syncytiotrophoblast cell layer of the placenta (58). However, CSA can also be found in the microvascular of the brain and lungs, although in these locations PfEMP1 acts as the predominant cytoadherent ligand (58). According to Rieger et al. (58), the reasoning for this specificity may be that placental CSA has at least six disaccharide repeats uncommon in other CSA. Another inference is that the concentration density of CSA in the placenta is much higher than that of the remaining microvasculature, thus facilitating cytoadherent interactions (58). Data has supported that VAR2CSA binds to CSA in a manner of shear-enhanced adhesion, in which the number of adhering cells first increases and then decreases as a result of increases in shear stress (R58). The authors also identify the role of catch bonds, in which the half-life of the ligand/receptor bond is increased due to strengthening of the bond by tensile force-induced allosteric effects (58).

The significance of this finding is that shear-enhanced adhesion has been noted in the rolling adhesion of PfEMP1 to ICAM-1 receptors (58). Interestingly, Rieger et al. (58) also identified that the geometric alignment of VAR2CSA matched that of CSA, indicating that knobs may be strategically placed by the parasite. This same pattern may be witnessed in other PfEMP1 ligands upon further study. It is necessary to study placental cytoadherence not only for the possibilities it provides in treating placental malaria, but also for the clues it may provide us in blocking the interaction between other PfEMP1 ligands with the endothelial vasculature.

In creating a vaccine to prevent placental malaria, the complexity of the VAR2CSA protein must be analyzed to determine whether a few domain fragments are responsible for CSA binding, or whether the entire ectodomain is needed for the high-affinity interaction (31, 57). In the case of VAR2CSA, it appears that the receptor/ligand binding site relies on at least four semi-conserved N-terminal domains to maintain specificity and affinity required for the interaction (31). It would be favorable to identify whether other PfEMP1 proteins follow similar binding patterns, although structural differences are likely. Moreover, we must recognize whether thalassemia and other hemoglobinopathies can be studied as a model for reducing cytoadherence of VAR2CSA to CSA. a thalassemia did not affect placental malaria in regards to birth weight, placental parasite density, maternal periphereal parasitemia, or maternal anemia (59, 60). Thus, although a few studies have supported that a thalassemia diminishes cytoadherence in the placental tissues, other findings indicate that no recognized effect on the development of placental malaria occurred in individuals with a thalassemia (31, 59). This finding puts into question the extent of which thalassemia protects against certain manifestations of malaria.

The most common form of severe thalassemia in populations across Asia has been identified as HbE ß thalassemia, in which Hemoglobin E and ß thalassemia are co-inherited (59, 61). Due to the frequency of HbE in countries such as Myanmar, Bangladesh, India, and Thailand, these areas show the highest prevalence of HbE/ß thalassemia co-inheritance with approximately 100,000 in Thailand, and approximately 200,000 in Bangladesh (59, 62). What has caught the attention of researchers, however, is the vast clinical diversity of the disease in its patients (59, 62). Theories have been investigated regarding the role of genetic modifiers found in the environment on the clinical development of HbE/ß thalassemia through phenotypic control (59). One such modifier has been identified as P. falciparum, which is rampant in Sri Lanka and has a known presence in various Asian countries as well (59). A study conducted in a region of Sri Lanka with low malarial transmittance, found that malarial antibodies were significantly higher in patients with HbE/ß thalassemia than in age-matched controls (59). The authors suggest that this may be due to an increased susceptibility to malaria in these patients (59). Increased red-cell turnover and bone marrow expansion associated with hypermetabolism are typical of these HbE/ß thalassemia cases, and when accompanied by the recurrent malarial fevers, may lead to changes in perspiration rates and body odor (59). Body odor may then lead to variable susceptibility to malaria through vector attraction, although other environmental factors may also play a role (59). Another possibility is that although P. falciparum invades RBCs of all ages, it has a preference for reticulocytes, which are abundant in HbE/ß thalassemia patients due to the high red-cell turnover rates (59).

Finally, splenomegaly is also common in these cases, and may leave the patient more prone to infection (59, 61). It was demonstrated that antibody frequency was higher in splenectomized HbE/ß thalassemia patients than in HbE/ß thalassemia patients with functioning spleens (59). However, malarial antibody levels were still significantly elevated in spleen-positive HbE/ß thalassemia patients compared to spleen-positive patients with non-mutated hemoglobin genes, and thus, we cannot assume that the splenectomy alone caused the increase (59). Other studies have found that there is a general association between splenectomy and more severe malaria, regardless of Hb status, thus this association should be inspected carefully in relation to HbE/ß thalassemia (59). More research is needed on how a weakening of splenic function may leave an individual more susceptible to P. falciparum infection (59). The spleen plays a key role in thalassemia's protection against malaria. IRBCs that fail to cytoadhere in HbE/ß thalassemia individuals may then be eliminated from the body via splenic clearance, diminishing both sequestration of the vital organs and the onset of severe malarial symptoms. In this case, co-inheritance of HbE/ß thalassemia may lead to a loss in the protection against malaria each disorder provides (59, 63). This negative epistasis is the dependence of an allele at a certain locus on another genotype co-inherited at a distinct locus to maintain fitness (64). This would help to explain the findings of O'Donnell et al. (59) that malarial antibodies were higher in patients with the co-inheritance trait, in that it may not only diminish protection, but may also increase susceptibility. Additionally, it may explain why patients splenectomized and with fully intact spleens both showed higher antibody levels (59). While its mechanism it still unknown, the co-inheritance of certain hemoglobinpathy appear to antagonize the benefits conferred when the mutation is inherited by itself (63).

O'Donnell et al. (59) suggest a fascinating concept on the interaction of P. vivax and P. falciparum in regions of the world in which both malarias are present in high frequencies. In these areas, the co-inheritance of HbE/ß thalassemia may increase patients' chance of survival (59). HbE/ß thalassemia patients have been shown to be more susceptible to P vivax than P falciparum, and the authors predict that an infection by the less lethal P vivax may serve as a form of pre-immunization against P. falciparum (59). As P falciparum typically is characterized by a higher mortality rate, the chance of survival for patients with HbE/ß thalassemia may increase (59, 65).

In a similar manner to HbE/ß thalassemia, while individually, sickle trait and a thalassemic traits offer protection against malaria, co-inheritance of the disorders has been shown to lead to a loss of protection, reversing the reduction of cytoadhesion, rosetting, and expression of PfEMP1 levels on the IRBCs (64, 66, 67). In fact, these phenotypes were reduced to levels characteristic of normal IRBCs (66). While the mechanism behind this occurrence has not yet been identified, the authors suggest that the concentration of HbS in HbAS individuals is negatively correlated with the number of a-globin deletions, indicating that the concentration of HbS is lowest in individuals suffering from a-thalassemia (64, 66, 67). They also state that lower concentrations of HbS have been associated with less disruption of the parasite's intracellular trafficking of proteins (66). Williams et al. (64) add that lower HbS concentrations may be associated with lower hemichrome binding of band 3 protein, lower opsonization by IgG and complement, and consequently, lower phagocytosis rates. Cytoadherence rates would thus remain stable and splenic clearance would be diminished. Williams et al. (64) also presume that merozoite invasion of the RBCs is dependent on hydration status, and thus upon membrane integrity. While the effects HbS and a thalassemia individually have on the membrane may be well-studied, their combined presence may alter such patterns (64).

The implications of negative epistasis lie in its ability to provide insight into the mechanisms of the individual hemoglobinopathies themselves (64). By identifying how the two disorders disrupt each other's anti-parasitic systems, we can gain understanding of the details of these systems.

Conclusion

Malaria has long decimated human populations in endemic regions. To ensure the fitness of the species, mutations have arisen to grant humans a higher chance of survival upon infection by the parasite. Erythrocyte stages of the Plasmodium's lifecycle are the stages in which parasite replication and development occur, and are the only stages which result in the severe manifestations of disease. Thus, the erythrocyte stages from a ring, to a trophozoite, and finally to a schizont are of particular interest to researchers. In recent years the concept of malarial cytoadherence has been more thoroughly analyzed and is believed to be a major factor in the survival of P falciparum in the human host. Data gathered from malaria endemic regions has provided insight into the protective role that hemoglobinopathies may play against malaria. In particular, my hypothesis applied to the thalassemias, as I correlated their mechanisms of protection to those of sickle cell. Both disorders are found in high frequencies throughout Africa, often in malaria endemic regions.

Data suggests the sickle cell and a thalassemia confer partial protection to severe malaria through the inhibition of cytoadherence. The mechanism of protection for ß thalassemia remains unclear. The literature contains data collected on the parasite's remodeling of the RBC through exported proteins, and how sickle cell and a thalassemia may alter this trafficking system. Irregular knob shape and density, as well as altered Maurer's clefts and lowered expression of PfEMP1 on the cell surface are all characteristics of IRBCs from a thalassemia and sickle cell patients.

Oxidative damage to the parasite has also been implicated as a mechanism that works in parallel with the inhibition of cytoadherence to mediate protection against severe disease. Mutations in hemoglobin production is found in sickle cell and both thalassemias, and hemoglobin instability gives rise to methemoglobin, reversible hemichrome, irreversible hemichrome, Heinz bodies, and free iron. All of these components may transform the parasite's intracellular trafficking of proteins, due to their interaction with spectrin, protein 4.1, actin, band 3 protein, and various lipids in the membrane. Cross-linkage of these components then alters membrane chemistry, making the cell more susceptible to autologous IgG and complement and thus, uptake by macrophages and monocytes. This appears to be particularly true of IRBCs containing ring stage parasites from ß thalassemic individuals, which are phagocytized at a higher rate than more mature forms. As previously mentioned, this may lower the burden of IRBCs which must be inhibited from cytoadhering.

Additionally, microcytosis may benefit cytoadherence inhibition in homozygous a thalassemia individuals. By producing a large density of RBCs carrying reduced levels of hemoglobin, the body forces the parasite to exert more energy to create severe symptoms, particularly cerebral anemia. Microcytosis has also been noted in ß thalassemia, and should be further studied in an effort to identify additional genetic conditions that may result in microerythrocytes in an effort to weaken the parasite's fitness.

All these mechanisms may act indirectly or directly to reduce cytoadherence. It is yet unknown how they interact with one another, and thus it is necessary to recognize the intricacies of protection. While individually the thalassemias may offer protection against malaria, co-inheritance with other hemoglobinopathies reduces said protection. Yet, in the case of HbE/ß thalassemia, this reduced protection allows for a pre-activation of innate or adaptive immunity towards P falciparum by way of an antecedent P vivax infection. What may at first appear to work against human survival, offers protection in a context-specific fashion.

Table 1. Various mechanisms incorporated by the blood disorders sickle cell and thalassemia against P falciparum

Mechanism	**Sickle Cell**	**α-Thalassemia**	**β-Thalassemia**
Cytoadherence Inhibition	+	+	-
Oxidative Damage	+	+	+
Microcytosis	-	+	+

These mechanisms are not necessarily independent, and may work synergistically to one another. Furthermore, data represented depicts only that which has been identified up until the present, with possibilities for amendment. (+) indicates that data has been collected supporting the use of the mechanism by the particular disorder. (-) indicates that no data or weak data has been collected supporting the use of the mechanism by the particular disorder.

This review of the literature has revealed that a thalassemia appears to follow many of the same mechanistic patterns of protection against malaria as sickle cell trait, whereas ß thalassemia remains more ambiguous in its relationship to malaria. Table 1 summarizes the protective mechanisms present in each of these hemoglobinopathies. While my hypothesis was supported, further analysis is needed to gain a more in depth understanding of the thalassemia variants. Future research should seek to understand differences in the oxidative potential and sensitivity among the different thalassemias. By assessing which form of thalassemia is more prone to the production of free heme and other oxygen species, we may understand at least one component of the protection against malaria. Further research should also be conducted in regards to the co-inheritance of multiple hemoglobinopathies. The literature indicates that any protection granted by any one hemoglobin variant is lost when more than one mutation is present. Where this co-inheritance is commonly observed in the world may give insight into how humans have evolved in regions where several hemoglobinopathies and malaria pathogens overlap.

As complicated as malarial mechanisms have proved to be, thalassemic and other hemoglobinopathic mechanisms of clearance have proved to be just as complex. Haldane offered his hypothesis on the blood diseases and their protective effect against malaria in 1949; we are still on the path towards establishing a systematic understanding of the many parts at play in this dynamic interaction.

REFERENCES

[1] Taylor SM, Cerami C, Fairhurst RM. Hemoglobinopathies: slicing the gordian knot of plasmodium falciparum malaria pathogenesis. PLoS Pathog 2013;9(5):1003327.

[2] Kilian N, Srismith S, Dittmer M, Ouermi D, Bisseye C, Simpore J, et al. Hemoglobin s and c affect protein export in plasmodium falciparum-infected erythrocytes. Biol Open 2015;4(3):400-10.

[3] Colah RB, Mukherjee MB, Martin S, Ghosh K. Sickle cell disease in tribal populations in india. Indian J Med Res 2015;141(5):509.

[4] Goncalves BP, Gupta S, Penman BS. Sickle haemoglobin, haemoglobin c and malaria mortality feedbacks. Mal J 2016;15:26.

[5] Cyrklaff M, Sanchez CP, Frischknecht F, Lanzer M. Host actin remodeling and protection from malaria by hemoglobinopathies. Trends Parasitol 2012;28(11):479.

[6] Wellems TE, Fairhurst RM. An evolving picture of the interactions between malaria parasites and their host erythrocytes. Cell Res 2012;22(3):453.

[7] Weatherall DJ, Williams TN, Allen SJ, O'Donnell A. The population genetics and dynamics of the thalassemias. Hematol Oncol Clin North Am 2010;24(6):1021.

[8] Muncie HL, Campbell JS. Alpha and beta thalassemia. Am Fam Physician 2009;80(4):339.

[9] Marengo-Rowe AJ.The thalassemias and related disorders. Proc Bayl Univ Med Cent 2007;20(1):27.

[10] Krause MA, Diakite SA, Lopera-Mesa TM, Amaratunga C, Arie T, Traore K, et al. a-thalassemia impairs the cytoadherence of plasmodium falciparum-infected erythrocytes. PLoS One 2012;7(5):37214.

[11] Tumian NR, Wong M,Wong CL. a-thalassemia-associated hydrops fetalis: A rare cause of thyrotoxic cardiomyopathy. J Obstet Gynaecol Res 2015;41(6):967.

[12] Cao A, Galanello R. Beta-thalassemia. Genet Med 2010;12:61.

[13] Haddad A, Tyan P, Radwan A, Mallat N, Taher A. ß-thalassemia intermedia: A bird's-eye view. Turk J Haematol 2014;31(1):5.

[14] Denic S, Nicholls MG. Genetic benefits of consanguinity through selection of genotypes protective against malaria. Hum Biol 2007;79(2):145.

[15] Akide-Ndunge OB, Ayi K, Arese P. The haldane malaria hypothesis: facts, artifacts, and a prophecy. Redox Rep 2003;8(5):311.

[16] Cholera R, Brittain NJ, Gillrie MR, Lopera-Mesa TM, Diakite SA, Arie T, et al. Impaired cytoadherence of plasmodium falciparum-infected erythrocytes containing sickle hemoglobin. PNAS 2007;105(3):991.

[17] Rug, M, Cyrklaff M, Mikkonen A, Lemgruber L, Kuelzer S, Sanchez CP, et al. Export of virulence proteins by malaria-infected erythrocytes involves remodeling of host actin cytoskeleton. Blood 2014;124(23):3459.

[18] Mayer C, Slater L, Erat MC, Konrat R, Vakonakis I. Structural analysis of the plasmodium falciparum erythrocyte membrane protein 1 (PfEMP1) intracellular domain reveals a conserved interaction epitope. J Biol Chem 2012;287:7182.

[19] Fairhurst RM, Bess CD, Krause MA. Abnormal PfEMP1/knob display on plasmodium falciparum-infected erythrocytes containing hemoglobin variants: fresh insights into malaria pathogenesis and protection. Microbes Infect 2012;14(10):851.

[20] Goel S, Muthusamy A, Miao J, Cui L, Salanti A, Winzeler EA, et al. Targeted disruption of a ring-infected erythrocyte surface antigen (RESA)-like export protein gene in plasmodium falciparum confers stable chondroitin 4-sulfate cytoadherence capacity. J Biol Chem 2014;289:34408.

[21] Sakaguchi M, Miyazaki N, Fujioka H, Kaneko O, Murata K.Three-dimensional analysis of morphological changes in the malaria parasite infected red blood cell by serial block-face scanning electron microscopy. J Struct Biol 2016;193(3):162.

[22] Ho M, White NJ. Molecular mechanisms of cytoadherence in malaria. Am J Physiol Cell Physiol 1999;276(6):1231.

[23] Hanssen E, Sougrat R, Frankland S, Deed S, Klonis N, Lippincott-Schwartz J, et al. Electron tomography of the maurer's cleft organelles of plasmodium falciparum-infected erythrocytes reveals novel structural features. Mol Microbiol 2007;67(4):703.

[24] Munwiler-Pachlatko E, Beck HP. Maurer's clefts, the enigma of plasmodium falciparum. Proc Natl Acad Sci USA 2013;110(50):19987-94.

[25] Maier AG, Rug M, O'Neill MT, Beeson JG, Marti M, Reeder J, et al. Skeleton-binding protein 1 functions at the parasitophorous vacuole membrane to traffic PfEMP1 to the plasmodium falciparum–infected erythrocyte surface. Blood 2007;109(3):1289.

[26] Spycher C, Rug M, Klonis N, Ferguson DJ, Cowman AF, Beck H, et al. Genesis of and trafficking to the maurer's clefts of plasmodium falciparum-infected erythrocytes†. Mol Cell Biol 2006;26(11):4074.

[27] Dearnley M, Chu T, Zhang Y, Looker O, Huang C, Klonis N, et al. Reversible host cell remodeling underpins deformability changes in malaria parasite sexual blood stages. Proc Natl Acad Sci USA 2016;113(17):4800.

[28] Das D, Patra M, Chakrabarti AC. Binding of hemin, hematoporphyrin, and protoporphyrin with erythroid spectrin: fluorescence and molecular docking studies. Eur Biophys J 2015;44(3):171.

[29] Davis SP, Amrein M, Gillrie MR, Lee K, Muruve DA, Ho M. Plasmodium falciparum-induced CD36 clustering rapidly strengthens cytoadherence via p130CAS-mediated actin cytoskeletal rearrangement. FASEB J 2012;26(3):1119.

[30] Ochola LB, Siddondo BR, Ocholla H, Nkya S, Kimani EN, Williams TN, et al. Specific receptor usage in plasmodium falciparum cytoadherence is associated with disease outcome. PLoS One 2011;6(3):14741.

[31] Dahlbäck M, Jorgensen LM, Nielsen MA, Clausen TM, Ditlev SB, Resende M, et al. The chondroitin sulfate A-binding site of the VAR2CSA protein involves multiple N-terminal domains. J Biol Chem 2011;286:15908.

[32] Doritchamou J, Sossou-tchatcha S, Cottrell G, Moussiliou A, Hounton Houngbeme C, Massougbodji A, et al. Dynamics in the cytoadherence phenotypes of plasmodium falciparum infected erythrocytes isolated during pregnancy. PLoS One 2014;9(6):98577.

[33] de Moraes LV, Dechavanne S, Sousa PM, Barateiro A, Cunha SF, Nuna-Silves S, et al. A murine model for pre-clinical studies on Var2CSA-mediated pathology associated to malaria in pregnancy. Infect Immun 2016.

[34] Li A, Lim TS, Shi H, Yin J, Tan SJ, Li Z, et al. Molecular mechanistic insights into the endothelial receptor mediated cytoadherence of plasmodium falciparum-infected erythrocytes. PLoS One 2011;6(3):16929.

[35] Kaul DK, Roth EF, Nagel RL, Howard RJ, Handunnetti SM. Rosetting of plasmodium falciparum-infected red blood cells with uninfected red blood cells enhances microvascular obstruction under flow conditions. Blood 1991;78(3):812.

[36] Davis SP, Lee K, Gillrie MR, Roa L, Amrein M, Ho M. CD36 recruits a5ß1 integrin to promote cytoadherence of P falciparum-infected erythrocytes. PLoS Pathog 2013;9(8):1003590.

[37] Jeney V, Ramos S, Berman M, Bechmann I, Tischer J, Ferreira A, et al. Control of disease tolerance to malaria by nitric oxide and carbon monoxide. Cell Rep 2014;8(1):126.

[38] Aidoo M, Terlouw DJ, Kolczak MS, McElroy PD, Kuile PO, Kariuki S, et al. Protective effects of the sickle cell gene against malaria morbidity and mortality. Lancet 2002;359(9314):1311.

[39] Arese P, Turrini F, Schwarzer E. Band 3/complement-mediated Recognition and removal of normally senescent and pathological human erythrocytes. Cell Physiol Biochem 2005;16:133.

[40] Kannan R, Labotka R, Low PS. Isolation and characterization of the hemichrome-stabilized membrane protein aggregates from sickle erythrocytes. Major site of autologous antibody binding. J Biol Chem 1988;263:13766.

[41] Hebbel RP. Beyond hemoglobin polymerization: the red blood cell membrane and sickle disease pathophysiology. Blood 1991;77(2):214.

[42] Carrell RW, Winterbourn CC. The unstable hemoglobins. Tex Rep Biol Med 1981;40:431.

[43] Kumar S, Bandyopadhyay U. Free heme toxicity and its detoxification systems in human. Toxicol Lett 2005;157(3):175.

[44] Slater AF, Swiggard WJ, Orton BR, Flitter WD, Goldberg DE, Cerami A, et al. An iron-carboxylate bond links the heme units of malaria pigment. Proc Natl Acad Sci USA 1991;88:325.

[45] Arruda MA, Rossi AG, de Freita MS, Barja-Fidalgo C, Graca-Souza AV. Heme inhibits human neutrophil apoptosis: Involvement of phosphoinositide 3-kinase, MAPK, and NF-κB. J Immunol 2004;173(3):2023.

[46] Kilian N, Srismith S, Dittmer M, Ouermi D, Bisseye C, Simpore J, et al. Haemoglobin S and C affect the motion of maurer's clefts in plasmodium falciparum-infected erythrocytes. Cell Microbiol 2013;15(7):1111.

[47] Veenemans J et al. a+-thalassemia protects against anemia associated with asymptomatic malaria: Evidence from community-based surveys in tanzania and kenya. J Infect Dis 2008;198(3):401.

[48] Destro-Bisol G, D'Aloja E, Spedini G, Scatena R, Giardina B, Pascali V. Resistance to falciparum malaria in a-thalassemia, oxidative stress, and hemoglobin oxidation. Am J Phys Anthropol 1999;109(2):269.

[49] De Franceschi L, Bertoldi M, Matte A, Santos Franco S, Pantaleo A, Ferru E, et al. Oxidative stress and ß-thalassemic erythroid cells behind the molecular defect. Oxid Med Cell Longev 2013;2013:985210.

[50] Ayi K, Turrini F, Piga A, Arese P. Enhanced phagocytosis of ring-parasitized mutant erythrocytes: a common mechanism that may explain protection against falciparum malaria in sickle trait and beta-thalassemia trait. Blood 2004;104(10):3364.

[51] Cappellini MD, Tavazzi D, Duca L, Graziadei G, Mannu F, Turrini F, et al. Metabolic indicators of oxidative stress correlate with haemichrome attachment to membrane, band 3 aggregation and erythrophagocytosis in ß-thalassaemia intermedia. Br J Haematol 1999;104:504.

[52] Kirschner-Zilber I, Setter E, Shaklai N. Association of hemoglobin chains with the cell membrane as a cause of red cell distortion in thalassemia. Biochem Med Metab Biol 1987;38(1):19.

[53] Premachandra BR. Interaction of hemoglobin and its component alpha and beta. chains with band 3 protein. Biochemistry 1986;25(11):3455.

[54] Fowkes FJ, Allen SJ, Allen A, Alpers MP, Weatherall DJ, Day KP. Increased microerythrocyte count in homozygous a+-thalassaemia contributes to protection against severe malarial anaemia. PLoS One 2008;5(3):56.

[55] Mockenhaupt FP, Bienzle U, May J, Falusi AG, Ademowo OG, Olumese P, et al. Plasmodium falciparum Infection: Influence on hemoglobin levels in a-thalassemia and microcytosis. J Infect Dis 1999;180(3):925.

[56] Williams TN, Wambua S, Uyoga S, Macharia A, Mwacharo JK, Charles RJ, et al. Both heterozygous and homozygous a+ thalassemias protect against severe and fatal plasmodium falciparum malaria on the coast of kenya. Blood 2005;106:368-71.

[57] Fernandez P, Petres S, Mecheri S, Gysin J, Scherf A. Strain-transcendent immune response to recombinant Var2CSA DBL5-e domain block P. falciparum adhesion to placenta-derived BeWo cells under flow conditions. PLoS One 2010;5(9):12558.

[58] Rieger H, Yoshikawa HY, Quadt K, Nielsen MA, Sanchez CP, Salanti A, et al. Cytoadhesion of plasmodium falciparum–infected erythrocytes to chondroitin-4-sulfate is cooperative and shear enhanced. Blood 2015;125(2):383.

[59] O'Donnell A, Premawardhena A, Arambepolad M, Samaranayaked R, Allen SJ, Petob TE, et al. Interaction of malaria with a common form of severe thalassemia in an Asian population. PNAS 2009;106(44):18716.

[60] Taylor SM, Parobek CM, Fairhurst RM. Impact of haemoglobinopathies on the clinical epidemiology of malaria: a systematic review and meta-analysis. Lancet 2012;12(6):457.

[61] Olivieri N, Muraca GM, O'Donnell A, Premawardhena A, Fisher CA, Weatherall DJ. Studies in haemoglobin E beta-thalassaemia. Br J Haematol 2008;141(3):388.

[62] Olivieri N, Pakbaz Z, Vichinsky E. HbE/ß-thalassemia: Basis of marked clinical civersity. Hematol Oncol Clin North Am 2010;24(6):1055.

[63] Fucharoen S, Weatherall DJ. The hemoglobin E thalassemias. Cold Spring Harb Perspect Med 2012;2(8):011734.

[64] Williams TN, Mwangi TW, Wambua S, Peto TE, Weatherall DJ, Gupta S, et al. Negative epistasis between the malaria-protective effects of a+-thalassemia and the sickle cell trait. Nat Genet 2005;37(11):1253.

[65] World Health Organizatiion. Malaria, 2016. URL:http://www.who.int/mediacentre/factsheets/fs094/en/

[66] Opi DH, Ochola LB, Tendwa M, Siddondo BR, Ocholla H, Fanjo H, et al. Mechanistic studies of the negative epistatic malaria-protective interaction between sickle cell trait and a+thalassemia. EBioMedicine 2014;1(1):29.

[67] Penman BS, Habib S, Kanchan K, Gupta S. Negative epistasis between a+ thalassemia and sickle cell trait can explain interpopulation variation in south Asia. Evolution 2011;65(12):3625.

In: Child and Adolescent Health
Editors: A Tenenbaum and J Merrick
ISBN: 978-1-53617-825-8

Chapter 10

FOOD INSECURITY AND BMI FOR CHILDREN AND ADOLESCENTS ACROSS SIX GRADE LEVELS

Oliver W Edwards**, PhD, BCBA-D and Whitney Shipman, EdS
Department of Counselor Education and School Psychology,
University of Central Florida,
Orlando, Florida, United States of America

ABSTRACT

Food insecurity and obesity are associated with adverse child health outcomes. Food insecure children demonstrate lower academic achievement and more behavioral difficulties than their peers. Among children and adolescents, obesity is strongly associated with diabetes, hypertension and heart disease. Objective: A dearth of data are available regarding food insecurity and Body Mass Index (BMI, a marker of obesity) among children at differing grade levels. This study examines the relationship between food insecurity and BMI among children across

* Corresponding Author's Email: owedwards@ucf.edu.

multiple grades. Study Group: The "Health Behaviour in School-aged Children" (HBSC) survey is administered in 42 countries around the world under the direction of the World Health Organization. It surveys the health-related of children and adolescents. This present study uses a nationally representative U.S. sample of 12,642 children in grades 5-10 from the HBSC. Methods: Kruskal-Wallis H tests were applied to examine whether BMI differs related to the 5th through 10th grade children's food insecurity. Mann-Whitney U tests were computed in order to follow-up Kruskal-Wallis H tests as a means of orthogonal pairwise comparisons. Results. Statistical analyses revealed food insecurity is associated with higher BMI scores when grade levels are combined. Pairwise comparisons suggest the difference is statistically significant in 9th grade, but the practical significance is limited. Conclusions: These results indicate reducing food insecurity is of greater importance than reducing BMI due to food insecurity.

INTRODUCTION

The numbers of children living in food insecure households in countries around the world is a public health concern (1). These food insecure households are found in countries across Africa, in Canada, in the United Kingdom and the United States (1-4). More than 15 million school-age children are part of the approximately 48 million persons who resided in food insecure households in the United States in 2014 (4). Food insecure households have ". . . limited or uncertain availability of nutritionally adequate and safe foods or limited or uncertain ability to acquire acceptable foods in socially acceptable ways"(5). Food insecure children demonstrate lower academic achievement, increased juvenile delinquency, and more behavioral difficulties than their peers (5, 6). In light of the importance of proper and sufficient nutrition in promoting health and school-related functioning, food insecurity is detrimental to all family members (7).

Research reveals a consistent connection between food insecurity and obesity among adults, particularly women (8). However, researchers have not reached consensus regarding the relationship between food insecurity and obesity in children. A comprehensive literature review indicates multiple studies report conflicting data regarding the association between food insecurity and obesity in children (9). Several recent studies show a connection between food insecurity and childhood obesity among preschool children and with heightened risk to be overweight among children and adolescents from Caucasian families and families with low SES (10, 11). However, these studies of older children and adolescents that report significant findings do not disclose statistical indices of practical significance such as standardized effect sizes (11). Moreover, when the results are converted to standardized effect sizes, the effect sizes are inconsequential. Conversely, other research studies do not reveal a relationship between food insecurity and obesity among children and adolescents using multiple measures of obesity and participant demographic characteristics (12). For example, a large-scale study revealed food insecurity and childhood obesity are unassociated for children between the ages of 8 and 17 based on gender and race/ethnicity (12). Unfortunately, however, none of the studies examines food insecurity and obesity across multiple grade levels.

Research suggests obesity is significant a national health concern (13). Overweight adults are at heighted risk for chronic diseases such as cardiovascular conditions, certain cancers, and overall low general well-being (13). Obesity consumes considerable financial and social resources and is one of the primary causes of preventable death in America (13). Additionally, overweight status and obesity are prevalent in schools because approximately 33% of school-age children in the United States are overweight and about 20% are obese (14).These children are at heighted risk to experience physiological difficulty, such as sleep apnea, hypertension, diabetes, and orthopedic challenges (13).In schools, obese children also tend to experience problems such as low engagement, more absences, and diminished academic performance (6).

Despite the association among food insecurity and adverse health and educational outcomes, a dearth of data are available regarding food insecurity and body mass index (BMI, a marker of obesity) among children at differing grade levels. More specifically, a paucity of research examines the labels of food insecurity among children in multiple grade levels and the children's associated BMI. This current research helps fill the gap in the knowledgebase. Analyzing the association between food security and BMI across grade levels adds specificity to knowledgebase and offers guidance regarding the need for prevention and intervention. By filling this gap in the literature, this research may offer stakeholders such as parents, school staff, and community agencies who work with families an opportunity to address a significant need of the children whom they serve. The goal is to determine whether labels of food insecurity are associated with BMI in connection to children's specific grade level. This study may help identify whether interventions to relieve food insecurity and obesity are particularly important for specific subgroups of children.

Food insecurity

The USDA introduced four labels to identify food security and food insecurity (15). High food security refers to no reported indications of problems or limitations accessing food. Marginal food security references one or two reports of anxiety about having insufficient food. In cases of marginal food security, there is no indication of having to change diet or limit the amount of food intake. Low food security refers to reduced access to quality of, and a variability in, diet. Very low food security refers to multiple indications of disrupted eating patterns and reduced food intake (4).

Not all households operating below the poverty level are food insecure and food insecure households can exist above the poverty level (4). That is, poverty is a necessary, but not sufficient condition for food insecurity. Income determines poverty level, but income and poverty do not reveal how households spend their financial resources. Thus, and of principal importance to this study, income and poverty are rather weak indicators of food insecurity and food insecurity and poverty are not interchangeable constructs. Some households may spend income disproportionately on housing, transportation, and entertainment and this may not leave sufficient funds to ensure the household is food secure (13).

Food insecurity affects children's functioning before they are born. Prenatal nutrition is vital for the development of the fetus. Food insecurity in pregnant women correlates with low infant birth weights and is associated with childhood health problems (5). They are twice as likely to be in poor health in comparison to their food secure counterparts (5). Children who are food insecure tend to earn lower scores on achievement tests and are more likely to have repeated a grade (5). Taken together, the research indicates food insecurity has direct and indirect implications for children's health and school functioning.

BMI

BMI is a relatively straightforward metric to classify overweight status and obesity in humans (16). In children, "[O]verweight is defined as a BMI at or above the 85th percentile and below the 95th percentile for children and teens of the same age and sex. Obesity is defined as a BMI at or above the 95th percentile for children and teens of the same age and sex. BMI is calculated by dividing a person's weight in kilograms by the square of height in meters. For children and teens, BMI is age- and sex-specific and is often referred to as BMI-for-age. A child's weight status is determined using an age- and sex-specific percentile for BMI rather than the BMI categories used for adults. This is because children's body composition varies as they age and varies between boys and girls. Therefore, BMI levels among children and teens need to be expressed relative to other children of the same age and sex" (17). A high BMI percentile ranking among children and adolescents identifies obesity. BMI at the 85th to less that the 95th percentile is considered overweight, and at the 95th or greater is considered obese for children and adolescents (17).

Among children and adolescents, obesity is strongly associated with diabetes, hypertension, and heart disease (18). Additionally, research suggests BMI is associated with bullying (16). High BMI predicts increased peer victimization and is associated with heightened rates of aggression against peers (16). The little data available regarding school variables and BMI classifications indicate schools with a large proportion of children from low SES communities tend to have a higher percentage of overweight children (19). Further, public schools and schools with large ethnic minority enrollment have higher average BMI values (19). Notwithstanding the aforementioned adverse health and school implications of food insecurity and BMI, no extant research examines multiple grade levels, food insecurity, and BMI as measured in this study.

Conceptual framework

Conceptually, food security infers easy and safe access to sufficient nutritious food. Healthful food consumption is important for school-age children since children who receive proper nourishment tend function better in school than children who do not receive proper nutrition (20). However, school-age children residing in food insecure households may primarily have easy access to unhealthful, highly processed foods, with high fat content and low levels of protein and nutrients (7). It is also likely that they have minimal access to the more expensive fruit and vegetables and other foods with necessary quantities of nutrients and minerals (7). These children may live in what is often known as food deserts. Researchers define food deserts as neighborhoods that lack foods that are nutritious, fresh, and reasonably priced (7). These communities are more likely to have food marts, corner stores, and fast food restaurants with sugary, fried, low nutritious foods than they have grocery stores within close proximity. Difficulty accessing nutritious foods is associated with harmful eating patterns, malnourishment, and health problems (5, 7, 20).

Although seemingly paradoxical, unhealthful diets and malnutrition may increase overweight status and promote obesity. The counterintuitive link between food insecurity and obesity among children and adolescents was initially advanced several years ago in a case study (21). It was hypothesized that this may occur due to "an adaptive process to food shortages whereby increasing the consumption of inexpensive energy dense foods results in increasing body mass" (21). Subsequent research consistently reveals that non-elderly adult women who live in food insecure households are at heightened risk to be obese when compared with their food secure peers (10). Plausible mechanisms that may explain this association include cheaper cost and overconsumption of energy-dense foods, overeating when foods become available, metabolic changes that may permit more efficient use of energy, fear of food restriction, and higher susceptibility to hunger, disinhibition, and environmental cues" (11). This potentially adaptive process of eating too much and eating poorly when food is available to stem hunger pangs later may contribute to increased weight gain and serve as the conceptual framework that guides this study.

Purpose of the study

Overall, food insecurity correlates with adverse outcomes (7). What's more, obesity is a significant concern in children due to its robust association with adverse health conditions and bullying (16, 18). However, the extant empirical literature offers a paucity of research that identifies the differences in labels of food insecurity and associated BMI. Thus, this study examines the relationship between a marker of obesity, BMI, and food insecurity among children across multiple grade levels. The findings may assist in developing interventions and policies to prevent and/or treat obesity among school-age children. The findings of this study will add specificity to the knowledgebase due to the discrete grade-level analyses.

The four labels of food security (1 = high food security, 2 = marginal food security, 3 = low food security, and 4 = very low food security) developed by USDA (2007) are used to investigate child and adolescents BMI categories among children. The primary research question is as follows: Will children in grades 5 through 10 manifest significantly different BMI scores in relationship to the four labels of food security identified by the USDA? The study operates under the hypothesis that across all of the six grade levels children's perceptions regarding their own food insecurity will be associated with higher BMI scores. This hypothesis may appear counterintuitive because it seems likely that children and adolescents living in food insecure households may not have sufficient food to consume. Thus, they should be underweight as opposed to overweight. However, the conceptual framework of this study asserts food security principally refers to having safe and acceptable access to sufficient nutritious food. It is unlikely that school-age children residing in food insecure households will have ready access to sufficient healthful foods. They may consume calorie-dense, inexpensive, fatty, and high-sodium foods resulting in increased body mass (20).

OUR STUDY

The "Health Behaviour in School-aged Children" (HBSC) survey is administered in 42 countries around the world under the direction of the World Health Organization. It is designed to investigate health-related and lifestyle behaviors among children enrolled in 5th through 10th grades. In the United States, it employs multistage area probability sampling techniques to obtain a representative group of school-age children in schools (22). Participants from the 2009-2010 cycle of the HBSC in the United States served as the sample for this study. "In the first stage of sampling Primary Sampling Units (PSUs) were stratified within each Census Division. These PSUs are comprised of one or more school districts of public schools. A total of 1,302 PSUs were created. A sample of 94 PSUs was selected. The total sample of PSUs was allocated to each Census Division in proportion to the total enrollment in the Census Division" (22).

Among the 475 schools that were eligible to participate in the survey, 314 consented to the survey administration. A total of 14,627 children in 5th through 10th grades were eligible to serve as participants. Not all eligible children gave assent to participate in the survey and other children were not at school during the first administration. This led to 301 children receiving administration of the survey on a different day. However, not all eligible children were available on the re-administration day. Overall,

12,642 children in grades 5 through 10 completed sufficient portions of the survey to serve as participants. This results in a participation rate of 90% (22).

Males comprise 51% and females 49% of the participants in this study. They include 5823 Caucasians, 2105 Black/African Americans, 460 Asians, 216 Native Americans/Alaska Native, 109 Hawaiian/Pacific Islanders, 819 with two or more ethnicities listed, and 2340 Hispanics. Participants can identify as Hispanic as well as a specific race/ethnicity. Self-reported family SES data reveal 89% of participants consider their family finances as average or better and 11% noted their family SES is below average.

Procedure

Various versions of the survey were written to be developmental appropriate for the 5th through 10th grade children. The survey was administered to children in a school classroom by school staff (e.g., counselors and nurses) and were usually completed in 45 minutes. Survey administrators were required to adhere to formal directions to explain the procedures to participants. Children completed their survey individually. "The Research Protocol includes detailed information and instructions covering the following: conceptual framework for the study; scientific rationales for each of the survey topic areas; international standard version of questionnaires and instructions for use (e. g., recommended layout, question ordering, and translation guidelines); comprehensive guidance on survey methodology, including sampling, data collection procedures. . ." (23). A comprehensive description of the HBSC history, design, and procedures are available from the developers and in numerous published studies (23).

In this current study, the independent variable of food insecurity is comprised of four levels aligned with the four labels of food security identified by the USDA: 1 = high food security, 2 = marginal food security, 3 = low food security, and 4 = very low food security. The HBSC identifies food insecurity using the following question: “Some young people go to school or to bed hungry because there is not enough food at home. How often does this happen to you? Always, Often, Sometimes, and Never.” For the purposes of this study, each participant is assigned into one of the four USDA food security labels dependent on their response to this question as follows: high food security = never hungry, marginal food security = sometimes hungry, low food security = often hungry, and very low food security = always hungry.

This study employs BMI as the dependent variable and it is computed based on the respondent's self-reported weight and height using the following formula: [Weight (lbs)/[Height (inches) * Height (inches)]. The developers of the HBSC also consider participants’ gender and age to determine BMI for children and adolescents. This is the case because “. . . a correct interpretation of a child's BMI requires factoring in the child's gender and age. This then places the child into a percentile and subsequent categorization. Coding was done based on percentiles from the year 2000 from the Centers for Disease Control” (22). Thus, participants’ gender and age are used to calculate the BMI categories for all children.

FINDINGS

Statistical analyses were conducted to determine whether participants’ BMI scores were higher in relation to their food insecurity category. In light of the categorical outcome data, non-parametric analyses were conducted (24). The Kruskal-Wallis H test examines whether BMI differs related to the 5th through 10th grade children’s four self-reported labels of food insecurity (i.e., 1 = high food security-never hungry, 2 = marginal food security- sometimes hungry, 3 = low food security-often hungry, and 4 = very low food security-always hungry). Assumptions of random sampling and independent observations are met in light of the robust standardization of the HBSC. The results reveal a statistically significant difference in BMI related to the four labels of food insecurity (Chi s quare = 25.236, df = 3, p = .000). Kruskal-Wallis (KW) Post Hoc analyses indicate the following rank order for BMI based on the four labels of food insecurity: 1. Often hungry (KW rank = 5351.66); 2. Sometimes hungry (KW rank = 5209.74); 3. Always hungry (KW rank = 5058.03); and 4. Never hungry (KW rank = 4950.22). Children who are often food insecure (i.e., low food security) evidence the highest BMI ranking.

The Mann-Whitney U test was computed in order to follow-up the Kruskal-Wallis H test as a means of orthogonal pairwise comparisons for each grade level separately based on the four food insecurity groups. To mitigate concerns with Type 1 error inflations because of the three comparisons (i.e., never hungry vs. always hungry, never hungry vs. often hungry, and never hungry vs. sometimes hungry), Bonferroni correction lowered the alpha level to .016. For the six grade levels, two statistically significant findings are evident. First, a statistically significant difference in BMI based on gender/age and food insecurity among the three pairs of groups occurred in 9th grade between children who never ($n = 1379$, $\bar{x} = 2.38$, $s = .71$) and often ($n = 63$, $\bar{x} = 2.63$, $s = .79$) experience food insecurity, $U = 35815$, $z = -2.906$, $p = .004$, $r = .08$. The effect size is very small using Cohen's classification indicating .1 is a small effect, .3 is a medium effect, and .5 is a large effect.(25) Second, the analysis reveals a statistically significant difference in BMI among 9th grade participants based on gender/age and food insecurity between children who never ($n = 1379$, $\bar{x} = 2.38$, $s = .71$) and sometimes ($n = 371$, $\bar{x} = 2.47$, $s = .75$) experience food insecurity, $U = 238453$, $z = -2.457$, $p = .014$, $r = .06$. The effect size accounts for a nominal amount of the variance.

DISCUSSION

In this research study, we examine nationally representative groups of children in six grade levels relative to their perceptions of their individual food insecurity along the following continuum: 1 = high food security-never hungry, 2 = marginal food security-sometimes hungry, 3 = low food security-often hungry, and 4 = very low food security-always hungry. The children's BMI, as a function of height and weight as well as their gender and age, was computed and statistically compared to their self-reported level of food insecurity. Omnibus statistical analysis generally supports the overarching hypothesis that children who report higher categories of food insecurity will evidence higher BMI scores. Nonetheless, more nuanced orthogonal pairwise analyses indicate it is only at the 9th grade level where children who perceive they experience food insecurity tend to have higher BMI scores than peers who do not experience food insecurity. Children in this grade who often or sometimes experience food insecurity have higher BMI scores than their peers who never experience food insecurity. However, small effect sizes account for nominal variance. Thus, although there is statistical support for differences in BMI in relationship to categories of food insecurity, these differences result in limited practical significance. The aforementioned notwithstanding, because entering high school is a major milestone in the transition to adulthood, the unpredictability and diversity of interpersonal relationships experienced in high school suggests adolescents they may require monitoring, if not targeted intervention, to ensure food insecure does not contribute to obesity in 9th grade.

A lack of consensus exists among researchers regarding the relationship between food insecurity and BMI among children and adolescents. However, studies do not examine the relationship among multiple grade levels or using the USDA's four labels of food insecurity. The findings of this study add to the literature that indicates food insecurity has minimal impact on children's BMI from grade 5 through 10. Although some research may support a connection between food insecurity and BMI, it does not appear to be a practically relevant relationship for 5th through 10th grade children (11). Other research suggests the relationship is stronger among preschool children as well as among adults.

Limitations

This study has several strengths including the use of a large-scale, nationally representative sample, comparisons across multiple grade levels, and findings that supplement the literature regarding the targeting of the limited prevention and intervention resources of schools. However, the findings are restricted because the survey uses self-report methodology to determine children's perceptions of their food insecurity. The children also self-reported their height and weight in order for the survey developers to compute the BMI. The children's perceptions and self-reports may not reflect reality. However, food insecurity is an undesirable circumstance that the children may be more prone to understate than overstate. In addition, the anonymous nature of the survey should preclude the need for social desirability in self-reports of height and weight. In light of the fact that HBSC is a decades-long, rigorously standardized survey, it is doubtful that the limitations lead to specious results. The field may benefit from longitudinal research in the future to help ascertain whether food insecurity predicts overweight status among preschool and young school-age children. In addition, future research may offer insight into whether perceptions of food insecurity differ from actual, physical food insecurity in BMI outcomes.

Implications for practice

As outlined in the literature review, food insecurity is associated with multiple adverse health and school-related outcomes (8). Food insecurity is particularly harmful to school-age children because children who are food insecure tend to demonstrate low mathematics achievement, grade retention, absenteeism, tardiness, psychoeducational referrals, anxiety, aggression, and difficult peer relationships (7). Several studies indicate a robust relationship between food insecurity and obesity among adults as well as preschool children (10). However, the results of this current study support other research showing food insecurity is not a strong predictor of markers of obesity (i.e., BMI) among children and adolescents (12). Therefore, it does not appear food insecurity results in significant weight gain for this population. These children may not require specialized intervention to moderate weight gain and BMI due to food insecurity.

A particularly important implication of this study is that it suggests the scarce prevention and intervention resources may be better directed toward eradicating food insecurity itself than decreasing BMI due to food insecurity. Taken together, the results of this investigation suggest substantial numbers of 5th through 10th grade children may benefit from home, school, and community prevention and intervention strategies to end their food insecurity, but that they may not need assistance with obesity as a result of food insecurity.

References

[1] Aberman N, Rawat R, Drimie S, Claros J, Kadiyala S. Food security and nutrition interventions in response to the AIDS epidemic: Assessing global action and evidence. AIDS and Behavior [serial on the Internet]. (2014, Oct), [cited November 22, 2016]; 18(Suppl 5): S554-S565.

[2] Tarasuk V, Cheng J, de Oliveira C, Dachner N, Gundersen C, Kurdyak P. Association between household food insecurity and annual health care costs. Canadian Medical Association Journal [serial on the Internet]. (2015, Oct 6), [cited November 22, 2016]; 187(14): E429-E436

[3] Harvey K. 'When I go to bed hungry and sleep, I'm not hungry': Children and parents' experiences of food insecurity. Appetite [serial on the Internet]. (2016, Apr 1), [cited November 22, 2016]; 99235-244.

[4] Coleman-Jensen A, Rabbitt M, Gregory C, Singh A. Household food security in the United States in 2014. USDA ERS. Available at: http://www.ers.usda.gov/media/1896841/err194.pdf

[5] Cook JT, Frank DA. Food security, poverty, and human developmental in the United States. Ann NY Acad Sci 2008;1136:193-209.

[6] Carey F, Singh G, Brown H, Wilkinson A. Educational outcomes associated with childhood obesity in the United States: Cross-sectional results from the 2011–2012 National Survey of Children's Health. Int J Behav Nutr Phys Activity [serial on the Internet]. (2015, Dec), [cited November 22, 2016];12.

[7] Edwards O, Cheeley T. Positive youth development and nutrition: Interdisciplinary strategies to enhance student outcomes. Child Sch 2016;38(3):170-7.

[8] Silverman J, Krieger J, Kiefer M, Hebert P, Robinson J, Nelson K. The relationship between food insecurity and depression, diabetes distress and medication adherence among low-income patients with poorly-controlled diabetes. J Gen Intern Med 2015; 30(10) 1476-80.

[9] Dinour L, Bergen D, Yeh M. Research: The food insecurity–obesity paradox: A review of the literature and the role food stamps may play. J Am Dietetic Assoc 2007;1071952-61.

[10] Speirs K, Fiese B. The relationship between food insecurity and bmi for preschool children. Matern Child Health J 2016;20(4):925-33.

[11] Casey P, Simpson P, Gossett J, Bogle M, Champagne C, Weber J, et al. The association of child and household food insecurity with childhood overweight status. Pediatrics 2006; 118(5):1406-13.

[12] Gundersen C, Garasky S, Lohman B. Food insecurity is not associated with childhood obesity as assessed using multiplie measures of obesity. J Nutrition 2009;139(6):1173-8.

[13] An R. Health care expenses in relation to obesity and smoking among US adults by gender, race/ethnicity, and age group: 1998–2011. Public Health 2015;129(1):29-36.

[14] Ogden C, Carroll M, Kit B, Flegal K. Prevalence of obesity and trends in body mass index among US children and adolescents, 1999-2010. JAMA 2016;307(5):483-90.

[15] US Department of Agriculture. (Food Security in the US. URL: http://www.ers.usda.gov/topics/food-nutrition-assistance/food-security-in-the-us.aspx.

[16] Piko B, Keresztes N, Pluhar Z. Aggressive behavior and psychosocial health among children. Pers Individ Diff 2006;40(5):885-95.

[17] Centers for Disease Control. National Health and Nutrition Examination of Survey Data. Hyattsville, MD: US Department of Health and Human Services, Centers for Disease Control and Prevention, National Center for Health Statistics, 2010.

[18] Freedman D, Mei Z, Srinivasan S, Berenson G, Dietz W. Cardiovascular risk factors and excess adiposity among overweight children and adolescents: The Bogalusa Heart Study. J Pediatrics 2007;150:12-17.e2.

[19] O'Malley P, Johnston L, Delva J, Bachman J, Schulenberg J. Variation in obesity among American secondary school students by school and school characteristics. Am J Prev Med 2007;33(4,Suppl):S187-94.

[20] Edwards O, Pratt H. Family meal participation as a corollary of positive youth development: Opportunities for counseling services. Int J Adv Couns 2016;38(2):89-96.

[21] Dietz W. Does hunger cause obesity? Pediatrics 1995;95(5):766-7.

[22] Iannotti RJ. Health behavior in school-aged children (HBSC), 2009-2010 – codebook: student survey. Hyattsville, MD: United States Department of Health and Human Services, National Institute of Child Health and Human Development, 2010.

[23] Roberts C, Freeman J, Samdal O, Schnohr C, Looze M, Rasmussen M, et al. The Health Behaviour in School-aged Children (HBSC) study: methodological developments and current tensions. Int J Public Health 2009;54(Suppl 2):140-50.

[24] Tabachnick B, Fidell L. Using multivariate statistics., 5th ed [monograph on the Internet]. Boston, MA: Allyn Bacon/Pearson Education, 2007.

[25] Cohen J. Statistical power analysis for the behavioral sciences, Rev. ed. Hillsdale, NJ: Lawrence Erlbaum, 1977.

In: Child and Adolescent Health
Editors: A Tenenbaum and J Merrick
ISBN: 978-1-53617-825-8

Chapter 11

FOOD FOR THOUGHT: A REVIEW OF SEVERE ACUTE MALNUTRITION RESEARCH IN THE 21ST CENTURY

Michael T Kody*, MS and Shannon Elizabeth Kody
School of Medicine, New York Medical College,
Valhalla, New York, United States of America

ABSTRACT

In this chapter we introduce the current guidelines regarding diagnosis and treatment of severe acute malnutrition (SAM), survey the current research in the field, and finally discuss actionable changes and future areas of research within this disease. Background: SAM is a misunderstood condition that is deeply interconnected with acute morbidity as well as long-term health problems. The survival rates for SAM without clinical intervention typically are 70-80% for marasmus and 40-50% for kwashiorkor. Not only can SAM kill directly, but it also dramatically increases the risk of fatalities through normally self-limiting health problems. Unfortunately, current guidelines and WHO

* Correspondence: Michael T Kody, MS, Medical Student, New York Medical College, Valhalla, New York, United States. Email: mkody@nymc.edu.

recommendations rely on physical exam indicators that may miss up to two-thirds of patients presenting with the kwashiorkor subtype of SAM. Results: Recent evidence demonstrates outpatient management of SAM increases time to nutritional resuscitation but is a less expensive option that does not increase mortality. The evidence on antibiotic use remains mixed, but guidelines suggest coverage should be properly evaluated and tailored to the individual. SAM complicated by HIV is not only more challenging to treat, but the decreased nutritional state may affect the efficacy of antiviral regimens and other medications. Conclusion: This field requires both comprehensive, specific research and combined medical, public health, and volunteer training to be appropriately addressed. With adequate funding and incentive, it is reasonable to attack SAM from scientific, political, and economic fronts with the goal of eradicating this problem and improving global health.

Introduction

Severe acute malnutrition (SAM) is a misunderstood condition that is deeply interconnected with acute morbidity as well as long-term health problems. Surprisingly, there is a lack of overall information as well as contradictory guidelines for managing individuals suffering from this condition. SAM is a global health issue that predominately affects children under the age of five (1). The World Health Organization (WHO) estimates that SAM affects over 20 million children globally and remains most prevalent in economically underdeveloped countries throughout Asia and sub-Sahara Africa (1). SAM is defined as an exceedingly low ratio of weight to height, yet this deficiency can also manifest itself through other forms (1). Although there are many different methods of assessing SAM status, a simple guided band tool can be used to measure the circumference of a child's arm at a mid-upper level (1). In the age range of six to sixty months, a mid-upper arm circumference of fewer than 110 millimeters can be used as an indicator of a SAM emergency (1).

During states of malnutrition, the physiologic adaptations that take place are crucial for individual survival, but during continued starvation these adaptations eventually decrease the individual's ability to deal with other stressors (2). To this point, all types of SAM can cause developmental deficiencies manifesting in delayed physical, mental, and psychological growth, plus more acute problems such as wasting, malabsorption, low protein synthesis, and chronic infection due to immune system impairment (3). There are two distinct, classical forms of SAM, each with their own ramifications on treatment and effects. Marasmus, or energy deficiency, is probably what is most commonly associated with SAM, as it is the state of severely lacking all nutrient categories (3). This is also described as classical wasting. A more silent type of SAM is known as kwashiorkor. Kwashiorkor presents in a different way than marasmus because it is a severe protein-only deficiency in which the individual still has sufficient carbohydrates for energy needs (3). Because of the lack of protein synthesis, the individual is likely to suffer from nutritional edema causing generalized ascites (3). To an untrained eye, this abdominal edema can give the appearance of a well-fed individual when in actuality; this represents severe malnourishment. Even to the trained professional, kwashiorkor can be more difficult to diagnosis because the patient may present with adequate fat and hepatomegaly that both obscure wasting (3). In this disease, the carbohydrate intake is meeting or even exceeding the caloric requirements of the individual, but that does not make this disease any less lethal. In fact, the survival rates for SAM without clinical intervention typically are 70-80% for marasmus and 40-50% for kwashiorkor (2).

Not only can SAM kill in a direct manner, but also it greatly increases the risk of fatalities through other, normally self-limiting health problems (1). The WHO estimates that SAM increases mortality by a factor of 5-20 times when compared to mortality rates of well-nourished children (1). Ultimately this increase causes mortality rates to surpass 20% in especially impacted areas like the Democratic Republic of the Congo (1). Due to the interconnectivity of this condition, the actual burden of SAM may be harder to estimate. Specifically, SAM is implicated as the primary cause of immunodeficiency worldwide, and recent work is uncovering the association between these two conditions (4). Even uncomplicated SAM can lead to the development of numerous other disease states which ultimately are documented as the cause of death (4). Not only does uncomplicated SAM diminish the immune system and lead to disease development, but also pre-existing diseases can severely impact the individual's capacity to fight infection while malnourished (4).

More so than in other diseases, severe malnutrition is propagated by a combination of economic, political, and environmental factors. At first glimpse, SAM may not be thought of as a contagious disease, yet, from an epidemiology perspective, it is human interaction that directly destabilizes a region or a population to the point that malnutrition becomes endemic. The classical method of SAM treatment involved in-patient care, but it is becoming increasingly apparent that this treatment simply is not sufficiently elastic to adjust with the sporadic, unpredictable nature of episodic SAM (1). Luckily, community-based management is starting to gain traction as an appropriate method of combatting the devastating effects of SAM (1).

It appears that early detection, advances in treatment, as well as a community-based method of treatment can all contribute to greatly decrease the overall mortality rate of SAM (1). As more is discovered about the immense interconnectivity of this pathology with other disease states, even more delicate and specific protocols must be established for proper treatment and resuscitation (1). The most common, current treatment for SAM is to supplement ready-to-use therapeutic food (RUTF) until an adequate weight to height ratio has been reached (1). According to the WHO, a child suffering from uncomplicated SAM will need to be supplemented over a period of 6-8 weeks with RUTFs, and this requires approximately 10-15 kg (costing to 30 - 45 dollars) of therapeutic food (1). Recent advances in RUTFs have helped to develop energetic, simple, and storable foods for proper resuscitation (1). Micronutrient and antibiotic supplementation, along with a clean water supply also remain crucial to restoring a healthy body weight (1). There remain differing viewpoints as to the role of antibiotics during SAM treatment, but most agree that SAM complicated by preexisting immunodeficiency requires antibiotic prophylaxis to properly treat the patient (1).

While this paper's focus is on the current diagnostic and treatment research for treating children with SAM in low socioeconomic areas, it is important to note that SAM is a problem in even the most developed nations. Parkinson's disease, anorexia, chemotherapy side effect and numerous other ailments can commonly cause severe malnutrition in the developed world (3).

Diagnosis

As previously mentioned, kwashiorkor and marasmus are two different types of malnutrition: marasmus is wasting where kwashiorkor is edematous wasting (3, 5). The difference between the two is nontrivial. Specifically, both WHO guidelines and the most practical resources for diagnosing SAM status rely heavily on classical wasting (weight to height ratio and arm circumference), but the question remains how much kwashiorkor type SAM do these types of tools miss (1, 5)? A recent study investigated this question and determined that a large number of children suffering from kwashiorkor did not meet the classical diagnostic criteria for SAM (5). Of children suffering from SAM in the form of protein deficiency, 62% of children measured by mean upper arm circumference and 66% of children measured by weight to height ratio would not qualify as moderately malnourished (5). This underestimation in the prevalence of SAM causes missed patients, missed communities with a higher SAM burden, and from a global perspective, a significant misestimation of the effects and number of those affected by SAM.

Acute Treatment

Once diagnosis has been established, current treatment focuses on restoring a nutritional state to the individual. The food choice must have high-energy content, adequate micronutrients, and be safe for consumption by individuals in SAM status (1). The gold standard food for malnutrition is known as F100, but due to its water content, careful preparation and refrigeration are critical in order to make sure that the F100 does not spoil(1). Recently, RUTFs have been utilized in the field because they have a very low water content while providing all the necessary supplementation to increase nutritional status (1). The low water content is particularly important because it allows safe storage and much less care to be given to the preparation of food, which is beneficial in community-based care (1).

Community-based care

In a study from the London School of Medicine and Tropical Hygiene, the benefits of in-patient, day care, and domiciliary care were compared in Bangladesh (6). Specifically, 573 children aged 12-60 months with no complicating factors pertaining to their SAM status were randomly assigned into three different groups (6). The in-patient group was provided antibiotics, micronutrient supplementation, and small, frequent food supplementation while staying in a 60-bed clinic until their weight to height ratio exceed 0.80 (6). The day care group was cared for in a clinical environment from 8 am to 5 pm, 6 days a week until the weight to height ratio exceed 0.80 (6). The third group -- the domiciliary care group -- was treated for one week at the day care center then returned home with weekly visits from trained health care professionals (6). Within the three groups, in-patient care provided the quickest recovery and domiciliary care the slowest recovery, but the mortality rate was statistically equal between all three groups (6). Notably, the cost of in-patient treatment was over five times more expensive than the cost of domiciliary care. This led to the conclusion that in uncomplicated SAM cases, the most cost-effective treatment is community-based, domiciliary care (6).

Antibiotics

The use of prophylactic, broad-spectrum antibiotics remains a controversial subject in management of SAM. Naturally, there is a strong correlation between poor nutritional status and an impaired immune system. In the previous (1999) updated World Health Organization, "Management of severe malnutrition: A manual for physician and other senior health workers" all potential SAM cases were to be treated in an in-patient manner with broad-spectrum antibiotics (7). Both of these recommendations are currently being challenged by new research.

In a recent study from Niger, 2,399 children with SAM were treated through a community-based-method and were randomized into groups receiving amoxicillin or placebo during their treatment (8). In this study, there was no significant difference in the nutritional recovery between the two groups (65.9% with amoxicillin vs. 62.7% with placebo), but it is noted that amoxicillin slightly decreased the number of patients that had to be transferred to in-patient care during their treatment (8). Therefore, this research lends itself to the conclusion that antibiotics are not necessary in nutritional recovery if healthcare infrastructure is put in place to monitor patients for development of diseases (8). Adding to the growing evidence for reducing antibiotic use, a retrospective study looked at a similar group of SAM patients (Malawian children, age 6-59 months, and being treated through a community based method) found a decreased recovery rate for patients treated with amoxicillin compared to those that did not receive any antibiotic treatment (9). The only conclusion drawn is that additional prospective studies need to be completed, but as more investigation is occurring, there is growing evidence against the use of antibiotics in uncomplicated SAM.

One of the few prospective investigations of antibiotic use in SAM used a similar population (Malawian children, age 6-59 months, and being treated through a community-based method), and randomly assigned them into groups that received amoxicillin, cefdinir, or placebo for a week while being treated for SAM (10). In this study, the antibiotic groups had a higher rate of recovery, a lower mortality rate, and a faster rate of weight gain when compared to the group that did not receive antibiotics (10). Overall the use of antibiotics remains a controversial treatment in uncomplicated SAM cases.

Complicated SAM

As treating uncomplicated SAM cases is already difficult, matters are made more confounding when SAM cases are complicated. Specifically, in areas where malnutrition is commonplace there is often a high prevalence of HIV, malaria, tuberculosis, and other diseases. In fact, in a recent study looking at a very similar population of Malawian children, researchers found that "in sub-Saharan Africa, mortality is three times higher in HIV-infected children with severe malnutrition than in non-infected children" (11). One of the critical questions in HIV complicated SAM treatment is when is the best time to start antiretroviral therapy (11)? WHO guidelines recommend starting antiretroviral only after adequate nutritional status has been reached, but a recent study found that greater than one-third of HIV positive malnourished children would have benefited from antiretroviral therapy even before they reached an adequate weight (11).

The question of when to start a drug therapy in SAM afflicted individuals may seem relatively straightforward, but it is complicated by two different factors. Not only must one consider the impact that drugs will have on the individual in a nutritionally deprived state, but also one must consider the whole-system physiological changes that may affect the fundamental pharmacodynamics of the necessary drugs. For example, in clinical trials of anti-malaria therapies, WHO standard protocol systematically excludes severely malnutrition individuals, yet there is a large overlap in the areas of SAM and malaria (12). Current trials are investigating changes in drug dynamics, after a study conducted on the efficacy of artemether-lumefantrine showed that 123 out of the 124 patients in the study were cured of falciparum malaria (13). The only treatment failure was in a single malnourished child who was included in the study (13). While there are multifactorial circumstances that affected why this failure occurred, SAM is such a physiologically distinct condition that it may be implicated in decreasing drug efficacy (13).

LONG TERM EFFECTS

Severe acute malnutrition's effects on virtually all physiological functions tend to cause lifelong changes in a patient's health. These long-term effects not only cause a variety of problems but also may even predispose individuals to be more prone to future SAM.

Gut microbiota

In one particular study, which has ramifications in both treatment and disease development, the microbiota of gut bacteria was analyzed in 317 pairs of twins. In this study approximately half of the twin pairs became malnourished and were treated with RUTF (14, 15). While RUTF supplementation worked to restore nutritional status, the microbiota's maturation in these individuals significantly lacked that of the persistently nourished group (14). Next, fecal samples from 3 of the healthy twins and 3 of the malnourished twins were transplanted into mice that had been fed a typical Malawian diet. Interestingly, the combination of a Malawian diet and fecal microbiota from malnourished individuals caused significant weight loss during the 3-week posttransplant time period during which the study was conducted (14). While the transplantation part of this study is a small sample, it does call for more research into the idea of malnutrition affecting physiologic functions in a manner that perpetuates recurrent malnourished states.

Permanent effects

Acute malnutrition – especially during early life – has been tied to numerous long-term problems that manifest much later in life (16, 17, 18). A study evaluated the development of diabetes in populations that survived the 1959 to 1962 famine in China (16). They found that famine exposure during childhood – especially in female subjects – significantly increased the chance of developing type II diabetes later in life (16). Another study conducted on prisoners of war from World War II surmised that not only did acute malnutrition caused the expected immunodeficiency, but it also caused acute, neurological impairments (17). Further, this acute malnutrition left a significant fraction of the patients with long-lasting (surpassing the 36-year time period of the study) neurological problems (17). Lastly, a study compared the health status of 70 European Jews born under Nazi rule to 230 Israeli born individuals of the same age range (18). A variety of general health factors were affected with statistically significant increases in hypertension, diabetes, angina pectoris, heart failure, and decrease in bone health (18). Naturally all of these studies have a multitude of other potential factors affecting their results – differing ancestry, culture, small sample size, but they do serve a call to action for more research into the long-term effects of acute nutritional insults.

DISCUSSION

SAM is an exceedingly complicated nutritional state that manifests itself through a multitude of physiologic effects and is even further burdened by preexisting conditions. Complicating factors exist in the fact that times of severe malnutrition can be catalyzed by environmental, economic, political, and general destabilization in populations. Due to the complex inter-workings that precipitate SAM, policy and surveillance may be the most useful tools for preventing malnutrition. Diagnostically speaking, striking a balance between cost-effectiveness, amount of training required, and ease of distribution has come at the expense of underdiagnosing kwashiorkor type SAM. Further research must be conducted in the area of diagnosis. Not only are there ethical considerations when the gold standard diagnostic tool misses affected individuals, but the exclusion of patients also causes an underestimation of the number of individuals affected with SAM. This underestimation may directly affect policy and inter-government assistance because SAM is likely a larger problem than it seems.

Unfortunately, due to inherent constraints of areas affected, cost of treatment has to be a primary concern in treating SAM. Community-based methods of management provide similar outcomes at a lower cost, and they allow patients to be treated in the comfort of their own community. Naturally, SAM treatment is often funded by non-governmental organizations, and through cost-effective delivery of the same outcomes, these NGOs will have more power and outreach to limit the global burden of SAM. Further, by identifying HIV positive patients and those with other preexisting conditions that can beget SAM, it is likely that the global incidence of SAM would greatly decrease.

The use of antibiotics in uncomplicated SAM cases remains controversial. Retrospective studies serve to guide where future research should investigate, but they must not be given too much value due to the magnitude of extenuating factors -- patient adherence to antibiotic regimen, undiagnosed complicating factors, consistency of antibiotic prescriptions, et cetera -- that obscure their data. Further, it is reasonable to conclude the misuse of antibiotics in areas affected by SAM could lead to resistance and quickly become a global health issue. By continuing to research the efficacy of broad-spectrum antibiotics in SAM resuscitation, more effective treatments can be developed while simultaneously decreasing the incidence of resistant bacteria.

Antibiotics are not the only area needing further research. Even in locations where SAM is a constant problem there is systematic exclusion of malnourished individuals from studies. There is evidence for pharmacodynamic changes in drugs when used on SAM individuals, and if future research does not include these people, it will decrease global disease eradication efforts. Also, SAM tends to manifest itself when newborns are weaned off of milk, and due to this, most studies on resuscitation are for age ranges 6 - 60 months. This again systematically excludes an entire population of malnourished people under the age of 6 months, who have little to no recommendations for treatment.

Unfortunately, not only does SAM need more research, but also due to the number of factors that can cause SAM, there remains academic and applicative confusion on how to manage endemic SAM. The actual process of resuscitation is a delicate balancing act that requires medical training, yet many academic institutions still treat SAM as solely a public health issue. By offering an interdisciplinary medical and public health course that deals with SAM, institutions could take a step forward in eradicating this problem for future generations.

Malnutrition is a disease state that has existed as long as life has. Its multifactorial nature both in development and treatment means that bringing an end to malnutrition will be a complicated task. At the same time, nearly all SAM can be prevented with access to an adequate supply of food. In this time of advanced innovation and technological development, it is easy to pass simple problems for the allure of solving more sophisticated challenges, yet some of the most elementary of problems can have the largest effect on the health of our global society. With adequate funding and incentive, it is reasonable to attack SAM from scientific, political, and economic fronts with the goal of eradicating this problem and improving global health.

Acknowledgments

The authors have no financial interest or benefit associated with this paper. The authors report no conflicts of interest. Special thanks to Dr Larry Thomas, Chairman and Founder of Tropical Health Alliance Foundation.

References

[1] Community-based management of severe acute malnutrition. A joint statement by the World Health Organization, the World Food Programme, the United Nations System Standing Committee on Nutrition and the United Nations Children's Fund. Geneva: World Health Organization, 2007.

[2] Collins S, Dent N, Binns P, Bahwere P, Sadler K, Hallam A. Management of severe acute malnutrition in children. Lancet 2006;368:1992-2000.

[3] McCance KL, Huethe SE. Pathophysiology: the biology basis for disease in adults and children. 7th ed. St Louis, MO: Mosby, 2014.

[4] Katona P, Katona-Apte J. The interaction between nutrition and infection. Clin Infect Dis 2008;46:1582-8.

[5] Frison S, Checchi F, Kerac M. Omitting edema measurement: how much acute malnutrition are we missing? Am J Clin Nutr 2015;102:1176-81.

[6] Ashworth A, Khanum S. Cost-effective treatment for severely malnourished children: What is the best approach? Health Policy Plann 1997;12:115-21.

[7] Management of severe malnutrition: A manual for physicians and other senior health workers. Geneva: World Health Organization, 1999.

[8] Isanaka S, Langendorf C, Berthe F, Gnegne S, Li N, Ousmane N, et al. Routine amoxicillin for uncomplicated severe acute malnutrition in children. New Engl J Med 2016;374:444-53.

[9] Trehan I, Amthor RE, Maleta K, Manary MJ. Evaluation of the routine use of amoxicillin as part of the home-based treatment of severe acute malnutrition. Trop Med Int Health 2010;15:1022-8.

[10] Trehan I, Goldbach HS, LaGrone LN, Meuli GJ, Wang RJ, Maleta KM, et al. Antibiotics as part of the management of severe acute malnutrition. New Engl J Med 2013;368:425-35.

[11] Chinkhumba J, Tomkins A, Banda T, Mkangama C, Fergusson P. The impact of HIV on mortality during in-patient rehabilitation of severely malnourished children in malawi. T Roy Soc Trop Med H 2008;102:639-44.

[12] Methods for surveillance of antimalarial drug efficacy. Manual. Geneva: World Health Organization, 2009.

[13] Valecha N, Srivastava P, Mohanty SS, Mittra P, Sharma SK, Tyagi PK, et al. Therapeutic efficacy of artemether-lumefantrine in uncomplicated falciparum malaria in india. Malaria J 2009;8:107.

[14] Smith MI, Yatsunenko T, Manary MJ, Trehan I, Mkakosya R, Cheng J, et al. Gut microbiomes of malawian twin pairs discordant for kwashiorkor. Science 2013;339:548-54.

[15] Reyes A, Blanton LV, Cao S, Zhao G, Manary M, Trehan I, et al. Gut DNA viromes of malawian twins discordant for severe acute malnutrition. Proc Natl Acad Sci USA 2015;112:11941-6.

[16] Wang N, Wang X, Han B, Li Q, Chen Y, Zhu C, et al. Is exposure to famine in childhood and economic development in adulthood associated with diabetes? J Clin Endocrinol Metabol 2015;100:4514-23.

[17] Gill GV, Bell DR. Persisting nutritional neuropathy amongst former war prisoners. J Neurol Neurosurg Psychiatry 1982;45:861-5.

[18] Bercovich E, Keinan-Boker L, Shasha SM. Long-term health effects in adults born during the holocaust. Isr Med Assoc J 2014;16:203-7.

In: Child and Adolescent Health
Editors: A Tenenbaum and J Merrick
ISBN: 978-1-53617-825-8

Chapter 12

FOOD ADDITIVES: AN OVERVIEW OF HEALTH IMPLICATIONS AND REGULATION AND CONTROL IN THE UNITED STATES

Sharmeen Samuel, MD, Kelly Brown, MD and Dilip R Patel*, MD, MBA, MPH
Department of Pediatric and Adolescent Medicine,
Western Michigan University Homer Stryker MD School of Medicine,
Kalamazoo, Michigan, United States of America

ABSTRACT

Numerous ingredients are added to food that we consume daily. This practice is not new; in fact, it dates back hundreds of years. In its broadest sense a food additive is any ingredient that is added to the food in order to preserve, flavor, blend, thicken and color foods. Food additives have played a useful role in reducing serious nutritional deficiencies, and help

---

* Correspondence: Professor Dilip R Patel, MD, MBA, MPH, Chair, Department of Pediatric and Adolescent Medicine, Western Michigan University Homer Stryker MD School of Medicine, 1000 Oakland Drive, D48G, Kalamazoo, MI 49008-1284, United States. Email dilip.patel@med.wmich.edu.

ensure the availability of flavorful, nutritious, safe, convenient, colorful and affordable foods that meet consumer expectations year-round. In the United States, food and color additives are evaluated, regulated and monitored primarily by the United States Food and Drug Administration (FDA). The United States Food and Drug Administration has come under increased scrutiny by the public and elected officials with regards to its ability to ensure safe food supply, adequately monitor the food industry, and potential conflicts of interest with food industry. Multiple disciplines of study contribute to the advancement of the science of food additives, and their manufacturing, monitoring and regulation for safe use by public. Among these disciplines are toxicology, epidemiology, food science, environmental science, chemistry, and bioengineering. This paper provides an overview of key aspects of food additives as these relate to their human and environmental health implications and regulations in the United States.

INTRODUCTION

The United Stated Food and Drug Administration (FDA) defines a food additive as, "any substance the intended use of which results or may reasonably be expected to result -- directly or indirectly -- in its becoming a component or otherwise affecting the characteristics of any food" (1). This definition includes any substance used in the production, processing, treatment, packaging, transportation or storage of food. The FDA definition, therefore, requires a premarket approval for any additive. The definition excludes three categories of food ingredients: (1) ingredients whose use is generally recognized as safe (GRAS) by experts, based on their extensive history of use in food before 1958 or based on published scientific evidence (1). Examples of GRAS substances include salt, sugar, spices, vitamins and monosodium glutamate (MSG); (2) those ingredients approved for use by FDA or the US Department of Agriculture prior to the food additives provisions of law (1-3). Examples include sodium nitrite and potassium nitrite used to preserve luncheon meats; and (3) color additives and pesticides where other legal premarket approval requirements apply. A food additive that is added to the food for a specific purpose is considered a direct food additive and most such additives are identified in the ingredients label of foods (1). An indirect food additive is any substance that becomes part of the food in trace amounts due to its packaging, storage or other handling (1).

A color additive is a type of food additive defined as "any dye, pigment or substance which when added or applied to a food, drug or cosmetic, or to the human body, is capable (alone or through reactions with other substances) of imparting color" (1, 4). FDA approved food color additives are subject to certification or exempt from certification. All synthetic color additives are subject to FDA certification. Dyes are a type of certified color additives that dissolve in water and are manufactured as powders, granules, liquids or other special-purpose forms (1, 5). They can be used in beverages, dry mixes, baked goods, confections, dairy products, pet foods and a variety of other products (1, 5). Lakes are also a type of certified color additives that are water insoluble dyes and because of their relatively higher stability are preferred for coloring products containing fats and oils or items lacking sufficient moisture to dissolve dyes (1, 5). Typical uses include coated tablets, cake and donut mixes, hard candies and chewing gums. Color pigments derived from natural sources such as vegetables, minerals or animals are exempt from FDA certification (1). Examples of exempt colors include annatto extract (yellow), dehydrated beets (bluish-red to brown), caramel (yellow to tan), beta-carotene (yellow to orange) and grape skin extract (red, green) (1).

FOOD ADDITIVES

Food additives can be added to the food at any stage of its production, preparation, or consumption (1). Based on their main intended use or function, the food additives are divided into the following five broad categories: 1) taste enhancers, 2) antioxidants, 3) preservatives, 4) stabilizers and emulsifiers and 5) coloring agents (1, 6). The wide range of food additives, their functions and examples of use are provided in table 1 (1).

Table 1. Uses of food additives

Food Additive	Function	Examples of Use
Preservatives	Prevent food spoilage from bacteria, molds, or yeast (antimicrobials); slow or prevent changes in color, flavor, or texture and delay rancidity (antioxidants); maintain freshness	Fruit sauces and jellies, beverages, baked goods, cured meats, oils and margarines, cereals, dressings, snack foods, fruits and vegetables
Sweeteners	Add sweetness with or without the extra calories	Beverages, baked goods, confections, table-top sugar substitutes
Color additives	Offset color loss due to exposure to light, air, temperature extremes, moisture and storage conditions; correct variations in color; enhance colors that occur naturally; provide color to colorless food	Candies, snack foods, margarine, cheese, soft drinks, pudding and pie fillings
Flavors and spices	Add specific flavors, either natural or synthetic	Pudding and pie fillings, gelatin desert mixes, cake mixes, salad dressings, candies, soft drinks, ice cream
Flavor enhancers	Enhance flavors already present in foods	Many processed foods
Fat replacers	Provide expected texture and a creamy feel in reduced-fat foods	Baked goods, dressings, frozen desserts, confections, cake and desert mixes
Nutrients	Replace vitamins and minerals (enrichment); add nutrients that may be lacking in diet (fortification)	Flour, breads, cereals, rice, milk, energy bars
Emulsifiers	Allow smooth mixing of ingredients, prevent separation, keep emulsified products stable, reduce stickiness, control crystallization, keep ingredients dispersed, and help products dissolve more easily	Salad dressings, peanut butter, chocolate, margarine, frozen desserts

Food Additive	Function	Examples of Use
Stabilizers and thickeners; binders, texturizers	Produce uniform texture, improve mouth-feel of the food	Frozen desserts, dairy products, cakes, pudding and gelatin mixes, dressings, jams, jellies, sauces
Leavening agents	Promote rising of baked goods	Breads and other baked goods
Anti-caking agents	Keep powdered foods free-flowing, prevent moisture absorption	Salt, baking powder, confectioner's sugar
Humectants	Retain moisture	Shredded coconut, marshmallows, soft candies, confections
Yeast nutrients	Promote growth of yeast	Breads and other baked goods
Dough strengtheners and conditioners	Produce more stable dough	Breads and other baked goods
Firming agents	Maintain crispness and firmness	Processed fruits and vegetables
Enzyme preparations	Modify proteins, polysaccharides and fats	Cheese, dairy products, meat
Gases	Serve as propellant, aerate, or create carbonation	Oil cooking spray, whipped cream, carbonated beverages

Source: United States Food and Drug Administration, 2015.

Food additives have been used over hundreds of years for a variety of purposes, such as use of salt to preserve meats and fish, added herbs and spices to improve the flavor of foods, preserved fruit with sugar, and pickled cucumbers in a vinegar solution (1, 6). With scientific and technological advances, thousands of new food ingredients are being introduced for human consumption making it necessary for the government to provide oversight of food industry to ensure public safety. Major events in the food industry regulatory history in the United States are summarized in table 2 (1, 2, 6-9).

The FDA is the main regulatory agency for food additives. The key functions of the FDA, its Science Board and its Advisory Committee are summarized in Table 3 (1, 7). The FDA, regulates and monitors the administrative, chemical, and toxicological information on food additives through a program called Priority-based Assessment of Food Additives (PAFA) (1). PAFA program categorizes food additives in an informational database called Everything Added to Food in the United States (EAFUS) based on available toxicological information, the uses of substances in food production, and the presence of banned substances (1). The FDA maintains a list of over 3,000 ingredients in its data base EAFUS (1).

Prior to marketing a new food or color direct additive, a manufacturer or other sponsor needs to first file a petition with the FDA for a formal review and approval (1,4,7). The petition must provide sufficient evidence of safety of the additive relative to its proposed use (1). Once a petition is received by the FDA the adequacy of filling is evaluated by the Office of Food Additive Safety and parts of petition are distributed to experts for further evaluations that include chemistry review, toxicology review, environmental review, evaluation by other government experts and evaluation by non-government expert (1, 4, 7). Following this review process advisory committee input is received, a final safety evaluation is made, the administrative record is complied, and a Federal Register final rule is drafted (1, 7). The final regulation is published in the Federal Register and the regulation appears in the Code of Federal Regulations (1).

Table 2. Food regulatory history in the United States

Year	Regulatory Event
1906	President Theodore Roosevelt signed into law the original Food and Drugs Act. This law prohibited interstate commerce in mislabeled or adulterated drugs, foods, and drinks.
1913	The Gould Amendment of 1913 required the plain and conspicuous marking of weight, numerical count, or measure on the outside of food packages.
1927	Reorganization of the US Bureau of Chemistry in 1927 resulted in the formation of the Food, Drug, and Insecticide Administration (later shortened to the Food and Drug Administration) as a regulatory agency.
1938	The passage of the Food, Drug, and Cosmetics Act of 1938 established mechanisms for providing safe tolerances for unavoidable toxic substances in food, and this act authorized standards on the identity and quality of foods.
1940	In 1940, the FDA transferred from the Department of Agriculture to the Federal Security Agency, and Walter G. Campbell became the first Commissioner of Food and Drugs.
1958	Congress passes the Food Additives Amendment of 1958
1960	Congress passes the Color Additives Amendment of 1960. The Food Additives Amendment (1958) and the Color Additive Amendment (1960) included the Delaney clause, stating, "No additive shall be deemed to be safe if it is found to induce cancer when ingested by man or laboratory animals or if it is found, after tests which are appropriate for the evaluation of the safety of food additives, to induce cancer in man or animals." The Delaney clause authorizes the FDA to permit continued use of certain additives on a provisional basis during safety evaluations.
1969	President Nixon orders a review of FDA's food additive decisions.
1973	FDA revises food additive and GRAS regulations.
1982	Select Committee on GRAS Substances completes its review. FDA issues guidance (known as Redbook) based on comprehensive assessment of program. FDA launches its Priority-Based Assessment of Food Additives program.
1997	FDA launches voluntary GRAS notification program.
1999	FDA began to consult with US Department of Agriculture during the review process for ingredients that are proposed for use in meat and poultry products.
2000	FDA launches food contact substance notification program.
2010	Government Accountability Office issues report finding flaws with GRAS program.
2011	Congress passes the FDA Food Safety Modernization Act of 2011.
2012	FDA issued draft guidance on nanotechnology and food; it provides guidance for evaluation of nanomaterials. New nano-engineered substances, whether direct food additives or food contact substances, cannot be GRAS

Table 3. Agencies responsible for regulating food additives

Agency	Functions
US FDA	Protect the public health by ensuring that foods are safe, wholesome, sanitary, and properly labeled. Promote the public health by promptly and efficiently reviewing clinical research and taking appropriate action on the marketing of regulated products in a timely manner. Participate through appropriate processes with representatives of other countries to reduce the burden of regulation, harmonize regulatory requirements, and achieve appropriate reciprocal arrangements. Where appropriate, carry out its mission in consultation with experts in science, medicine, and public health, and in cooperation with consumers, users, manufacturers, importers, packers, distributors, and retailers of regulated products.
US FDA Science Board	Provides advice to the FDA Commissioner and other appropriate officials on a wide variety of food and drug related issues including: specific complex scientific and technical issues important to the agency and its mission; emerging issues within the scientific community; keeping pace with technical and scientific developments, including regulatory science; agency research; and upgrading the agency's scientific and research facilities and training opportunities.
US FDA Food Advisory Committee	Provides advice to the FDA Commissioner and other appropriate officials on emerging food safety, food science, nutrition, and other food-related health issues and may be tasked with making recommendations on matters including: broad scientific and technical food or cosmetic related issues; the safety of new foods and food ingredients; labeling of foods; nutrient needs and nutritional adequacy; and safe exposure limits for food contaminants.

Source: United States Food and Drug Administration.

Indirect additives are approved via a premarket notification process requiring the same data that is required for approval of direct additives by petition (1). Under the Food Additives Amendment, two groups of ingredients were exempted from the regulation process: (1) Prior-sanctioned substances are substances that FDA or USDA had determined safe for use in food prior to the 1958 amendment, and, (2) GRAS (generally recognized as safe) ingredients (6, 8).

Based on the findings of its evaluation, the FDA determines an appropriate level of use of an additive that includes a built-in safety margin (1). Because of inherent limitations of scientific evidence available at any given point in time, FDA must determine if there is a reasonable certainty of no harm to consumers when an additive is used as proposed (1,10). Once an additive is approved, the FDA issues regulations that may include the types of foods in which it can be used, the maximum amounts to be used, and how it should be identified on food labels (1). Because new information becomes available based on research, the FDA continues to re-evaluate the safety of food additives on an ongoing basis. If new information suggests either real or potential harm from the food additive, the FDA may prohibit its use or conduct further evaluation (1). Regulations known as Good Manufacturing Practices (GMP) limit the amount of food ingredients used in foods to the amount necessary to achieve the desired effect. Food manufacturers are required to list all ingredients in the food on the label (1).

FOOD ADDITIVES AND HUMAN HEALTH

Concerns over adverse health effects of food additives have been a subject of ongoing scientific inquiry (5, 6, 11-15). Reactions to food additives can be either dose dependent or idiosyncratic. The idiosyncratic responses to food additives are non-dose dependent and non-immunological.

The dose dependent effects of food additives in humans are evaluated by the acceptable daily intake (ADI) and estimated daily intake (EDI) (6). ADI and EDI estimations are primarily utilized for the evaluation of chronic effects of additives, such as carcinogenesis and mutagenesis (6). The maximum allowable dietary exposure to a food additive is related to ADI (6). ADI index is based on effects of food additives observed in animal models, specifically, the no-observed-adverse-effect level (NOAEL) determined in animal studies from their lifetime exposure the substance (6). Because EDI is based on lifetime exposure, it is an indication of cumulative exposure to a given substance, and reflects the concentration of that substance in the food itself as well as the amount of consumption of the particular food (6). In order to determine ADI, NOAEL is simply divided by 100 (6). Both, the ADI and EDI are determined for each food additive (6). To take into account the addition of new additive or food, the concentration of a food additive is adjusted accordingly (6). FDA approval of a food additive is contingent upon the stipulation that the sum of all EDIs of a food additive from all sources must not exceed the ADI (6). There has been some debate about the application of such a standard in children and adolescents.

It is estimated that 2% of the US population develops sensitivity or an adverse reaction to food additives (6). A subset of population is at a higher risk to hypersensitivity or allergic reactions; for example, in children who have asthma the incidence of hypersensitivity reactions to food additives is estimated to be 10% (6). According to recommendations from the American Academy of Allergy, Asthma, and Immunology, patients who experience an adverse reaction to food additives should specifically be evaluated for sensitivity to annatto and carmine. In addition, to annatto and carmine, the following additives have been reported to cause anaphylaxis: erythritol, guar gum, psyllium, carrageenan, lupine, pectin, gelatin, mycoprotein, and certain spices (15).

Kobylewski and Jacobson (5) published an in-depth review of human and animal studies that looked at each of the currently used food dyes and artificial coloring agents (5). Based on their extensive analysis they found that all of the nine currently FDA approved dyes are associated with adverse health reactions in either animals or humans. These adverse health effects include allergic hypersensitivity reactions, carcinogenicity, and genotoxicity.

The evidence either supporting or refuting such an association between food additives and hyperactivity in children is inconclusive at best and current guidelines do not recommend elimination diet for children who have hyperactivity (15). However, studies show that a small subset of children may be more sensitive to certain food additives (13). For example, a small number of preschool children who are sensitive to tartrazine may benefit from eliminating foods that contains tartrazine (13). Whether or not children with hyperactive behavior should be screened for food/chemical intolerance is still debatable. The current guidelines do not recommend testing the children with hyperactive or other psychiatric disorders for food/chemical hypersensitivity as there is not much evidence that eliminating such dietary components from the diet would change the management of these children (15).

RECOMMENDATIONS

As new chemical substances are synthesized and new naturally occurring ingredients are identified, research should continue on an ongoing basis to ensure safe use of these substances as food additives. Because clinical manifestations of chronic toxicity may be subtle and take several years to develop, long-term surveillance of these substances is important. In addition to studying the acute and chronic health effects from use of additives in humans, their effects on animals and environment should also be closely monitored (2, 3, 12). Research should also focus on safe and sustainable packaging of food as the use of packaged and stored food is common and often necessary (1, 16).

Application of nanotechnology is a rapidly advancing field of study and its application in food industry should also be a focus of future research (9). Advances in biotechnology have made it possible to produce additives in novel ways, not possible before, and is an area of active research. For examples certain biotechnology techniques allow the use of simple microorganisms to produce food additives (1). These additives are essentially the same as naturally occurring food ingredients. In fact, the

FDA first approved the production of bioengineered enzyme rennin back in 1990 (1).

The current regulatory process for food by the FDA has been a subject of debate and experts have suggested a careful review and reform in certain areas (6-10). The regulation or lack of regulation of substances that are considered as generally regarded as safe (GRAS) has come under increased scrutiny. Neltner et al. (2013) looked at some concerns regarding this issue (8). The current regulation allows manufacturers to determine when an additive is GRAS. The manufacturers are not required to submit their review and determination of an additive as GRAS.

In their analysis of food additives Neltner et al. (2013) estimated that of more than 10'000 additives are allowed in food, 43% were GRAS additives (8). The study further found that the manufacturers have made GRAS determinations that allow the use of an estimated 1000 of these additives, without notifying the FDA (8).

In 2010, the US Government Accountability Office (GAO) also scrutinized the GRAS program, concluding that the FDA should strengthen its oversight of GRAS determinations by manufacturers, minimize the potential for conflicts of interest between the FDA and manufacturers, and require the manufacturers to provide the FDA with basic information about their GRAS determination (10). Maffini et al. (10), based on their review of the FDA's food additives safety assessment process, recommended that a further review of FDA's science and decision making and development of a path to modernize food additives safety assessment (10). The authors specifically identified the following as areas of concern: toxicology test guidelines, tools used to predict health outcomes, conflict of interest in manufacturers' decisions, lack of a reassessment strategy, and lack of a definition of harm (10).

CONCLUSION

Food additives are an essential part of today's food production, supply and consumption. Although, it is difficult to be absolutely sure of the safety of each food additive, the food supply in the United States is generally considered safe. FDA, as the main food regulatory agency in the USA continues to provide fairly reassuring oversight of the food industry. However, in the United States, the food additive regulatory agencies and processes have been subject of ongoing criticism and scrutiny in recent years.

REFERENCES

[1] Food and Drug Administration. Food additives. URL: http://www.fda.gov/Food/IngredientsPackagingLabeling/FoodAdditivesIngredients/ucm094211.htm.

[2] Moeller DW. Food, In: Moeller DW. Environmental health, Fourth Edition, Cambridge, MA: Harvard University Press, 2011:113-36.

[3] United States Department of Agriculture. Food safety and inspection service. URL: http://www.fsis.usda.gov/wps/portal/fsis/home.

[4] Kumar A, Madan AK. Color additives: Legislative perspective in the United States, Europe, Australia, and India. Int J Pharma Comp 2014;18(4):293-300.

[5] Kobylewski S, Jacobson MF. Toxicology of food dyes. Int J Occup Environ Health 2012;18(3):220-46.

[6] Rangan C, Barceloux DG. Food additives and sensitivities. Dis Mon 2009;55(5):292-311.

[7] Magnuson B, Munro I, Aboot P, Baldwin N, Lopez-Garcia R, Ly K, et al. Review of the regulation and safety assessment of food substances in various countries and jurisdictions. Food Addit Contam Part A Chem Anal Control Expo Risk Assess 2013;30(7):1147-220.

[8] Neltner TG, Alger HM, O'Reilly JT, Krimsky S, Bero LA, Maffini MV. Conflicts of interest in approvals of additives to food determined to be Generally Recognized as Safe: out of balance. JAMA Intern Med 2013;173(22):2032-6.

[9] Zhang M, Jin J, Chang YN, Chang X, Xing G. Toxicological properties of nanomaterials. J Nanosci Nanotech 2014;14(1):717-29.

[10] Maffini MV, Alger HM, Olson ED, Neltner TG. Looking back to look forward: a review of FDA's Food Additives Safety Assessment and recommendations for modernizing its program. Compr Rev Food Sci Food Safety 2013;12:439–53.

[11] Bledza D, Gromadzinska J, Wasowicz W. Parabens: from environmental studies to human health. Environ Int 2014;67:27-42.

[12] Marshall BM, Levy SB. Food animals and antimicrobials: impacts on human health. Clin Micro Rev 2011;24:718-33.

[13] Martyn DM, McNulty BA, Nugent AP, Gibney MJ. Food additives and preschool children. Proc Nutr Soc 2013;72:109-116.

[14] Oplatowska-Stachowiak M, Elliott CT. Food colors: existing and emerging food safety concerns. Crit Rev Food Sci Nutr 2017;57(3):524-48.

[15] Sampson HA, Aceves S, Bock SA, James J, Jones S, Land D, et al. Food allergy: a practice parameter update – 2014. J Allergy Clin Immunol 2014;134:1016-25.

[16] Russell DAM. Sustainable (food) packaging: An overview. Food Addit Contam Part A Chem Anal Control Expo Risk Assess 2014;31(3):396-401.

Section three: Adolescent health

In: Child and Adolescent Health
Editors: A Tenenbaum and J Merrick
ISBN: 978-1-53617-825-8

Chapter 13

THE RELATIONSHIP BETWEEN BILINGUALISM AND COGNITIVE DEVELOPMENT AMONG SAUDI ARABIAN SCHOOL-AGED CHILDREN

Salman Elbedour**, PhD, Manal Ahmad Sawan, PhD, Joseph A Bawalsah, PhD, Anan Abu Mariam, PhD, Hussien Tarawneh, PhD and Gregory Reed, PhD
Psychology and Special Education Program,
Al-Ahliyya Amman University, Amman, Jordan,
Human Development and Psychoeducational Studies,
Howard University and Human Development and Psychoeducational Studies, Howard University, Washington, DC,
United States of America

* Correspondence: Salman Elbedour, PhD, Psychology and Special Education program, Al-Ahliyya Amman, Amman 19328, Jordan. Email: Selbedour@Howard.edu.

ABSTRACT

The relationship between second language acquisition and cognitive abilities (IQ) has long been the focus of research in the West, yet none had been conducted in Arabic speaking parts of the world. This study gathered data from female high school students in Saudi Arabia to explore the relationship between second language acquisition and IQ. An analysis of covariance revealed a difference between the two language acquisition groups in the Raven's total raw scores, with bilingual students attaining statistically significant and practically significant (i.e., moderate effect size) higher raw scores, on average, than their monolingual peers. Analysis of scaled scores revealed statistically significant differences on all Wechsler Intelligence Scale for Children–Fourth Edition IQ scale subtests (Similarities, Picture Completion, Digital Span, Symbol Search, and Arithmetic). Speaking more than 1 language has linguistic benefits and, as this research confirms, general cognitive benefits. The findings support the benefits of bilingual education programs.

INTRODUCTION

The study of how bilingualism is related to cognitive ability has its roots in the study of how language is related to thought. Jean Piaget (1896-1980) (1) posited that thinking is primary and is manifested initially in overt action and not with words. Language affords the representation of thought (2) and permits the development of higher cognitive operations in the cognitive stage termed formal operations.

An opposing view is the Whorf-Sapir hypothesis, which held that language determines and shapes thought (3). A third view is that of Lev Vygotsky (1896-1934) (4), who proposed that language and thought are initially independent, but later merge as a child begins to socialize. In early childhood, the child has some concepts or thoughts that are not necessarily connected to specific words. To Vygotsky, humans do not experience the world directly, but through the use of psychological tools or signs such as counting systems, writing and diagrams, maps, and language. Those who learn more than one language may gain the advantage of greater cognitive flexibility (4).

Defining bilingualism has presented challenges for researchers, resulting in a wide variation in definitions. Bilingualism has been defined as equal native fluency in two or more languages as well as trying to learn a second language in school. Bialystok (5) argued that bilingualism is a continuum between these two end points. Often bilingual ability is an outcome of a colonial history. For instance, Pakistan and India are members of the Commonwealth, and their legal systems are in English. In addition, a local language (Urdu or Punjabi in Pakistan) is used as in education. Children are educated in both languages from an early age. In Lebanon, French and Arabic are used, and Syria used either French or English as a counterpoint to Arabic. Saudi Arabia never had a colonial history but has had strong ties with both Great Britain and the United States English is widely taught, but Arabic dominates Saudi education. For the purposes of this study we invoke the broadest definition of bilingualism: learning two or more languages while in school.

The threshold theory developed by Cummins (6) contends that bilingualism could have a positive cognitive effect when bilingual students accomplish high levels of linguistic proficiency in both languages. Low levels of proficiency in both languages will have a negative influence on cognitive development. Finally, high proficiency in one language and lower proficiency in the other language could have either a positive or negative effect on a bilingual's cognitive development (6).

Hakuta and Garcia (7) stated, "recent studies suggest that all other things being equal, higher degrees of bilingualism are associated with higher levels of cognitive attainment." Rather than "competition over mental resources by the two languages…there are even possible cognitive advantages to bilingualism" (7). Barac and Bialystok (8) found bilingual children's performance on an executive control task "exceeded monolinguals."

A study by Diaz (9) lends "some support to the claim that bilingualism fosters the development of cognitive abilities, especially during the initial period of second-language learning"; most importantly, results indicated "no negative consequences as a result of an early bilingual experience." In trying to lay the debate to rest, Diamond (10) argued, "Children raised bilingually develop a specific type of cognitive benefit during infancy, and that bilingualism offers some protection against symptoms of Alzheimer's dementia in old people." The "specific cognitive development," according to Diamond (10), is related to "superior executive function," the ability to accommodate a switch in rule change.

The debate over the effects of bilingualism is not simply academic. Funding for various bilingual programs is at risk depending upon the results. Thus research on the cognitive effects of bilingualism has substantial theoretical as well as practical significance.

Peal and Lambert (11) published a seminal study on bilingualism in which they used carefully selected samples that controlled for socioeconomic status (SES). They found that balanced bilingual children, in fact, scored higher on verbal portions of the Stanford-Binet and Wechsler tests and on other tests of cognitive ability, especially those with a strong verbal focus (11, 12). Further, Hakuta and Diaz (12) found that as children became more confident and fluent in the second language, their cognitive abilities and mean IQ scores improved.

This study extends the investigation of the cognitive effects of bilingualism by comparing intellectual abilities between monolingual Arabic and bilingual female Saudi students in Grades 7–11 with a sample of native female Arabic-speaking students in Riyadh, Saudi Arabia. Although significant research has been conducted on the relationship between second language acquisition and intellectual abilities, most of this research has been carried out in developed Western countries. Some research has been conducted in China, Taiwan, and India, but very limited research has been conducted in the Arabic-speaking Middle East, and none in Saudi Arabia.

Saudi Arabia presents a particularly interesting laboratory for study. First, the country is officially (and practically) monolingual in Arabic of the Saudi dialect. Guest workers speak different Arabic dialects or other languages. For native-born Saudi students, however, other languages are taught as foreign languages, sometimes early in the education process. Because the Saudi economy is tightly integrated with the rest of the world, it is in the government's interest to have substantial populations of English,

French, Spanish, Chinese, and Japanese speakers. These languages are taught in Saudi schools teaching native Saudi students who are, by and large, from high SES families. The children of guest workers, to the extent that they live in Saudi Arabia rather than in their homelands, study in separate schools. It is also worth noting that all schools in Saudi Arabia are segregated by gender, with boys and girls studying separately.

Second, many native-born Saudis study European languages (especially English) extensively in school, constituting Fishman's (13) "elite bilingualism" and Lambert and Taylor's (14) "additive bilingualism." To Fishman (13), elite bilingualism occurs when a child with high SES parents becomes fluent in another high-status language in addition to a majority language. To Lambert and Taylor (14), additive bilingualism occurs when a second language is used along with the first in education and economic life.

Third, a large population of nonnative Arabic speakers work and live in Saudi Arabia, but use of their native languages is discouraged, as is the use of nonnative Arabic dialects (15), conditions constituting Fishman's (13) "folk bilingualism" and Lambert and Taylor's (14) "subtractive bilingualism." To Fishman (13), folk bilingualism occurs when a child of low SES parents learns the majority language on the streets. To Lambert and Taylor (14), subtractive bilingualism occurs when a second language replaces a first language in education and economic life.

With this in mind, the main purpose of this study was to explore the extent to which second language learning and acquisition is correlated with higher intellectual abilities of children in Saudi Arabia. For this study, folk and bilingual students (the children of non-Saudi guest workers) were not included in the sample.

Most of the empirical studies cited above investigated the correlation between bilingualism and cognitive development for developed countries. Fewer studies have explored the validity of this relationship in the context of developing countries, including those in the Middle East. Therefore, more research is needed to investigate the relationship between intelligence/cognitive ability and language in developing countries.

In this study, intellectual ability was measured by scaled scores pertaining to the Raven IQ scale and the five subtests of the Wechsler Intelligence Scale for Children–Fourth Edition (WISC-IV; 16) subtests, which were translated to Arabic. The subtests from the WISC-IV scale used were (a) Similarities (measure of verbal comprehension), (b) Picture completion (measure of processing speed), (c) Digit span (measure of working memory), (d) Symbol search (measure of processing speed), and (e) Arithmetic (measure of working memory). The current study addressed two research questions:

- Do Arabic/English-speaking bilingual female students attain higher scores on cognitive development tasks as measured by the Raven test than do Arabic-speaking monolingual female students?
- Is female students' knowledge of more than one language (Arabic/English) associated with higher cognitive intellectual development as measured by WISC-IV subtests (Similarities, picture completion, digital span, symbol search and arithmetic)?

Brody (17) argued that bilingual students increase the average IQ of the population and people with higher IQs (a) perform better at school, (b) are attracted to occupations with greater complexity, (c) learn job-related knowledge more quickly, (d) are able to work more accurately and quickly, and (e) learn nonacademic knowledge more quickly. This implies causality, but our study only explores the correlation between second language acquisition in school and IQ and makes no specific claims about causality in the process of second language acquisition.

These benefits are in addition to the substantial benefits to Saudi Arabia that come directly from having a multilingual population. The Saudi economy is driven by oil and finance. Because both industries are, at their cores, multinational, business often is conducted in languages such as English and Japanese, and having a population educated in these languages allows for the better conduct of business.

OUR STUDY

There were 207 participants in this study: (a) 107 bilingual female Saudi students and (b) 100 monolingual Arabic female Saudi students. All participants were in Grades 7–11. The ages of these participants ranged from 10.8 years (i.e., 10 years and 10 months) to 15.8 years (i.e., 15 years and 10 months), with an average age of 13.48 years (SD = 1.35). The following grades were represented: Grade 7 (n = 29; 14.0%), Grade 8 (n = 43; 20.6%), Grade 9 (n = 52; 25.1%), Grade 10 (n = 38; 18.4%), and Grade 11 (n = 45; 21.7%). Of the 107 bilingual female participants, 10 (9.3%) had been studying English for 1–3 years, 65 (60.7%) for 3–5 years, and 28 (26.2%) had been studying English for 5–10 years. As previously noted, these students tend strongly to come from high SES environments.

After Institutional Review Board report of approval was issued, the primary researcher contacted 10 schools from Riyadh, Saudi Arabia, to request their participation in the study. From the list of female high schools in Riyadh, four high schools were randomly selected to elicit the participation of 207 female students. The principal investigator held a meeting with the school principals with the aim of recruiting a pool of approximately 200 female students (approximately 100 monolingual female students and approximately 100 bilingual female students), to be chosen randomly from Grades 7–11 in the four schools. The student selection process resulted in the selection of 100 bilingual female students and 107 monolingual female students.

The principal investigator strictly complied with all Institutional Review Board rules and from Saudi educational agencies in working with the participants. Selected students who chose not to participate were replaced by a random selection of other eligible students. The bilingual students, again, tended to be elite, additive, high SES bilinguals.

Instruments

Participants were administered the following five subtest measures from the WISC-IV scale (16): Similarities, picture completion, digital span, symbol search, and arithmetic. Participants also completed Raven's (18) Progressive Matrices Test, Standard Version.

Procedure

The tests were administered in a group setting within each school (e.g., school library, or lecture hall) and required approximately 1 hour and 45 minutes to complete. Students receive a detailed description of the study, the importance of the study, measures designed to protect confidentiality, and the implications of this study for future intervention with students. In addition, each student received a consent form for his or her parents and for the student to sign to allow participation. All participants completed all tests/subtests in the same order. Participants followed our instructions, and the principal investigator and a research assistant carefully monitored the administration of the tests.

The principal investigator instructed participants to complete the cognitive tests without assistance from their peers. Participants were instructed not to indicate any personal data that would disclose their identity. Participants did not receive any compensation for participation.

The surveys administered in this study are cognitive-based with less bearing on emotional dimensions. The Raven instruments (Colored Progressive Matrices, Standard Progressive Matrices, and Advanced Progressive Matrices) have been repeatedly studied and found to be reliable measures of Spearman's psychometric g across language and culture and gender groups (19–21).

Hambleton (22) argued that the purpose of translation should be providing productive validity for different languages. He suggested that in order to confirm the accuracy of the translation, two professional translators should translate the test back to English (22). Translated versions of the selected WISC subtests were given to two different Arabic professional translators in Saudi Arabia to validate the accuracy of translation. Some minor changes were made to the translated subtests as a result. Moreover, to confirm the accuracy of the translated version of the subtests, two other professional translators translated these subtests back to English.

OUR FINDINGS

The total Raven test raw score was used in this study. Unfortunately, this raw score could not be converted to a scaled score, because the 29 items used were the same 29 items used by Elbedour, Hur, and Bouchard (23) and DeFries, Plomin, Vandenberg, and Kuse (24) from a shortened version of the Raven test (19) for which no scaled scores are available. Thus the Raven raw total scores were used to compare the two groups.

The 207 participants varied in age, from 10.8 years to 15.8 years ($M = 13.48$, $SD = 1.35$), thus we conducted an analysis of covariance that involved adjustment for age. Results revealed that after adjusting for age, the bilingual group of female Saudi high school students (estimated marginal M [EMM] = 16.06, SE = 0.42) attained statistically significantly higher raw scores, on average, than did the monolingual group of female Saudi high school students (EMM = 13.16, SE = 0.44), $F(1, 204) = 21.11$, $p < .0001$. The effect size, as measured by partial eta-squared, associated with this difference was .09, which, as before, indicated a moderate effect size (25). Nevertheless, caution should be exercised in interpreting this finding because the two groups being compared represented intact (nonrandomized) groups (26).

To examine differences in intellectual abilities scores, the raw scores pertaining to all five WISC-IV scale subtests were converted to scaled scores. Because Digital Span comprised two subtests—Digit Forward and Digit Backward—six WISC-IV subtest scaled scores were analyzed. Table 1 presents the mean, standard deviation, and range for each of the six subtest scaled scores as a function of second language acquisition (i.e., monolingual Arabic vs. bilingual female Saudi high school, Grades 7–11).

Table 1. Mean, standard deviation, and range for each of six WISC-IV subtest scaled scores as a function of form of language acquisition among female Saudi students grades 7-11

Subtest	Bilingual				Monolingual			
	N	*M*	*SD*	Range	*N*	*M*	*SD*	Range
Similarities	107	10.43	2.10	4-14	100	7.67	1.87	4-16
Digit Forward	107	2.86	1.51	1-7	100	1.73	1.18	1-6
Digit Backward	107	1.71	0.94	1-5	100	1.13	0.53	1-4
Symbol Search	107	14.37	4.33	1-19	100	10.96	4.51	1-19
Picture Completion	107	11.64	4.68	1-19	100	9.39	4.14	1-19
Arithmetic	107	5.62	2.39	1-23	99	4.22	1.62	1-13

According to Onwuegbuzie and Daniel (27), variables for which either the standardized skewness coefficient (i.e., skewness coefficient divided by its standard error) or the standardized kurtosis coefficient (i.e., kurtosis coefficient divided by its standard error), or both, are outside the +3 range suggest extreme departure from normality. An examination of the skewness and kurtosis coefficients revealed a serious departure from normality for five of the subtests: Similarities, digital forward, digit backward, symbol search, and arithmetic (see Table 2).

As can be seen in Table 2, for the bilingual group of female Saudi high school students, both the standardized skewness and standardized kurtosis coefficients were outside the + 3 range of normality for Arithmetic (i.e., large positive skew and a leptokurtic distribution that was characterized by a more peaked shape), whereas for Digit Backward (i.e., large positive skew) and Symbol Search (i.e., large negative skew), the standardized skewness coefficient was outside the range of normality. For the monolingual group of female Saudi high school students, both the standardized skewness and standardized kurtosis coefficients were outside the range of normality for Similarities (i.e., large positive skew and a leptokurtic distribution that was characterized by a more peaked shape), Digit Forward (i.e., large positive skew and a leptokurtic distribution that was characterized by a more peaked shape), and Arithmetic (i.e., large negative skew and with a leptokurtic distribution that was characterized by a more peaked shape), whereas, for Digit Backward, the standardized skewness coefficient was outside the range of normality (i.e., large positive skew). Thus, these two sets of standardized skewness and standardized kurtosis coefficients (i.e., for both groups) indicated that only Picture Completion had standardized skewness and standardized kurtosis coefficients that were within the + 3 range of normality, suggesting that this was the only subtest that yielded scores that were (approximately) normally distributed. Caution should be exercised, however, in interpreting this finding.

Table 2. Skewness, kurtosis, and standardized values for each WISC-IV subtest scaled scores as a function of second language acquisition among female Saudi students grades 7–11

Subtest	Bilingual				Monolingual			
	Skewness (*SE*)	**Standardized skewness**	**Kurtosis (*SE*)**	**Standardized kurtosis**	**Skewness (*SE*)**	**Standardized skewness**	**Kurtosis (*SE*)**	**Standardized kurtosis**
Similarities	-0.52 (0.23)	-2.26	-0.06 (0.46)	-0.13	1.07 (0.24)	4.46[a]	3.09 (0.48)	6.44[a]
Digit Forward	0.53 (0.23)	2.30	-0.26 (0.46)	-0.57	1.64 (0.24)	6.83[a]	1.93 (0.48)	4.02[a]
Digit Backward	1.24 (0.23)	5.39[a]	0.86 (0.46)	1.87	4.42 (0.24)	18.42[a]	19.74 (0.48)	1.13
Symbol Search	-0.88 (0.23)	-3.83[a]	0.40 (0.46)	0.87	-0.09 (0.24)	-0.38	-0.30 (0.48)	-0.63
Picture Completion[b]	-0.27 (0.23)	-1.17	-0.50 (0.46)	-1.09	0.37 (0.24)	1.54	0.01 (0.48)	0.02
Arithmetic	3.85 (0.23)	16.74[a]	26.40 (0.48)	55.00[a]	1.69 (0.23)	-7.34[a]	8.53 (0.48)	17.77[a]

Note. Standardized skewness = skewness/standard error (*SE*) of skewness; standardized kurtosis = kurtosis / *SE* of kurtosis.

[a]Denotes a coefficient greater than Onwuegbuzie and Daniel's (2002) cut point of ±3, thereby indicating a serious departure from normality.

[b]Denotes a WISC IV subtest that is (approximately) normally distributed for both language acquisition groups.

Because of the nonnormal nature of the data and heterogeneity of variance, a series of nonparametric independent sample t tests—specifically Mann-Whitney's U—was conducted to examine differences in intellectual abilities, as measured by six sets of WISC-IV subtest scores, between monolingual Arabic and bilingual female Saudi high school students, Grades 7–11. In addition, the Bonferroni adjustment was applied to accommodate the fact that six Mann-Whitney's U were conducted, such that the total experiment-wise error rate did not exceed 5% (28). This correction was undertaken by dividing the nominal alpha value by 6 (i.e., .05/6 = .0083). Therefore, the adjusted level of statistical significance was .0083. After applying the Bonferroni adjustment, the series of Mann-Whitney U tests revealed a statistically significant difference between the two language acquisition groups for all six subtest scores: Similarities, $U = 1704.00$, $p < .0001$; Digit Forward, $U = 2930.00$, $p < .0001$; Digit Backward, $U = 3355.00$, $p < .0001$; Symbol Search, $U = 3000.50$, $p < .0001$; Picture Completion, $U = 3744.00$, $p < .0001$; and Arithmetic, ($U = 2728.00$, $p < .0001$.

It can be seen from Table 1 that for all six subtest scaled scores, the bilingual group of female Saudi high school students attained statistically significantly higher scores than did the monolingual group of female Saudi high school students. The Cohen's (25) d effect size associated with these six sets of differences were as follows: Similarities, $d = 1.38$; Digit Forward, $d = 0.83$; Digit Backward, $d = 0.75$; Symbol Search, $d = 0.77$; Picture Completion, $d = 0.51$; and Arithmetic, $d = 0.68$. According to Cohen's criteria, $d = .2$ represents a small effect size, $d = .5$ represents a moderate effect size, and $d = .8$ represents a large effect size. Thus, the aforementioned effect sizes suggest that Similarities yielded an extremely large effect size; Digit Forward, Digit Backward, and Symbol yielded large effect sizes; Arithmetic yielded a moderate-to-large effect size; and Picture Completion yielded a moderate large effect size.

In the previous section, the bilingual group of female Saudi high school students were compared to the monolingual group of female Saudi high school students, one WISC-IV subtest at a time via a series of univariate analyses, the Mann-Whitney's U. In this section, these two groups are compared with respect to all six sets of scaled scores simultaneously. Specifically, a discriminant analysis was used to conduct this analysis, to further validate the findings obtained from the Mann Whitney U analyses.

Because five of the six scaled scores departed from normality, caution should be exercised in interpreting results stemming from the discriminant analysis. In addition, prior to conducting the discriminant analysis, Box's M test was conducted to assess the homogeneity of the variance-covariance matrix involving the six variables of interest (29). Box's M statistic was 31.76, which suggested heterogeneity of the variance-covariance matrix, $F(21, 151117.49) = 62.22$, $p < .0001$. Because of the presence of heterogeneity, caution should be exercised in interpreting the results of the discriminant analysis.

The discriminant analysis revealed a statistically significant canonical function, Chi-square(6) = 103.91, $p < .0001$, Wilks's Lambda = 0.60. The corresponding canonical correlation was .64, which suggested a moderate to large effect size (25). In addition, the group centroid (the average score on the discriminant function for students in both groups) for this function was 0.79 for the bilingual group of female Saudi high school students and -0.85 for the monolingual group of female Saudi high school students. These statistics indicated that the discriminant function maximally separated these two groups.

Table 3. Standardized and structure coefficients for the six WISC-IV subtest scaled scores

Subtest	**Standardized coefficient**	**Structure coefficient**
Similarities	.79[a]	.85[a]
Digit Forward	.27	.51[a]
Digit Backward	.27	.48[a]
Symbol Search	.24	.46[a]
Picture Completion	-.10	.41[a]
Arithmetic	-.04	.32[a]

[a]Coefficients with effect sizes larger than .3.

An examination of the standardized canonical discriminant function coefficients (Table 3) revealed that, using a cutoff loading of 0.3 (29), the Similarities subtest was practically significant. Further, the structure coefficients (i.e., structure matrix) between the independent variable set and the standardized canonical discriminant function (Table 3) indicated that, using a cutoff loading of 0.3, all six scaled scores discriminated the two language acquisition groups. The Similarities subtest was the most significant predictor of language acquisition group, followed by digit forward, digit backward, symbol search, picture completion, and arithmetic.

DISCUSSION

The findings of the current study broadly fit into the spectrum of recent studies on bilingualism and cognition (11). Our findings, researched in relatively prosperous high school environments in Saudi Arabia, clearly support a positive view of bilingualism. Comparisons were made between the cognitive performances of monolingual and bilingual groups of Saudi students on different cognitive IQ tasks derived from the Raven IQ scale and the five subtests of the WISC-IV translated into Arabic. The IQ tasks were administered in Arabic, the native language of both the monolinguals and bilinguals. Because English proficiency was not assessed, we can offer no discussion of the effects of high proficiency in English but only of the effects of studying English.

The bilingual students attained statistically significantly higher scores on all IQ tasks than did the monolingual students. More specifically, the series of Mann-Whitney U tests revealed a statistically significant difference between the two language acquisition groups for all six subtest scores. The similarities subtest was the most pronounced effect of language acquisition, followed by digit forward, digit backward, symbol search, picture completion, and arithmetic, respectively.

The results for all six subtest scaled scores showed that the bilingual high school students performed significantly better than the monolingual students on IQ subtests. The results of this study provide strong evidence for the plasticity of cognitive systems in response to language experience and provide data showing that female Saudi Arabian students with bilingual backgrounds outperformed their peers on cognitive tasks. Other studies on bilingual families have reached similar conclusions (c.f., 30).

In another survey of studies on bilingualism and intelligence, Barac and Bialystok (31) insisted that bilingualism may have no effect on intelligence, but it does have positive effects on metalinguistic awareness. For example, Michael and Gollan (32) found that bilingual speakers demonstrated improved nonverbal cognitive abilities but more restricted receptive vocabulary in comparison to monolingual natives. Weil (33) also found that native bilingual adults displayed "superior performance" to monolingual adults on a task that measures social cognition, which required subjects to identify emotion from facial expressions.

These findings are somewhat counterintuitive, in that the consequences of an expanded linguistic experience produce better nonverbal processing but poorer verbal processing. However, even these findings have been disputed. When Peal and Lambert tried to replicate their 1960s findings in the early 1990s in Montreal schools in order "document how bilingualism negatively affected intellectual performance so that appropriate solutions could be developed to solve the existing problems of bilingual education," they instead discovered that "the bilingual group performed significantly better than the monolingual group on most of the measures, including verbal intelligence" (cited in 34).

One intriguing implication of this study relates to the issue of full bilingualism (where a person is an equally and natively fluent speaker of two or more languages) versus second (foreign) language acquisition. Because our data do not measure competence in two languages, the findings suggest certainty that the act of learning a second language is associated with higher IQ scores. It may be that simply being a student of another language broadens the intellectual capability of the language learner.

A second implication has to do with national educational policy. If it is in the interest of a nation to have intelligent (high IQ) citizens, then promoting bilingualism as a national educational policy is in order. Of course, the greater the capacity of a population to speak other languages the greater their capacity to engage in trade with other countries. Thus, the substantive value of bilingualism in increasing the ability to economically contribute must be noted, but the effect of learning or acquiring other languages can generate a more intelligent population more capable of prospering in the world.

One prominent limitation needs to be considered when making inferences from this study. The bilingual students were elite and additive bilingual. Further research is needed to examine whether folk bilinguals and/or subtractive bilinguals would also register higher intelligence scores when compared to comparable monolinguals.

In summary, this study provides evidence affirming the merits of bilingual education. But additional research is needed to determine the specific features of bilingual education that affect the various aspects of intellectual functioning.

ACKNOWLEDGMENT

This study is based on the doctoral dissertation of the second author, entitled "The relationship between bilingualism and cognitive development among Saudi Arabian school-aged children," Howard University, Washington, DC, United States.

REFERENCES

[1] Piaget J. The origins of intelligence in children. New York: International Universities Press, 1952.

[2] Piaget J. Adaptation and intelligence: Organic selection and phenocopy. Chicago, IL: University of Chicago Press, 1974.

[3] Whorf B J. Language, thought and reality: Selected writings of Benjamin Lee Whorf. Cambridge, MA: MIT Press, 1956.

[4] Vygotsky L. Thought and language, Rev ed. Cambridge, MA: MIT Press, 2012. (Original work published 1962).
[5] Bialystok E. Reshaping the mind: The benefits of bilingualism. Can J Exp Psychol 2011,65:229-35. doi:10.1037/a0025406.
[6] Cummins J. The influence of bilingualism on cognitive growth: A synthesis of research finding and explanatory hypotheses. Bilingual Education Project 1976,9:1-43.
[7] Hakuta K, Garcia E. Bilingualism and education. Am Psychologist 1989,44:374-9.
[8] Barac R, Bialystok E. Bilingual effects on cognitive and linguistic development: Role of language, cultural background, and education. Child Dev 2012,83(2):413-22.
[9] Diaz R M. Bilingual cognitive development: Addressing three gaps in current research. Child Dev 1985,56:1376-88.
[10] Diamond J. The benefits of multilingualism. Science 2010,330:332-3.
[11] Peal E, Lambert M. The relation of bilingualism to intelligence. Psychol Monogr 1962,76(27):1-23.
[12] Hakuta K, Diaz R. Relationship between the degree of bilingualism and cognitive ability: A critical discussion and some new longitudinal data. In: Nelson K, ed. Children's language, Vol. 5. Hillside, NJ: Erlbaum, 1985:319-44.
[13] Fishman J, ed. Bilingual education: Current perspectives, Vol. 1. Arlington VA: Center for Applied Linguistics, 1977.
[14] Lambert W E, Taylor D M. Language minorities in the United States: Conflicts around assimilation and proposed modes of accommodation. In: Van Home W A, Tonnesen T V, eds. Ethnicity and language, Vol. 6. Madison, WI: Institute on Race and Ethnicity, 1987:58-89.
[15] Rosenhouse J, Goral M. Bilingualism in the Middle East and North Africa: A focus on the Arabic-speaking world. In: Bhatia T, Ritchie W, eds. The handbook of bilingualism. Malden, MA: Blackwell, 2004.
[16] Wechsler D. Wechsler Intelligence Scale for Children, 4th ed. San Antonio, TX: PsychCorp, 2003.
[17] Brody N. Intelligence, schooling, and society. Am Psychologist 1997,52:1046-50.
[18] Raven J C. Standard progressive matrices. London: Lewis, 1958.
[19] Abdel-Khalek A, Raven, J. Normative data from the standardization of Raven's standard progressive matrices in Kuwait in an international context. Soc Behav Pers 2006,34:169-80.
[20] Carlson J, Jensen C M. Reliability of the Raven colored progressive matrices test: Age and ethnic group comparisons. J Consult Clin Psychol 1981;49:20-2.
[21] Kazem A, Alzubaidi A, Yousif YH, Aljamali FA. Psychometric properties of Raven's colored progressive matrices for Omani children aged 5 through 11 years. Soc Behav Pers 2007;35: 1385-98.
[22] Hambleton R. Translating achievement tests for use in cross-national studies. Eur J Psychol Assess 1993;9(1):57-68.

[23] Elbedour S, Hur Y-M, Bouchard T J Jr. Similarity in general mental ability in Bedouin full and half siblings. Intelligence 1997;25(2):71-82.

[24] DeFries JC, Plomin R, Vandenberg SG, Kuse AR. Parent–offspring resemblance for cognitive abilities in the Colorado Adoption Project: Biological, adoptive, and control parents and one-year-old children. Intelligence 1981,5:245-77. doi:10.1016/S0160-2896(81)80012-8.

[25] Cohen J. Statistical power analysis for the behavioral sciences, 2nd ed. Hillsdale, NJ: Erlbaum, 1988.

[26] Onwuegbuzie A J, Daniel L G. Typology of analytical and interpretational errors in quantitative and qualitative educational research. Curr Issues Educ 2003;6(2):1-34. URL: http://cie.asu.edu/volume6/number2.

[27] Onwuegbuzie A J, Daniel L G. Uses and misuses of the correlation coefficient. Res Schools 2002;9(1):73-90.

[28] Ho R. Handbook of univariate and multivariate data analysis and interpretation with SPSS. London: Chapman Hall, 2006.

[29] Tabachnick BG, Fidell LS. Using multivariate statistics, 5th ed. Boston, MA: Allyn Bacon, 2007.

[30] Bain B, Yu A. Cognitive consequences of raising children bilingually: One parent, one language. Can J Psychol 1980;34(4):304-13.

[31] Barac R, Bialystok E. Cognitive development of bilingual children. Language Teacher 2011;44(1):36-54. doi:10.1017/S0261444810000339.

[32] Michael EB, Gollan, TH. Being and becoming a bilingual: Individual differences and consequences for language production. In: Kroll JF, De Groot AMB, eds. Handbook of bilingualism: Psycholinguistic approaches. New York: Oxford University Press, 2005:389-941.

[33] Weil M. Bilingualism and social cognitive development: The effect of dual-language acquisition on nonverbal communication. Dissertation. College of Wooster Libraries, 2012. URL: http://openworks.wooster.

[34] edu/cgi/viewcontent.cgi?article=6454&context=independentstudy.

[35] Crosby R, Prescod R. Effects of bilingualism on cognitive abilities. Anna Gifu Shotoku Gakuen University Faculty of Foreign Language 2009;48:15-21.

In: Child and Adolescent Health
Editors: A Tenenbaum and J Merrick
ISBN: 978-1-53617-825-8

Chapter 14

SCHOOL PSYCHOLOGY: A CASE STUDY AND NEEDS ASSESSMENT IN RIYADH, SAUDI ARABIA

Mona I Alsoqaih[1], PhD, Salman Elbedour[1,*], PhD, Gregory Reed[1], PhD, Kamilah Woodson[1], PhD and Joav Merrick[2-6], MD, MMedSc, DMSc

[1]Department of Human Development and Psychoeducational Studies, School of Education, Howard University, Washington, DC, United States of America
[2]National Institute of Child Health and Human Development, Jerusalem
[3]Office of the Medical Director, Health Services, Division for Intellectual and Developmental Disabilities, Ministry of Social Affairs and Social Services, Jerusalem
[4]Division of Pediatrics, Hadassah Hebrew University Medical Center, Mt Scopus Campus, Jerusalem, Israel
[5]Kentucky Children's Hospital, University of Kentucky School of Medicine, Lexington, Kentucky, United States of America

---

* Correspondence: Professor Salman Elbedour, Department of Human Development and Psychoeducational Studies, School of Education, Howard University, 2441 Fourth Street, NW, Washington, DC 20059, United States. E-mail: selbedour@howard.edu.

[6]Center for Healthy Development, School of Public Health, Georgia State University, Atlanta, Georgia, United States of America

Abstract

This chapter is the first initiative to examine the status of the field of school psychology in the Kingdom of Saudi Arabia. Data was obtained from 150 Saudi school principals, 150 teachers, and 10 chairs of Riyadh-based schools of education or psychology programs. Findings showed a significant lack of university-level training in school psychology, with none of the 10 Riyadh universities surveyed offering any program at any level in school psychology, and only 3 universities offering a PhD program in counseling psychology. The study also revealed a corresponding concern by Riyadh-area school educators that they needed more training in fundamental school psychology functions such as student assessment, diagnosis, intervention, and overall preparedness in serving children who face significant psychological challenges. For example, 83.3% to 99.3% of teachers felt that they were either not able or only able to a limited degree to identify or diagnose any developmental, social, emotional, academic, or mental challenges, and that they needed training. Across the 16 types of challenges, teachers' ability to provide assessment was less than 5% (4.7% in writing and reading problems; 4% in physical disabilities, attention problems, and classroom disciplines; and 3.3% in speech disorders and hearing problems. At least 93% of all teachers said they were not able or able only to some degree to design intervention plans for students' social, academic, mental, emotional, or cognitive challenges. This study provides valuable data on the strengths and deficits of school psychology programs and school psychologists in the Kingdom of Saudi Arabia.

Introduction

School psychology is a scientific field that has gained much attention as it has gained maturity and multifaceted applications and usage over time. According to Merrell et al. (1) school psychology is a crucial player in the educational and mental health processes of various stakeholders, children, and their families, seeking to affect positive change. The role of the school psychologist has transitioned from an initial philosophical base to an evolving scientific database. School psychology originated in the 1890s and soon became a subfield under the American Psychological Association (APA). In 1899, the first school-based psychological clinic was created in the Chicago public schools (2). As a result, school psychology emerged to aid with the identification and placement of students through the development of achievement tests. Proven to be beneficial to the educational field, school psychology became a means for the United States (US) government to reinforce children's rights for education, protection, and safeguarding, as articulated by United Nations Convention on the Rights of the Child; in fact, 2014 was the 25th anniversary of the United Nations Convention on the Rights of the Child.

As the field has evolved, a chief mission of psychology, and school psychology in particular, is to build a strong foundation for children's rights for education and safeguarding. In the US, two organizations, the American Psychological Association (APA), the National Association of School Psychologists (NASP), campaign for children's rights to education, health, and safety through designing school curricula to increase attention to children's rights to fulfill their potential, follow their academic aspirations, and become competent and responsible citizens. School psychologists must make critical decisions to aid in the educational process to enable children of various abilities to reach their potential.

This paper brings to light the need for school psychology as an essential field in the Kingdom of Saudi Arabia. In particular, this study focuses on the importance of in-school psychological services, the individuals who could benefit, and the future of school psychology as the Saudi nation progresses in the 21st century.

Who needs school psychologists and why?

To place the evolving field of school psychology in context, especially as it develops in highly varying cultures around the world, a brief examination of the definition and role of school psychology will be helpful. In the

United States, where school psychology services in public school systems have been established for some time, the American Psychological Association defines school psychology as follows:

> School psychology is a general practice and health service provider specialty of professional psychology that is concerned with the science and practice of psychology with children, youth, families; learners of all ages; and the schooling process. The basic education and training of school psychologists prepares them to provide a range of psychological assessment, intervention, prevention, health promotion, and program development and evaluation services with a special focus on the developmental processes of children and youth within the context of schools, families, and other systems.
>
> School psychologists are prepared to intervene at the individual and system level, and develop, implement, and evaluate preventive programs. In these efforts, they conduct ecologically valid assessments and intervene to promote positive learning environments with which children and youth from diverse backgrounds have equal access to effective educational and psychological services to promote healthy development (1).

Similarly, the US-based National Association of School Psychologists has described the role of school psychologists in this way:

> School psychologists help children and youths succeed academically, socially, behaviorally, and emotionally. They collaborate with educators, parents, and other professional to create safe, healthy, and supportive learning environments that strengthen connections between home, school, and the community for all students.
>
> School psychologists are highly trained in both psychology and education, completing a minimum of a specialist-level degree program (at least 60 graduate semester hours) that includes a yearlong supervised internship. This training emphasizes preparation in mental health and education interventions, child development, learning behavior, motivation, curriculum and instruction, assessment, consultation, collaboration, school law, and systems. School psychologists must be certified and/or licensed by the state in which they work. They also may

> be nationally certified by the National School Psychology Certification Board (NSPCB). The National Association of School Psychologists sets ethical and training standards for practice and service delivery (1)

As these descriptions indicate, school psychology is a subfield of psychology that seeks to apply psychological principles within an educational profession in an educational setting. As a profession, school psychology is a field that has gone through and will continually go through metamorphosis. Zimbardo (3) maintained that psychology and its applied mental health fields such as school psychology have transcended an era of skepticism and entered a new era of validation for societal values. These attitudes and values are incorporated and influenced by psychological research.

Historically, the school psychologist held the role of the gatekeeper within the educational system and "became inextricably linked to intelligence testing and individual assessment and classification" (1). Traditionally, IQ assessment has been a major activity for school psychologists. For example, the Binet-Simon test (Alfred Binet (1857-1911) and Theodore Simon (1872-1961)) was originally developed in France in 1905 to detect "mental retardation" and determine whether students were capable of following the regular school curriculum. The Binet-Simon IQ test has paved the way for a multitude of intelligence tests. Today, educational assessment has turned into a billion-dollar industry that can influence college placement, affect workplace job skills assessments, validate program funding, monitor students on a local, state, national and global level, and aid in the detection of learning deficiencies/disabilities and mental illness.

Slowly, the field has shifted from IQ assessment to the proactive advancement of a healthy environment and the well-being and mental health of individuals. School psychology has shifted from a study of the limited and impaired (i.e., treatment to fix that which is broken) to the integration of professional service delivery that emphasizes "improved academic competence, social and emotional functioning, family-school partnership, classroom instruction, and school-based child and family health and mental health services for all learners" (4).

Bagnato (5) notes that the role of school psychologists in recent years has evolved to include approaches to early intervention, prevention, and providing students with diverse needs, thus strengthening communication skills and relationships with students. The field has also seen shifts to address prevention, intervention, and early screening for children and adolescents – important steps for the improvement of schools' mental health programs as well as the field's transition from epistemology to practicality.

According to Merrell et al. (1), school psychology has struggled, yet has managed to arrive at a place of credibility as a scientific discipline. The number of school psychologists has tripled, and the field's growth has had an enormous impact on the level of research, training, and professional practice (1). According to the NASP and APA, the majority (60 -70%) of school psychologists are found in public institutions of higher education. The rate of female to male graduation is approximately four to one. Narrowing the statistics to doctoral students, based on National Science Foundation (NSF) findings, 71% of psychology doctoral graduates are female. Of these female doctoral students, the NSF found that 75% are counseling psychologists, 76% are clinical psychologists, and 76% are school psychologists. The US Bureau of Labor Statistics' Employment Projections Program projects that between 2010 and 2020, school psychologists will account for 22% of the employed psychologists, an increase of over 30,000 jobs (from 154,300 in 2010 to 188,000 projected for 2020) (6).

As the field of school psychology evolves, school psychologists will increasingly be called upon to: (a) focus on prevention and youth development in place of assessment or diagnosis; (b) increase collaboration with educators and other child service specialties; (c) integrate computerized technology into prevention and intervention activities; (d) increase home–school collaboration; (e) develop culturally sensitive and culturally appropriate services; (f) focus on problem-solving models and professional flexibility; (g) focus on indirect psychological service models;

(h) work to enhance the development, health, and mental health of all children; (i) decrease special education service involvement and increase regular education service participation; (j) become educational curriculum and program evaluation experts; (k) serve as safe school initiative coordinators; (l) serve as performance assessment and outcome specialists; (m) develop self-reflection and recursion; and (n) become proactive in place of being reactive (7).

School psychology: A global view

Recent academic publications have highlighted an increased awareness of the globalization or internationalization of school psychology. However, while school psychology services appear to emerging to a limited degree in many countries around the globe, the majority of the world's 2.2 billion children do not have access to school psychology services (8). Based on data from a 2008 study by Jimerson et al. (9) among the 192 member states of the United Nations, 109 countries (57%) showed no evidence of school psychologists, compared to 83 countries (43%) that did. However, among the 43% countries that did show evidence of having school psychology professionals, only 29 (35%) required "school psychology" to be licensed; 56 countries (67%) had university programs that prepared school psychologists, and only 19 countries (23%) had university programs providing doctoral level preparation in the field.

Nonetheless, there is a clear need for school psychologists in the international arena. Globally, there are far too few school psychologists to serve potentially needy populations. For example, among the 20 nations with the world's largest populations, 80% do not offer any form of school psychological services. As of 2008, these countries were identified as China, India, Indonesia, Pakistan, Bangladesh, Russia Nigeria, Japan, Mexico, Philippines, Vietnam, Egypt, Ethiopia, Iran, Thailand, and the Democratic Republic of Congo (10). As stated earlier, globally an estimated 2.2 billion children lack access to school psychological services (10).

OUR STUDY

This research is presented as the first needs assessment study to be conducted in the city of Riyadh, Saudi Arabia, about the field of school psychology. According to McCawley (11) and Thompson et al. (12), a needs assessment is a methodical approach to epistemology encompassing the learning abilities, interests, or attitudes of a defined group of individuals based on a specific subject matter over a given period of time. Needs assessment has two goals: 1) comprehension of the body of knowledge that already exists in the field in order to determine what educational product or services are needed, and 2) comprehension of what can be done to impart the knowledge to a clientele in a manner that is accessible, acceptable, and useful. Thompson et al. (12) provided six crucial, fundamental components to be provided by a needs assessment: (1) impact on the audience in the form of education and training; (2) approaches that are educationally most effective; 3) awareness of existing programs and deficiencies that allow for training and efficient utilization of resources; 4) outcomes that are generated based on information due to the current situation; 5) demand for future research programs and products; and 6) credibility in the program for serving the targeted audience and communicating to the funding authorities in a competent and professional manner.

The intent of this survey-based needs assessment was to collect data to examine a variety of objectives.

Objective 1 (university and college level)

Here the purpose was to survey the availability and type of degrees (masters and doctoral level) of professional psychology programs including school psychology in Saudi Arabian universities and colleges.

Sample: A descriptive survey (Survey I) was administered to university chairs of the ten leading schools of education or psychology programs in the Kingdom of Saudi Arabia. The chairs of the programs were asked to provide responses regarding the availability of professional psychology programs devoted to the delivery of psychological services to students in schools. For example, the chairs were instructed to indicate if whether their institutions offered clinical, school, counseling, developmental, educational, experimental, general, industrial/ organizational, personality, psychometrics, social and physiological psychology. Chairs were asked to indicate if their institutions offered special education, social work, or school counseling. They were also asked to indicate the modal degree the department offers (master's degree or PhD). The survey was emailed or mailed to the chairs of the 10 departments, and they were instructed to complete the survey and return it to the investigator.

Research question: Do Saudi Arabian universities and colleges offer appropriate professional service delivery psychology programs to address the needs and challenges (e.g., developmental, academic, social, emotional, intellectual) of school-aged children in Saudi Arabian schools?

Objective 2 (school level- school administrators)

We wanted to survey the availability, degree types (masters and doctoral level) and identity of service providers in Riyadh schools (e.g., school psychologist, school counselor, educational psychologist, social worker, clinical psychologist).

Sample: 150 Riyadh-area principals were randomly selected to participate in this study. Of the principals surveyed, 85% held a bachelor's degree and about 11% held a master's degree.

Survey II was administered to school administrators to determine the specialization of service providers of psychological services within their schools. For example, the school administrator was asked if he/she had a service provider in the field of psychological services and the identity of the provider. These providers may include clinical psychologists, counseling psychologists, educational psychologists, general psychologists, and/or personality and school psychologists. In addition, participants were asked if their school had social workers, school counselors, and special educators. The survey also asked whether the psychological service provider held a master's or PhD level degree. The result of this survey presented a picture of availability and status of school psychologists, compared to other related professional service providers in their respective schools.

Research question: Are the present number of mental professional health providers, (e.g., school psychologists, social workers, clinical psychologists) in Riyadh schools sufficient to address the population of Saudi Arabian children with exceptionalities and special needs?

Objective 3 (teacher level)

To assess the knowledge base of teachers in Riyadh schools in areas pertaining to school psychology in particular assessment, diagnosis and intervention as well as the training needs of teachers in regard to specific population with challenges in schools.

Sample: Of the 150 teacher participants, 93.3% held BA degrees and 6.7% held MA degrees. There were only marginal differences between females and males in educational achievement; specifically, 92% of males had BA degrees, compared to 94.7% among females. However, males had slightly higher proportions of master's degrees than did females (8% compared to 5.3%).

Survey III made of three parts were administered to teachers is to determine the knowledge base of 150 teachers who were randomly selected to participate in this study. The survey included three areas/parts: (a) assessment; (b) identification; (c) instruction and intervention. Teachers were instructed to complete all three portions of the survey. The survey sought to identify whether the teacher was adequately trained in areas across the three domains (1-diagnosis, 2-assessment, and 3- intervention and instruction) of service to students with challenges (i.e., learning disabilities, visual impairments or blindness, deafness or being hard of hearing, physical disabilities, speech and communication disorders, and writing problems). Teachers were asked to rate their level of knowledge with respect to assessment, intervention, and instruction (three surveys) of students who have developmental, learning or educational challenges. Teachers were also asked to rate their knowledge on each survey in the following ways: adequately trained; generally adequately trained; and needing significant training in this area. Furthermore, teachers were asked if they had received professional development training in these areas. Responses from teachers across the three domains were used to determine the level of preparation and competencies that teachers demonstrated in the field of psychological services of school-aged children. The survey took participants 20-30 minutes to complete.

Research question: To assess the knowledge base of teachers in Riyadh schools in areas pertaining to school psychology, in particular (1) assessment, (2) diagnosis, and (3) intervention, the following research question was proposed: Is the knowledge base of teachers in Riyadh adequate in order to identify, assess, provide instruction and intervention to students with specific disabilities and exceptionalities?

Recruitment procedure

After the Howard University Institutional Review Board (HUIRB) report of approval was issued, the first survey was emailed or mailed to the chairs of the 10 departments that were randomly selected to participate in this study, and they were instructed to complete the survey (Survey I) and return it to the investigator. A second survey (Survey II) was administered individually to 150 school principals who were randomly selected from school principals to participate in this study and who completed a survey via email, taking participants 20-30 minutes to complete. From the list of schools that agreed to participate (whose principals also volunteered to participate; see above), a random sample of 150 teachers were recruited to complete the teacher survey (Survey III) in the library hall.

Participating schools' program chairs, school principals, and teachers were apprised of the importance of the study. The confidentiality procedures of the study were fully explained to participants. The fact that participation was on a voluntary basis was stressed. To assure as much consistency as possible, all participants (chairs, school principals, and teachers) were given the same directions. Just as with the department chairs, each subject was given a brief description of the study's importance, the format of the study, and ethical research guidelines outlined by the American Psychological Association in 1992 to maintain subject's confidentiality. As part of those guidelines, subjects were assured that no background or personal information would be shared, that all data was aggregated, and no data was collected on a personal level. To guarantee this, subjects were reminded not to disclose any personal information. In addition, it was made clear to survey subjects that they would receive no direct benefit for participating in the study.

Table 1. Degrees offered in professional psychology programs in Saudi Arabian universities

Psychology specialty	Master's	PhD	Any degree
Clinical psychology	0	1	1
Counseling psychology	5	3	8
Development psychology	1	2	3
Educational psychology	2	1	3
Experimental psychology	0	0	0
General psychology	0	1	1
Industrial psychology	1	0	1
Personality psychology	1	1	2
Physiological psychology	0	0	0
Psychometrics	0	0	0
School psychology	0	0	0
School counseling	0	0	0
Special education	2	0	2
Social psychology	3	2	5
Psychiatrics psychology	1	1	2
Social work	3	1	4

FINDINGS

Table 1 depicts the availability and type of degree (master's and doctoral level) of professional psychology programs, including school psychology, in Saudi Arabian universities and colleges. The following tables represent the responses of ten chairs of psychology or education. None of the ten universities has any program at any level in these fields of psychology: school psychology, experimental, physiological, psychometrics, and school counseling. Only three universities offer a PhD program in counseling psychology, only two universities offer a PhD program in development and social psychology, and six universities offer only a PhD program in psychology: clinical, educational, general, personality, psychiatrics, and social work psychology.

The distribution of master's degrees is similar to that of PhDs. Five universities have a master's degree level program in counseling psychology, three universities have a master's degree program in social psychology and social work; two universities have a program in educational and special education; and four universities have only one program at the master's level, including developmental psychology, industrial psychology, personality psychology, and, psychiatrics psychology. None of the ten universities offer a master's degree in the remaining seven specialties.

As shown in Table 2, out of the 150 principals, 88.7% hold a bachelor's degree and about 11% hold master's degrees. When viewed by gender, 85% of males and 92% of females hold bachelor's degrees, while 15% of males and 8% of females hold master's degrees. None of the participants in the sample hold Ph.D. degrees. The different geographical regions have almost the same distribution of principals' education degrees. The percentages of bachelor's degree holders range from 83% in the north to 93% in the west and south.

The second research question examined the availability of degree types (master's and doctoral level) and identity of service providers in Riyadh schools (e.g., school psychologist, school counselor, educational psychologist, social worker, clinical psychologist, etc.). Based on school principals' reports, the results (see Table 2) showed that only three types of specializations exist in their schools. These are general psychology (20%), with 14.7% holding BA degrees and 5.3% holding master's degrees; special education (39%), with 33.7% holding BA degrees and 5.3% holding master's degrees; and social work (41%), with 38.9% holding BA degrees and 2.1% holding master's degrees. The schools have no representations from the other related fields such as clinical psychology, school psychology, counseling psychology, school counseling, or psychiatry.

As Table 2 shows, in nine out of the twelve specialties, all the schools lack specialists in any field. In only three fields – general psychology, special psychology, and social work – about a quarter of the service providers hold a bachelor degree. Based on this data, the present number of mental professional health providers is insufficient to address the population of Saudi Arabian children with exceptionalities and special needs.

Table 2. Distribution of specialties by degree according to reporting by school principals

Type of specialty of professional health provider in school	University degree			
	No degree	Bachelor's	Master's	PhD
Clinical psychology	100.0%	0.0%	0.0%	0.0%
Counseling psychology	100.0%	0.0%	0.0%	0.0%
Development psychology	100.0%	0.0%	0.0%	0.0%
Educational psychology	100.0%	0.0%	0.0%	0.0%
General psychology		14.7%	5.3%	0.0%
Physiological psychology	100.0%	0.0%	0.0%	0.0%
School counseling	100.0%	0.0%	0.0%	0.0%
Special education		33.7%	5.3%	0.0%
School counseling	100.0%	0.0%	0.0%	0.0%
Personality psychology	100.0%	0.0%	0.0%	0.0%
Psychiatrics psychology	100.0%	0.0%	0.0%	0.0%
Social work		38.9%	2.1%	0.0%

School level: Teachers

The third research question examined the knowledge base of teachers in three major school psychology areas: diagnosis, assessment, and providing intervention plans.

The sample included 150 teachers from five different regions, with 30 teachers from each region divided equally between females and males and between school levels: elementary, middle and high. Of the teachers surveyed, 93.3% held a BA degree and 6.7% held MA degrees, with marginal differences between females and males in educational achievements; specifically, 92% of males had obtained BA degrees, compared to 94.7% of females. However, males achieved a slightly higher number of master's degrees than females (8% compared to 5.3%).

In Table 3, we can see that the percentage of teachers who are either not able or able to some degree to identify any of the difficulties and need training ranges from 83.3% for classroom disciplines to 99.3% in sexual assault victims. The distribution is not uniform among the different difficulties. The most striking figure is the 84% who said they were not able to identify characteristics of sexual assault; this number, combined with another 15.3% who said they were able to identify sexual assault victims "to some degree" yields a glaring 99.3% of teachers who believe they are in need of training and preparation to identify characteristics of sexual assault victims. Similarly, 99.3% of teachers also show very limited competency to identify victims of crises situations. For example, 97.3% and 96% of teachers felt they were not able to identify motivational and attitudinal or anxiety and depression symptoms, respectively. These figures attest to the limited preparation and competency of teachers in identifying and diagnosing emotional, academic, behavioral, biological, personality disabilities or challenges.

Table 3. Teachers' identification of student difficulties and level of training

Type of difficulty	Ability to diagnose the following difficulties			Did you receive training in this field?	
	Not able & need training	Able to some degree & need training	Very able & no need for additional training	Never	Yes
Learning disabilities all	24.7%	66.7%	8.7%	94.0%	6.0%
Visually impaired/blind all	32.0%	60.0%	8.0%	99.3%	0.7%
Deaf/hard of hearing all	33.3%	57.3%	9.3%	99.3%	0.7%
Physical disabilities all	25.3%	58.7%	16.0%	97.3%	2.7%
Speech and communication disorders	44.7%	44.7%	10.7%	95.3%	4.7%
Writing problems all	16.7%	68.0%	15.3%	88.7%	11.3%
Reading problems all	20.7%	62.7%	16.7%	92.7%	7.3%
Mathematics problems all	35.3%	52.7%	12.0%	94.0%	6.0%
Attention problems all	54.0%	36.7%	9.3%	99.3%	0.7%
Mental retardation all	46.7%	43.3%	10.0%	98.0%	2.0%
Anxiety/depression all	66.0%	30.0%	4.0%	99.3%	0.7%
Conduct delinquency all	58.7%	37.3%	4.0%	98.7%	1.3%
Motivational/attitudinal problems	76.7%	20.7%	2.7%	99.3%	0.7%
Sexual assault victims all	84.0%	15.3%	0.7%	100.0%	0.0%
Crises situations all	69.3%	30.0%	0.7%	100.0%	0.0%
Classroom disciplines all	14.0%	69.3%	16.7%	81.3%	18.7%

The percentage of teachers who believe they are very able and do not need any training barely exceeds 15%. Only in the following difficulties does the competency percentage exceed 10%: 16.7 in classroom disciplines, 16% in physical disabilities, 16.7% in reading problems, 15.3% in writing problems, 12% in mathematical problems 10.7% in communication disorders, and 10% in mental retardation, in declining order. Interestingly, the percentages of males who are able to some degree to diagnose the different difficulties but feel the need for extra training was always higher than those of females. For example, among male teachers, those who felt they needed extra training totaled 30.7% in communication disorders, 28% in the case of mental retardation, and 24% in the case of learning disabilities and conduct delinquency. However, the percentage of females who felt very able to diagnose problems and felt they needed no more training were higher, in general, than those of males: 21.3% in the case of physical disabilities, 18.7% in the case of communication disorders, 17.3% in reading and writing problems, and 16% in attention problems.

Regarding the question of whether teachers received training in identifying any of the difficulties in different fields, in almost all the listed fields in Table 3, most teachers (both male and female) received no training or preparation, ranging from 81.3% receiving no training regarding classroom disciplines, to 100% receiving no training in cases of sexual assault victims and crises situations. In the case of classroom disciplines, 18.7% reported that they had received training. The differences between males and males were marginal.

Table 4 presents the knowledge base of the same teachers assessment, the ability to use reliable and valid tools to assess in the area of assessing of disabilities, exceptionality, and challenges (e.g., academic, behavioral, emotional, and social). Results show that across all areas of challenges, at least 96% of the teachers are not able or able only to some extent to assess disabilities and challenges, and therefore need training. Across the 16 types of challenges presented to teachers (see Table 4), the ability of teachers in the area of assessment does not exceed 4.7% (e.g., 4.7% in the areas of writing and reading problems; 4% in the areas of physical disabilities, attention problems, and classroom disciplines; and 3.3% in the areas of speech and communication disorders and deafness and hearing problems). These results convey strong evidence that teachers are not able to assess any of the problems and feel the need to obtain training.

Table 4. Teachers' competence in student assessment, compared to level of training

Type of difficulty	Ability to diagnose the following difficulties			Did you receive training in this field?	
	Not able & need training	Able to some degree & need training	Very able & no need for additional training	Never	Yes
Learning disabilities	89.3%	8.7%	2.0%	99.3%	0.7%
Visually impaired/blind	88.7%	8.0%	3.3%	99.3%	0.7%
Deaf/hard of hearing	90.0%	6.7%	3.3%	99.3%	0.7%
Physical disabilities	90.0%	6.0%	4.0%	100.0%	0.0%
Speech and communication disorders	90.7%	6.0%	3.3%	100.0%	0.0%
Writing problems	88.0%	7.3%	4.7%	100.0%	0.0%
Reading problems	90.0%	5.3%	4.7%	99.3%	0.7%
Mathematics problems	90.0%	7.3%	2.7%	99.3%	0.7%
Attention problems	92.7%	3.3%	4.0%	100.0%	0.0%
Mental retardation	92.0%	5.3%	2.7%	100.0%	0.0%
Anxiety/depression all	93.3%	6.0%	0.7%	100.0%	0.0%
Conduct delinquency all	94.7%	4.7%	0.7%	100.0%	0.0%
Motivational/attitudinal problems	93.3%	6.0%	0.7%	100.0%	0.0%
Sexual assault victims	91.3%	7.3%	1.3%	100.0%	0.0%
Crises situations	91.3%	6.7%	2.0%	100.0%	0.0%
Classroom disciplines	85.3%	10.7%	4.0%	100.0%	0.0%

Table 5. Teachers' competence in intervention, compared to level of training

Type of difficulty	Ability to diagnose the following difficulties			Did you receive training in this field?	
	Not able & need training	Able to some degree & need training	Very able & no need for additional training	Never	Yes
Learning disabilities	85.3%	14.0%	0.7%	98.0%	2.0%
Visually impaired/blind	89.3%	8.7%	2.0%	100.0%	0.0%
Deaf/hard of hearing	90.0%	7.3%	2.7%	100.0%	0.0%
Physical disabilities	91.3%	7.3%	1.3%	99.3%	0.7%
Speech and communication disorders	86.7%	12.7%	0.7%	98.7%	1.3%
Writing problems	50.0%	43.3%	6.7%	85.3%	14.7%
Reading problems	46.0%	48.0%	6.0%	90.7%	9.3%
Mathematics problems	62.0%	32.7%	5.3%	91.3%	8.7%
Attention problems	87.3%	11.3%	1.3%	100.0%	0.0%
Mental retardation	92.7%	6.0%	1.3%	100.0%	0.0%
Anxiety/depression	91.3%	8.0%	0.7%	100.0%	0.0%
Conduct delinquency	86.7%	13.3%	0.0%	99.3%	0.7%
Motivational/attitudinal problems	92.7%	6.7%	0.7%	99.3%	0.7%
Sexual assault victims	95.3%	4.7%	0.0%	100.0%	0.0%
Crises situations	88.7%	11.3%	0.0%	99.3%	0.7%
Classroom disciplines	39.3%	54.0%	6.7%	77.3%	22.7%

In Table 5, results show that at least 93% of all teachers are not able or are able only to some degree to design intervention plans when faced with students' exceptionality, challenges, disabilities (e.g., developmental, learning, social, emotional, biological, or mental). For example, none of the teachers in three areas – conduct delinquency, sexual assault victims, and crises situations – show any evidence of competency in designing or building intervention programs, and are therefore in need of training in these areas. Less than 1% of the teachers felt they were able to provide intervention psychological services in the following areas: learning disabilities (0.7%), anxiety and depression (0.7%), speech and communication disorders (0.7%), and motivational/attitudinal problems (0.7%). Again, these results are strong evidence that teachers are not able to intervene in solving any of these problems, and they feel the need to get training.

Regarding the question of whether teachers received training in intervening in any of the difficulties in different fields, it is safe to say that none of teachers, males or females, ever had any specific training in these areas.

To sum up the findings from Tables 3-5, we can conclude with high confidence that teachers in Saudi Arabian schools feel unable to identify, assess, or intervene in any of the above psychological difficulties facing their students. Even more disturbing, despite the absence of any training, high percentages of teachers intervene to deal with some of these difficulties (54% in the case of classroom discipline). The clear message is that much more effort needs to be put into training teachers to identify, assess, and intervene in solving the psychological difficulties facing Saudi schoolchildren.

DISCUSSION

International school psychology is a relatively young field. Venezuela formed the first freestanding school psychology professional association in 1968. Since then, school psychology associations have been created in at least 23 countries (8). The United Nation's declaration of 1979 as the Year of the Child helped advance the status of international school psychology. Before this UN Convention, the field of psychology had always been a "strong supporter of children's rights in words and deeds." In the last quarter century since the announcement of the Year of the Child, school psychology in particular has played a leading role "in actualizing the Convention" (13) as well as continuing to monitor its adherents. One country that could benefit from the creation of school psychology training programs is Saudi Arabia. The findings demonstrated that none of the ten Saudi universities in a random survey of graduate programs in psychology or education had either master's or PhD programs in school psychology.

However, just when turbulence around the globe has caused children and families to be "on the move in unprecedented numbers" (14), leading to a greater need for psychological services, funding for school psychologists is threatened by budget cuts, even in relatively wealthy countries like Saudi Arabia. Across the 16 types of challenges presented to teachers, the ability of teachers to perform formal assessment did not exceed 4.7% (e.g., 4.7% in the areas of writing and reading problems; 4% in the areas of physical disabilities, attention problems, and classroom disciplines; and 3.3% in the areas of speech and communication disorders and deafness and hearing problems). These findings of this study conveyed strong evidence of the limited competencies of teachers in diagnosis, assessment, and intervention and then expressed need of Saudi teachers to obtain training in this area.

The recent worldwide Great Recession has forced school districts in the United States to find budget cuts. And even though federal special education law requires students be evaluated for services, some school districts are cutting positions, not filling vacancies, and shortening the hours of psychologists on staff. Before these cuts, the United States was second in the world in the ratio of school psychologists to students, with one practitioner for every 1,506 schoolchildren. Turkey ranked first, with one school psychologist for every 1,267 students. Japan was third. These were the only three countries with ratios smaller than 1 to 5,000 (15). The findings certainly demonstrate that the Saudi School don't have teachers who are professionally equipped to assess, identify and intervene nor have the number of school psychologists that we feel is necessary to address the academic, developmental, cognitive or socioemotional challenges faced by Saudi school-aged children.

For example, Turkey is currently facing political and economic turmoil. For May 2016, the number of tourists to arrive in the country "fell 34.7 per cent, year-on-year – the biggest drop in 22 years. Each month this year has registered a double-digit percentage point fall, apart from January where visitors fell just 6.4 per cent" (16). With tourism providing almost 13% of Turkey's GDP in 2015 (Turkey), such a drop will have a dramatic ripple effect across the economy as tensions over relations with the Kurds, Russia, Syria, ISIL and other actors continue to simmer. (By comparison, tourism in the US contributes 8% to the GDP, according to the World Travel and Tourism Council in 2015). Turkey has done "a commendable job in welcoming the Syrian refugees, setting up entire cities equipped with clinics and schools" (17), but it may be difficult to continue helping at that pace.

Draguns (18) was already speaking out for the strengthening of international school psychology because of the plight of refugees long before the current global refugee crisis, with "approximately half of the 19.5 million registered refugees globally" being children and youth (14). To enhance international school psychology, the author focuses on language, since much of the exchange of information currently occurs in English, while many of the problems are occurring in non-English-speaking countries. "It has been proposed," Draguns wrote, "that all psychotherapy is embedded in the cultural milieu in which it occurs" (18). Given that observation, Draguns (18) insisted it would be best if somehow psychologists could "overcome the linguistic isolation from psychologists for whom English is not the principal language" including psychological service delivery professional from Saudi Arabia and Middle-East. Although admitting it would be costly, Draguns proposed translating non-English papers at conventions and expanding the foreign language options for school psychology journal papers (18).

Almost as if in response to Draguns' concerns, Jimerson (13) indicated in the publication School Psychology Quarterly that "there is particular interest in featuring informative scholarship from colleagues around the world, including multisite national and international projects, with a focus on empirical work that has the potential to be adapted to and implemented around the globe" (13), while stressing every manuscript is subject to same policies and guidelines.

Despite the economic hurdles, the increase in turmoil world-wide, the over-emphasis on English, and the potential saturation of the subject in academia, school psychology continues to be of great importance. As Oakland (19) wrote, "Schools often provide the only stable and accessible portal to boys and girls of every class and race. Schools are found in all countries and constitute the only universal institution with which psychology has had an abiding relationship" (19). Fortunately, despite its relative youth, school psychology has a robust training process. The ISPA (International School Psychologist Association) approved International Guidelines for the Preparation of School Psychologists in 1996. In addition, these guidelines outline a model curriculum for school psychology programs, one that includes supervised practica and internships (19).

While some signs of growth in the field of school services are apparent in large countries that had few school psychologists previously, such as the People's Republic of China and the Russian Federation, in most other countries expansion is not apparent (19). Still, school psychology has yet to emerge in many countries (20) such as Saudi Arabia and other countries of the Middle-East. Based on data from a 2008 study (9) it was found that among the 192 member states of the United Nations, 109 countries (57%) showed no evidence of school psychologists, compared to 83 countries (43%) that did. However, of the 83 countries that claimed to have school psychological services, only 29 countries (or 35%) required the licensing of school psychologists. That means the majority of the world's 2.2 billion children do not have access to school psychology services (9) or, if they do, those school psychologists may be inadequately trained. Only 19 countries (23%) have university programs providing doctoral level preparation in the field. Because cultural context and language is important, it would be best if school psychologists could be trained in the countries in which they practice. In Saudi Arabia, the finding of this study demonstrates lack of school psychology and other related professional special program offerings school counseling.

Therefore, one country that could benefit from the creation of school psychology training programs is Saudi Arabia. An average of 96% of the Saudi teachers surveyed for this study said they had received no special training that would help them recognize challenges faced by students in 16 areas ranging from sexual assault to reading problems. The good and bad news is that an average of almost 44% of these teachers understood that they could use some training in the various areas of challenge. The fact that they recognized their need is important because it shows a willingness to get help. The fact that the number is so high does not reflect well on the kinds of services students are getting in some areas.

The survey numbers of teachers who claimed to have some sort of training in assessing the challenges is even more telling, with an average of 98.6% of teachers admitting they had no training in assessing the challenges in the same 16 areas. Once again a significant average – a little under 91% – acknowledged they could use some help.

The survey numbers regarding the teachers' abilities to create intervention programs were very similar to the numbers for recognizing the challenges, with an average of 96.1% of the teachers saying they received no training for designing and implementing interventions and an average of almost 80% admitting they could use some training in the 16 areas of challenges.

Despite these shortcomings, Saudi Arabia seems well positioned to expand its educational offerings into the specialty of school psychology, for education has always been "valued, encouraged, and supported by Islam" (21). The Turks built famous schools on the Arabia peninsula after the Ottoman conquest of Arabs in 1517, but education stagnated from that point until after World War I. At the outbreak of World War I, only religious schools, a small regional education system set up by the Turks, and a few private schools existed in Arabia. The Directorate of Education took over the private schools in the Hijaz shortly after Abdulaziz al Saud unified the country in 1925 and established the first public elementary school (22). Although “Islam has no specific statement about separating men from women in the field of education and labour” (23), no formal public schooling for girls existed in Saudi Arabia for many years, although there is evidence that immigrants established the first private girls’ school in 1941 or 1942 (24).

The Ministry of Education was established in Saudi Arabia in the early 1950s. In 1957 the first university opened in Riyadh. By 1958, the government offered six years of elementary school and three years of intermediate and secondary school, much like the system in the U.S. of elementary, junior, and senior high school (25). Under specific guidelines, the first public school for girls started in Riyadh in 1960 and women were allowed to work for the government as teachers and school administrators. In the mid-1960s, fewer than 100 Saudi female college students were matriculating (22).

Much changed in the next decades. By 1990, women represented 47% of total undergraduate college enrollment (26). Within a dozen years, women accounted for a majority of college graduates (22). Over a quarter century after the first government-sanctioned education of women, more than 70% of all occupations held by Saudi women in Saudi Arabia involved teaching (25).

In 2005, the new leader of Saudi Arabia, King Abdullah, focused much energy on education. According to Arab News (2014 April 3), “When King Abdullah ascended the throne in 2005, there were seven public universities. Ten years later, there are 28 public and nine private universities. In addition, at least 10 more universities are expected to open within the next five years.” The private Prince Mohammad Bin Fahd University in the Eastern Province opened its doors in 2006, becoming “the first to enroll both male and female students in separate facilities” (27).

In 2011, the Princess Nora bint Abdulrahman University (PNU), the world’s largest university for women, opened in Saudi Arabia. Estimated to cost more than $11.5 billion and planned to house 15 colleges, the university is expected to enroll up to 50,000 women (27).

In 2016, the Saudi education system—the only Arab system ever to be thus honored—was rated "one of the top fifty [28 out of 50] educational systems in the world" in recognition of the hard work and resources that have gone into it (28). Media outlets such as US News and World Report now rank some Saudi universities in the top 400 universities worldwide.

Given the increasing excellence of Saudi higher education, its preponderance of female students, the fact that most school psychologists are women in their 30s (19), and the ability of Saudi females to get jobs in education, it would seem there is a perfect convergence of opportunities to begin programs in school psychology within Saudi Arabia's university system.

Both male and female school psychologists would be a great benefit to Saudi schools. According to the NASP, school psychologists can work with teachers in many of the areas in which Saudi teachers feel deficient, including data collection and analysis; assessment; progress monitoring; school-wide practices to promote learning; resilience and risk factors; consultation and collaboration with teachers and other staff and administrators; academic/learning interventions; mental health interventions; behavioral interventions; instructional support, prevention and intervention services; special education services; crisis preparedness; response and recovery to crises; family-school-community collaboration; diversity in development and learning; research and program evaluation; and professional ethics, school law, and systems.

Finally, the present survey research has inherent limitations and strengths. First, data for the current study was drawn primarily from Riyadh schools, and such limited sampling is likely to produce a sample that is not fully representative of the total school principals, teachers, and student population in the Saudi Arabia. Future researchers might wish to reproduce this study with more rigorous stratified sampling methods from different locations in Saudi Arabia that will better represent the whole community of school principals, teachers, and students. Because of the stigma associated with psychology, subjects may not have reported their responses to the survey questions in honest and genuine ways that may color their feelings and create a bias in the findings. Finally, this survey study represents the first study on this topic; therefore; baseline data does not exist to validate the findings of the present study.

Despite these potential flaws, this study is timely; its findings may serve as the foundation for understanding the nature, quality, and need of professional psychological services in Saudi schools.

REFERENCES

[1] Merrell WM, Ervin RA, Peacock GG. School psychology for the 21st century: Foundation and practices. New York: Guilford, 2012.

[2] Tharinger DJ, Miller JA, Pryzwansky WB. School psychology: A specialty of professional psychology with distinct competencies and complexities. Prof Psychol Res Pract 2008;39(5):529-36. doi: 10.1037/0735-7028.39.5.529.

[3] Zimbardo P. Does psychology make a significant difference in our lives? Am Psychol 2004;59(5):339-51.

[4] Ysseldyke J, Burns M, Dawson P, Brenna K, Morrison D, Ortiz S, et al. School psychology: A blueprint for training and practice III. Bethesda, MD: National Association School Psychologists, 2006.

[5] Bagnato SJ. Of helping and measuring for early childhood intervention: Reflections on issues and school psychology's role. Sch Psychol Rev 2006;35(4):615-20.

[6] US Department of Labor. Bureau of Labor Statistics. URL: http://www.bls.gov/ooh/Life-Physical-and-Social-Science/Psychologists.htm#tab-6.

[7] Sheridan SM, D'Amato RD. Partnering to chart our futures: School Psychology Review and School Psychology Quarterly Combined Issue on the Multisite Conference on the future of school psychology. Sch Psychol Quart 2003;18(4): 352–7.

[8] Oakland T, Jimerson S. Best practices in school psychology: History and current status of school psychology internationally. In: Thomas A, Grimes J, eds., Best practices in school psychology V. Bethesda, MD: National Association School Psychologists, 2008.

[9] Jimerson SR, Skokut M, Cardenas S, Malone H, Stewart K. Where in the world is school psychology: Examining evidence of school psychology around the globe. Sch Psychol Int 2008;29:131-44. Doi: 10.1177/0143034308090056.

[10] Thomas A, Grimes J, eds. Best practices in school psychology V. Bethesda, MD: National Association School Psychologists, 2010.

[11] McCawley PF. Methods for conducting an educational needs assessment: Guidelines for cooperative extension system professionals. Moscow, ID: University of Idaho Extension, 2009:3-23.

[12] Thompson DW, Loesch LC, Seraphine AE. Development of an instrument to assess the counseling needs of elementary school students. Am Sch Couns Assoc 2003;7(1);35-9.

[13] Jimerson SR. Enhancing science, practice, and policy relevant to school psychology around the world. Sch Psychol Quart 2014;29(1):1-6. doi: 10.1037/spq0000066.

[14] Save the Children. Refugee children crisis, 2016. URL: http://www.savethechildren.org/site/c.8rKLIXMGIpI4E/b.9311443/k.5C24/Refugee_Children_Crisis.htm.

[15] Jimerson SR, Stewart K, Skokut M, Cardenas S, Malone H. How many school psychologists are there in the each country of the world? International estimates of school psychologists and school psychologist-to-student ratios. Sch Psychol Int 2009;30(6):555-67. doi: 10.1177/0143034309107077.

[16] Morris H. Is Turkey safe for tourists? The Telegraph 2016 Jun 29. URL: http://www.telegraph.co.uk/travel/advice/is-turkey-safe-for-tourists/.

[17] Cagaptay S. The impact of Syria's refugees on southern Turkey. Washington, DC: Washington Institute Near East Policy, 2014.

[18] Draguns JG. Toward a truly international psychology: Beyond English only. Am Psychol 2001;56(11):1019-30.

[19] Oakland TD. International school psychology: Psychology's worldwide portal to children and youth. Am Psychol 2003;58(11):985-92.

[20] Cook CR, Jimerson SR, Begeny JC. A model for predicting the presence of school psychology: An international examination of sociocultural, sociopolitical and socioeconomic influences. Sch Psychol Int 2010;31(4):438-61. doi: 10.1177/0143034310377580.

[21] Saleh MA. Development of higher education in Saudi Arabia. Higher Education 1986;15(1/2):17-23.

[22] Rugh WA. Education in Saudi Arabia: Choices and constraints. Middle East Policy 2002; 9(2):40.

[23] Al-Hariri R. Islam's point of view on women's education in Saudi Arabia. Comparat Education 1987;23(1):51-7.

[24] Bubshait A. Saudi women's education: History, reality and challenges. In: Women in Saudi Arabia: Cross-cultural views. Riyadh, Saudi Arabia: Ghainaa Publications, 2008:18-29.

[25] Al Rawf HS, Simmons C. The education of women in Saudi Arabia. Comparat Education 1991;27(3):287-95.

[26] Hamdan A. Women and education in Saudi Arabia: Challenges and achievements. Int Educ J 2005;6(1):42-64.

[27] Profanter A. Achievements and challenges in the educational realm in Saudi Arabia. Eur Sci J 2014;1:207-22.

[28] Ratyan MAM, Mohammad AAM. Saudi higher education reality and prospects: Evaluating careers' dimensions of university teaching, scientific research and community service using Northern Border University as a model. Indian J Sci Technol 2016;96(4):1-16.

In: Child and Adolescent Health
Editors: A Tenenbaum and J Merrick
ISBN: 978-1-53617-825-8

Chapter 15

EXPLORING PHYSICAL ACTIVITY ENGAGEMENT IN SECONDARY SCHOOL STUDENTS IN MONTEVIDEO, URUGUAY: A QUALITATIVE STUDY

Irene Parobii[1], BS, MPH,
Andrew E Springer[2,*], BA, MPH, DrPH,
Melissa B Harrell[2], BS, MPH, PhD,
Lucía Martinez Gomensoro[3], BSc,
María Traversa Fresco[3], BSc, Nianest Alers[4], BS, MPH,
Cheryl L Perry[2], BA, MA, PhD
and Diego Estol[3], MD, DPH

[1]Colorado State University, Denver-Extension, 4-H Program, Denver, Colorado, United States, [2]Michael and Susan Dell Center for Healthy Living, University of Texas Health Science Center at Houston School of Public Health, Austin Campus, Austin, Texas, United States of America, [3]Centro de Investigación para la Epidemia del Tabaquismo (CIET), Montevideo, Uruguay and

* Corresponding Author's Email: Andrew.E.Springer@uth.tmc.edu.

[4]Hawaii State Department of Health and CDC/CSTE Applied Epidemiology Fellowship Program, Hawaii State Department of Health, Honolulu, Hawaii, United States of America

Abstract

Physical activity provides multiple health and educational benefits to children and youth, yet the majority of young people across the globe, including adolescents in Uruguay, do not participate in sufficient physical activity. This chapter aims to further inform intervention efforts for promoting adolescent physical activity in Uruguay by exploring physical activity perceptions and practices as well as physical activity barriers and opportunities in a sample of public and private secondary school students living in and around Montevideo, Uruguay. A total of n = 65 secondary school students, ranging in age from 11 to 15 years, participated in 12 focus groups. Despite generally favorable attitudes expressed by participants toward physical activity and identification of common physical activities, findings indicated several barriers for physical activity engagement in this sample of Uruguayan secondary school students -- which often vary by gender and SES, including: lack of access and availability of physical activity opportunities both within and outside of school time, lack of places as well as equipment and infrastructure for engagement in physical activity, and lack of time and competing activities such as video games. Key themes related to the importance of the social context for physical activity- especially for girls, as well as opportunities for physical activity, including the need for more afterschool programming, were also documented. These findings provide further context for understanding adolescent physical activity in Uruguay as well as direction for future intervention efforts.

Introduction

In Uruguay, non-communicable diseases that include cardiovascular disease, cancers, diabetes and other chronic diseases account for 85% of total deaths nationwide (1). As with their Southern Cone neighbors Argentina and Chile, obesity is one chronic disease condition that has become a pressing public health issue for Uruguay in recent years (2), with national prevalence estimates indicating that just over one in five adult males (21.1%) and just over one in four adult females (28.1%) are obese (1). In Uruguayan children between the ages of 6 and 15 years, estimates based on national data indicate that between 18.8% and 26.6% are obese (3). As children who are obese have a greater risk of overweight or obesity in adulthood (4), increased public health attention and interventions are warranted to prevent the onset of obesity in Uruguayan children.

Physical activity is a key behavior for the prevention of childhood obesity (4) and also provides multiple additional health benefits, including the prevention of hypertension, type 2 diabetes, cardiovascular disease, and some types of cancer (5). Beyond physical health benefits, physical activity has been found to positively impact young people's academic achievement and cognitive performance, including their time-on-task, concentration and performance on standardized tests (6). Despite the multiple benefits of physical activity, less than one third of adolescents (28.8%) in Uruguay have been found to meet World Health Organization (WHO) physical activity recommendations of 60 minutes of daily physical activity (7) -- a prevalence rate that reflects global trends of low physical activity engagement in young people (8).

In exploring approaches to support physical activity engagement in Uruguayan adolescents, research is needed to identify individual risk and protective factors related to physical activity as well as opportunities and barriers in young people's contexts that are amenable to intervention. To the authors' knowledge, no such research from Uruguay has been published to date, specific to young people, and qualitative research on adolescent physical activity from Latin America is sparse. As previous research has found disparities in leisure time physical activity by gender in Uruguayan adolescents, with boys being more active than girls (7), and with documentation of lower physical activity among adolescents of lower socioeconomic status (SES) based on internationally diverse adolescent studies (9), research is also needed on the roles that gender and SES may play in shaping physical activity behaviors in Uruguayan adolescents.

This study aims to address current gaps in the literature and further inform intervention efforts for promoting adolescent physical activity in Uruguay by exploring physical activity perceptions and practices as well as physical activity barriers and opportunities in a sample of public and private secondary school students living in and around Montevideo, Uruguay. Based on data collected via a series of focus group discussions, we specifically explore these factors by gender and school socioeconomic status among urban and semi-urban Uruguayan adolescents.

OUR STUDY

The study was conducted as part of a health needs assessment for the ¡Activate Ya! project, a National Institute of Health-funded study of tobacco use and physical activity in Uruguayan secondary school students being led by a partnership between the [name removed for blinded review], Uruguay, and the [name removed for blinded review], a public university in the United States. In contributing to a better understanding of adolescent physical activity engagement, focus group discussions were conducted in 2013 with students in Ciclo Básico 1 and 2 (equivalent to 7th and 8th grades in the U.S. and representing students between the ages of 12 and 15 years of age) attending public and private schools in and adjacent to Montevideo, Uruguay. A total of 12 focus groups stratified by gender and grade level (Ciclo Básico 1 and 2) were conducted at three schools: one private school that serves higher income students ("middle-high SES school"), one public school that serves middle income students ("middle SES school'), and one public school that serves middle-low income students ("middle-low SES school").

Study measures and procedures

A 14-item focus group discussion guide was developed by the research team aimed at eliciting input from adolescents about intrapersonal factors related to physical activity engagement (e.g., knowledge, attitudes, and perceived barriers), physical activity practices and preferences, and environmental factors such as opportunities for physical activity engagement. The development of the focus group interview guide was informed in part by constructs from the Health Belief Model (e.g., perceived barriers) (10), the Theory of Reasoned Action/Planned Behavior (e.g., subjective norms; attitudes) (11), and the Ecological Model of Active Living (e.g., opportunities and environments) (12).

Students were invited to participate in the focus group discussions via verbal and written invitations delivered in their school. Participation in the focus groups was voluntary, and both student assent and parental informed consent were required for participation. Privacy and confidentiality were made clear as conditions for participating in the focus groups via written and verbal informed consent procedures. Permission to conduct the focus groups was granted by the school directors, and the study protocols were reviewed and approved by the Committee for the Protection of Human Subjects of the University of Texas Health Science Center's School of Public Health and the Comité de Ética de la Facultad de Medicina (UDELAR) in Uruguay.

The focus groups were conducted in Spanish between April and May of 2013 by two trained Uruguayan research staff members from [Uruguayan partner organization. Name removed for blinded review]. Focus group discussions were digitally recorded, and notes were taken by the interviewers. Transcripts were stored in a password-protected computer upon the completion of focus groups. Focus groups were conducted by posing a question and allowing open discussion, using probes whenever necessary. Each session was approximately one hour in duration and took place at school. Research staff transcribed all focus group discussions. Once focus group discussions were transcribed, two research staff (a primary English speaker and primary Spanish speaker) translated the transcriptions to English.

Data analysis

Analysis of the focus group data was conducted separately by two independent analysts from our research team, which included an initial phase of coding by the two analysts, and then a centering phase in which the analysts -- with input from the broader research team -- discussed and confirmed the specific codes. Content analysis (13) guided the analysis of the data and was conducted to identify and compare common themes using the NVivo qualitative data analysis software (QSR International Pty Ltd. Version 10, 2012). Specifically, data were analyzed by attaching a descriptor, grouping into categories, and then developing themes to describe these categories. Themes were explored by gender and school SES, with gender coded based on the stratified research design, and school SES coded based on the primary income status of the student's school, as defined by the school principal.

FINDINGS

A total of n = 65 secondary school students participated in the 12 focus groups conducted, which included 34 girls (18 girls from 1° Ciclo Básico and 16 girls from 2° Ciclo Básico) and 31 boys (14 boys from 1° Ciclo Básico and 17 boys from 2° Ciclo Básico), ranging in age from 11 to 15 years. The participants from the middle-high income school included 12 boys and 11 girls; participants from the middle-low income school included 10 boys and 11 girls; and participants from middle income schools included 11 boys and 12 girls. Below, we share the key findings from the focus groups as organized by the following thematic content areas: *physical activity norms and types of activities; perceived benefits of physical activity; perceived barriers for physical activity;* and *physical activity engagement inside and outside of school.* Where relevant, differences observed by gender and school SES are noted. If not noted, no differences by these factors were observed.

Physical activity norms and types of activities

Girls and boys across middle-low, middle, and middle-high SES schools shared that leisure-time physical activity tends to be common among adolescents their age, yet important differences were noted by gender. While most girls said that they themselves were active, they also reported that girls generally should do more physical activity, mentioning physical appearance and a changing body as important reasons to engage in physical activity. Reasons for lower engagement in physical activity among girls included that they find other activities more important for girls of their age, such as taking care of younger family members and studying. Girls shared that boys are generally more active than girls, but expressed that some boys need to be more active because men are more likely to be obese than women. While boys seemed to agree that physical activity was common for boys their age, they did note that not all boys like physical activity, with some preferring to play video games and spend time on the computer. Findings were mixed when boys were asked about how common physical activity engagement was for girls, with some boys noting that girls are sedentary and need to be active, and others noting that girls are active and do not need to be more active.

Across both girl and boy groups, participants noted gender-specific differences in types of physical activities. For example, a male student (middle-high SES school) remarked:

> "En el liceo tenés hándbol, fútbol y básquetbol. A hándbol solo...los profesores dicen '*Solo pueden ir niñas...*' Fútbol y básquetbol que yo sepa no va ninguna niña *[In school there is handball, soccer and basketball. For handball only, teachers say 'Only girls can go (participate)'... Soccer and basketball, as far as I know, not one girl goes (participates)]."*

In addition, it was also mentioned by a female student (middle-high SES school) that:

> "Está dicho '*los varones juegan al fútbol, las chiquilinas juegan hándbol,'* que el hecho de que a todos los varones les gusta más el fútbol que el hándbol..." *[It is said that 'boys play soccer, girls play handball,' which makes all the boys like soccer more than handball*].

Despite these differences, both girls and boys commented that there were activities that they engaged in together, which included soccer, tag, tennis, and volleyball. An emerging theme common to both boys and girls regarding joint participation in physical activity was safety. Females commented that boys play rough ("bruto") and throw and push ("pechar"), with boys sharing the same concerns about girls: "Pero es peligroso jugar con ellas [But it is dangerous to play with them (girls)]" (Male student, middle-low SES school). Boys also mentioned that sports clubs have clear distinctions between "masculine" and "feminine" sports, and that there are boys or girls that cannot participate in certain sports at clubs.

An important theme that emerged among girls was the importance of doing physical activity with others, particularly for girls with other girls, and that being alone or not having friends in the neighborhood influenced their activity levels. One female participant from a middle-low SES school stated: "Y yo, por ejemplo, soy más tímida y en el barrio no tengo ningún amigo [*I, for example, am more timid and do not have a single friend in the neighborhood*]." Another girl (middle-high SES school) said: "Las niñas prefieren ir como juntas [*Girls prefer to go together*]" and that for boys: "No les importa mucho estar tanto solos o sea...solos con el ejercicio y eso.[*It doesn't matter much to boys to be alone with exercise and things like this*]."

Perceived benefits of physical activity

When asked about the benefits of physical activity, girls and boys cited social and health related reasons. For both boys and girls, participants thought that participating in physical activity helped them make new friends, socialize, and work as a team. Several middle school girls also cited that extracurricular activities outside of school provided opportunities to meet with friends and do activities they like. Regarding health, boys and girls across all social classes indicated that physical activity takes care of the body by promoting physical and mental health, although some gender-specific reasons were noted. For example, boys shared that physical activity is important for mobility and building strength ("fortaleciendo"). They also noted that physical activity contributes to one's character development. As shared by one boy from a middle-high SES school: "Yo creo que los deportes te dan más valores; también te ayudan a crecer [*I think that sports give you more values; they also help you grow*]." Girls mentioned more frequently than boys that physical activity helps to prevent obesity. In addition, girls more commonly cited mental health as an important reason for engaging in physical activity, as reflected in quotes from middle-high and middle SES school participants: "Te distraes [*You entertain yourself*]" and "Estás como libre, como que te tranquilizas cuando haces un deporte que te gusta [*You are free, it is like you calm yourself when you are playing a sport that you like*]."

Perceived barriers for physical activity

Time, competing activities & transportation. Boys and girls across all social classes mentioned time (or lack thereof) as a reason some may not engage in physical activity, which included insufficient time during the day outside of school as well as limited time during school, such as recess time. Common reasons also given by middle-high income students were that other activities compete with physical activity, such as hanging out with friends or studying. In addition, boys and girls across school SES levels agreed that transportation can be a barrier to physical activity, as some activities and places for physical activity were not located in their neighborhoods. In response to this barrier, some middle-low SES school students mentioned biking as an accessible means of transportation. Middle-low SES school students said that feeling tired was also a barrier more frequently than participants from the higher SES schools.

Availability and access to opportunities. While boys and girls identified opportunities for physical activity, important SES and gender-related barriers were noted in relation to the availability and accessibility of these opportunities. The inability to pay for opportunities for physical activity (e.g., health clubs or gyms), for example, was brought up among boys and girls from across school SES levels. It was also common among middle-low income students to say that places to participate in physical activity are expensive, and that there are no free options in their neighborhood. Middle-low SES school students were also more likely to cite barriers such as no space, dirty space, no equipment, broken equipment, or few places in the neighborhood to be physically active. In addition, not enough space or equipment at school were obstacles cited by mostly middle-low income students. One girl from a middle-low SES school noted: "[Los areas de juego del liceo] [s]on muy chicos y no tienen espacio [*The school play areas are very small and do not have space*]".

Gender-specific barriers. While barriers to access and availability were cited by both girls and boys, across the sample more girls than boys reported that either there are not very many places near them to be physically active, or if there are, they do not know about them. Girls, mostly from the middle SES schools, also mentioned embarrassment or shame as a barrier ("verguenza") for girls to participate in physical activity. On the other hand, more boys mentioned preference for electronics (i.e., video games, computers) over physical activity as a barrier, although some male participants said that boys play on the computer but also engage in sports. More middle and middle-high income students tended to note electronics as a barrier. Boys and girls also identified dislike for physical activity as a barrier for some, and more girls than boys mentioned having friends that do not like physical activity. Lastly, middle-high SES school boys and girls both cited parents not allowing them to engage in sports as a barrier to physical activity.

Physical activity engagement during and outside of school time

Although recess (break time) and PE were cited as opportunities for physical activity during school, both boys and girls and participants across all school SES groups emphasized that it is difficult to engage in physical activity in school due to limited time and lack of equipment. Below we explore some of the opportunities and barriers cited for physical activity during school.

Recess time. Although boys mentioned physical activities that they engaged in during recess, such as ping pong, soccer and basketball, lack of equipment was cited as a barrier for engaging in physical activity during recess. Boys also reported that recess is short, usually 10-15 minutes long, and is often a time to eat. Similarly, girls also said that they do not have equipment such as soccer balls to play with during this time, that there is not enough time to engage in activity, and that they usually use this time to eat as well. Something that was mentioned by girls more than boys was their enjoyment with taking time to talk to their friends during recess. Although limited time was cited as a barrier by students of all social classes, middle-low and middle income students cited lack of equipment as a more common barrier to active play during recess. Example quotes illustrating these themes include:

> "Como que me parece que el año pasado en el colegio teníamos más tiempo como para hacer deporte. [*It seems to me that last year in school we had more time to play sports*]." (Girl, middle-high SES school).
>
> "Pero un día queríamos jugar al fútbol y no podíamos porque no había pelotas; las pelotas que teníamos estaban todas pinchadas, ta y son cosas así [*But one day we wanted to play soccer and we could not because there were no balls; the balls that we had were flat...as such, there are things like this*]." (Boy, middle SES school).

Physical Education class. Boys and girls across all social classes specified physical education (PE) class as an important opportunity for physical activity in school. Overall, participants discussed more likes than dislikes for their PE class. Positive aspects expressed by boys for their PE class included the opportunity to play sports and engage in competition, with appealing activities that included soccer, basketball, and tag. Girls also liked activities that included sports as well, such as volleyball, gymnastics, handball, soccer, and tag, as well as racing games ("carreras"). However, it should be noted that some girls expressed that they did not like anything about PE class. Middle-low and middle income students said playing together more was an attraction for them, while middle-high income students mostly highlighted engagement in sports as an attraction. Both boys and girls expressed the importance of having variety in sports as attractive, which was more often cited by middle-high SES school students. A main dislike of PE class noted by participants was 'theoretical classes', which require being inside a classroom and completing written exercises. Male and female students across all three school SES levels said these classes were boring and involved no activity: "La clase teórica porque es muy aburrida y no te moves [Theoretical class (is an aversion) because it is very boring and you do not move]" (Female student, middle-low SES school).

Activity breaks during class time. Activity breaks during class time, which may include short bouts of movement or activity, were not commonly practiced as reported by students. One exception was a student who reported that they have an activity break in Spanish class, although others said that those breaks do not involve activity but rather an activity that involved resting/taking time to close their eyes, such as a meditation break.

Walking and biking to/from school. Participants were asked about active transportation to and from school by biking or walking. Overall, riding bikes to school was generally reported as uncommon, with many comments noting confusion about where to leave bikes and the possibility of getting bikes stolen. However, more middle and middle-low students tended to say riding bikes was more common than middle-high students, with boys in these social classes being more likely to cite riding bikes. Some girls highlighted the dangers associated with biking: "A mi me gustaría eh, venir en bici, pero es medio peligroso el cruce de acá [I like to come on my bike, but the crossing is a bit dangerous over here]" (Female student, middle-high SES school). When considering walking as a method of active transport, more girls than boys reported that it is common for the majority of students to walk to school. Both middle-low and middle-high income students acknowledged that it is common for students to walk to school if they live close. However, middle-high income students more frequently said that they take the bus or are dropped off at school by their parents.

Outside of school time

Physical activity outside of school time. Across all social classes, both boys and girls commonly identified swimming, playing soccer, and bicycling as common activities they do outside of school. Boys and girls also mentioned going to "La Rambla", or the boardwalk, to walk, go to the park, or bike. Boys talked more about activities such as basketball, skating, and karate as primary activities they engaged in outside of school, while girls talked more about other activities such as volleyball, dance, handball, and artistic gymnastics. A common activity mentioned by middle-high income girls specifically was "ritmos," also known as rhythms or dance, which is commonly done at gyms, as well as basketball and swimming.. Middle-high and middle SES school boys and girls also communicated that they often go to sports clubs to play sports outside of school time; students from middle-low SES school students noted that this was common for some students, but not for them. While not specific to physical activity, middle-low SES school students specifically mentioned the occasional opportunity to attend "talleres," or after school workshops, yet these talleres were stated to not always be available for public schools.

DISCUSSION

Given national estimates that indicate that more than half of Uruguayan adolescents do not meet recommendations for daily physical activity (7), research is needed to provide further context into both the barriers and potential facilitating factors for PA engagement in young people living in Uruguay. Despite important limitations of the current study -- which include the small sample of adolescents from three secondary schools, as well as a limited geographic representation of urban students from Montevideo and surrounding area, this qualitative study contributes to the literature by exploring physical activity perceptions, practices, barriers, and opportunities for physical activity engagement among Uruguayan secondary school students, including boys and girls attending socioeconomically diverse schools. While the Uruguayan adolescents who participated in this study identified a range of physical activities as common to young people their age and expressed various physical, mental and social health benefits of physical activity- as previously documents with adolescents in Brazil (14), important gender-specific and SES-specific barriers for physical activity emerged that offer potential areas for future study and intervention.

In exploring previously documented gender disparities in physical activity behaviors among Uruguayan adolescents (7), we identified several gender-specific factors that may inhibit physical activity participation in Uruguayan girls and boys. Both girls and boys in this study identified some sports activities as being more a “girl sport” or more a “boy sport”, with some participants indicating that these beliefs are reinforced by their teachers as well as by sports clubs that do not allow some gender groups to play a given sport. These gender-biased perceptions of physical activity and sports have been previously cited by groups that include *la Red Para la Actividad Física* and underscore an ongoing need to respond to calls to “desexuar” (“de-sex/de-gender”) physical activity in order to ensure an equitable teaching and promotion of sports and games to both girls and boys (15).

While girls and boys in this study generally expressed that physical activity was something their peers engage in, some female participants felt that girls should do more physical activity for their appearance and changing bodies, and that boys should do more physical activity as men are more likely to be obese than women. As obesity affects both males and females in Uruguay, with lower rates for Uruguayan girls (3) yet higher rates for Uruguayan women (1), continued efforts are needed to raise awareness about the importance of physical activity for promoting a healthy weight for both boys and girls in Uruguay. Girls in this study were also more likely to report general feelings of embarrassment as a reason for not engaging in physical activity. Research on adolescent girls from the U.S. (16) and Canada (17) has found that body image concerns are important barriers to physical activity participation; further research is needed to understand the role of embarrassment and the potential role of body-related concerns as barriers for physical activity participation in Uruguayan girls.

Other key barriers cited by girls included the need to take care of siblings after school or on the weekend, the lack of places and opportunities near them to participate in physical activity, the importance of engaging in physical activity with other girls, and concerns about joint participation in sports with boys due to rough play. Taking care of siblings is a barrier that has been previously cited by Hispanic middle school girls in the U.S. who report child care as a more common activity compared to their white and African American counterparts (16). A large body of research has documented the important role social support plays in physical activity engagement among young people, which includes evidence from South America (18). Our findings suggest that fostering social support may be especially important in supporting girls' physical activity. The potential lack of places and opportunities for girl participation in sports and physical activity, the importance of engaging in physical activity with other girls, as well as concerns about joint participation in sports with boys merit further confirmation and present potential targets for intervention efforts.

For boys, video game playing was cited across focus groups as a potential reason why some boys their age did not participate in physical activity or sports. While research on screen time use, which includes TV watching and video game playing, and physical activity engagement is either mixed or shows small negative associations (19), findings from a recent qualitative research review of diverse international studies underscore the important role that video games and computers play as part of daily life for adolescents of this generation, which may include serving as a vehicle for social interaction (20). Further research on the functional meaning of screen time and video games within the adolescent context in Uruguay as well as how to incorporate more physical activity in a way that delivers similar benefits of screen time, such as positive adolescent social interaction and entertainment, holds potential to further inform intervention efforts.

In the current study, middle-low SES school students cited various barriers to physical activity that included the financial cost of physical activity opportunities, lack of free options in their neighborhood, and a lack of space, dirty spaces, and/or lack of equipment or broken equipment in school. Previous research based on internationally diverse samples of adolescents indicates an inverse association between physical activity and SES (9), and research from the U.S. has found that lower SES populations may have less access to PA supportive environments and resources (21). Our findings suggest a need for enhanced investments to create safe and accessible spaces and program opportunities for physical activity for adolescents in Uruguay, with specific focus on lower SES adolescents and girls.

While physical education class was cited as an important time for physical activity during school – with generally positive comments for PE from students in this study, Uruguayan secondary school students often receive PE class on only two days a week (for 80 minutes and 40 minutes at each time, respectively). As such, other opportunities to help students meet daily physical activity recommendations merit exploration. Recess presents an important opportunity for unstructured active play, yet participants in this study indicated that time for recess was limited, with usually only 10-15 minutes scheduled, which was time also used for eating. Beyond time, students also cited lack of equipment and space as key barriers. Although classroom activity breaks were not a common practice cited by this sample of students, classroom activity breaks have been found to provide meaningful opportunities for physical activity engagement (22) and merit further exploration for supporting adolescent

PA in Uruguay. Outside of school, "talleres" (afterschool workshops), which may provide opportunity for physical activity, were noted by some students, yet these workshops were not always offered at public schools. Further research on strategies for increasing adolescent physical activity both within and outside of school is warranted such as exploration of community-school partnerships, which have been found to enhance physical activity opportunities and engagement among students (23).

In recent years, Uruguay has taken several important steps toward increasing physical activity (PA) in young people, including passage of legislation to make PE a requirement for all primary school students in 2007 (24), implementation of 'open-air gyms' (25), and awareness raising and mobilization of social networks around PA via efforts led by groups such as la Red de Actividad Física del Uruguay, among other efforts. In our work with the ¡Activate Ya! study, a school-based intervention study taking place in 16 schools in and around Montevideo, qualitative findings from the current study have informed several of our intervention strategies, which are designed to decrease barriers noted by study participants and increase PA opportunities while enhancing intrapersonal factors such as PA knowledge, attitudes, self-efficacy, and a healthy and active self-concept. Key components of the ¡Activate Ya! program include the creation of a university student-led afterschool component ("Espacio Adolescente") that provides games and activities, a classroom component that incorporates student-centered activities aimed at promoting PA social norms, social support and positive intrapersonal factors, a classroom activity break component to enhance PA opportunities during the school day, and student-led action to promote social norms and awareness for PA via a community-wide final event in partnership with community organizations. The ¡Activate Ya! study will conclude in 2017, and we look forward to sharing our lessons learned and recommendations based on our findings.

Physical activity is a key health promoting behavior that provides multiple benefits for adolescents (5). Despite generally favorable attitudes expressed by adolescents in this study toward physical activity, our findings indicate several barriers for adolescent engagement in PA in

Uruguay -- which often vary by gender and SES, including: lack of access and availability of PA opportunities both within and outside of school time, lack of places for engagement in PA as well as equipment and infrastructure for PA, limited time, and competing activities such as video games. These findings provide further context for understanding adolescent physical activity engagement in Uruguay and provide a foundation for the design and implementation of efforts aimed at promoting physical activity with Uruguayan adolescents.

Acknowledgments

We express our sincere gratitude to our three partner schools and participating students in Uruguay for sharing their insights about adolescent physical activity participation. Funding for this study was provided by the National Institute on Drug Abuse (NIDA) and National Cancer Institute (NCI) (1 R01 DA035157-01), as part of the TOBAC program sponsored by the Fogarty International Center (FIC) of the National Institutes of Health (NIH) in the United States. This study was partially funded by the Michael & Susan Dell Foundation through resources provided at the Michael & Susan Dell Center for Healthy Living, The University of Health Science Center School of Public Health in Austin.

References

[1] World Health Organization (WHO). Noncommunicable Diseases Country Profiles: Uruguay [Internet]. 2014 [cited 2016 Sep 20]. URL: http://www.who.int/nmh/countries/ury_en.pdf.

[2] Rubinstein AL, Irazola VE, Calandrelli M, Elorriaga N, Gutierrez L, Lanas F, et al. Multiple cardiometabolic risk factors in the Southern Cone of Latin America: A population-based study in Argentina, Chile, and Uruguay. Int J Cardiol 20155;183:82-8.

[3] Severi C, Moratorio X. Double burden of undernutrition and obesity in Uruguay. Am J Clin Nutr 2014;100(6):1659S-62S.

[4] Koplan JP, Liverman CT, Kraak VA, eds. Preventing childhood obesity: health in the balance. Washington, DC: National Academies, 2005.

[5] US Department of Health and Human Services (USDHHS). 2008 Physical Activity Guidelines for Americans. Washington, DC: DHHS, 2008.

[6] Castelli DM, Glowacki E, Barcelona JM, Calvert HG, Hwang J. Active Education: Growing evidence on physical activity and academic performance. Research Brief - Active Living Research January 2015. URL: http://activelivingresearch.org/sites/default/files/ALR_Brief_ActiveEducation_Jan2015.pdf.

[7] Ministerio de Salud Pública (MSP)/World Health Organization (WHO)-Uruguay. Global School-Based Health Survey: Uruguay 2012 Fact Sheet [Internet]. 2012. [cited 2016 Sep 20]. URL: http://www.who.int/chp/gshs/2012_Uruguay_GSHS_FS.pdf?ua=1.

[8] Sallis JF, Bull F, Guthold R, Heath GW, Inoue S, Kelly P, et al. Lancet Physical Activity Series 2 Executive Committee. Progress in physical activity over the Olympic quadrennium. Lancet 2016;388(10051):1325-36.

[9] Stalsberg R, Pedersen AV. Effects of socioeconomic status on the physical activity in adolescents: a systematic review of the evidence. Scand J Med Sci Sports 2010; 20(3):368-83.

[10] Champion VL, Skinner CS. The health belief model. In: Glanz K, Rimer BK, Viswanath K, eds. Health behavior and health education: Theory, research, and practice. San Francisco, CA: Jossey-Bass, 2008:45-65.

[11] Montano DE, Kasprzyk D. Theory of reasoned action, theory of planned behavior, and the integrated behavioral model. Health behavior: Theory, research and practice. San Francisco, CA: Jossey-Bass, 2008:67-96.

[12] Sallis JF, Cervero RB, Ascher W, Henderson KA, Kraft MK, Kerr J. An ecological approach to creating active living communities. Annu Rev Public Health 2006;27:297-322.

[13] Zhang Y & Wildemuth BM. Qualitative analysis of content. In: Wildemuth B, ed. Applications of social research methods to questions in information and library science. Westport, CT: Libraries Unlimited, 2009:308-19.

[14] Zieff SG, Guedes CM, Wiley J. Youth knowledge of physical activity health benefits: a brazilian case study. ScientificWorldJournal 2006;6:1713-21.

[15] Antúnez M. Actividad física y género. Red Para la Actividad Física y Desarrollo Humano/Año II. 2012. [cited 2012 Sep 20]. URL: http://www.redaf.gob.ar/articulos/actividad-fisica-genero_c28e.pdf.

[16] Grieser M, Vu MB, Bedimo-Rung AL, Neumark-Sztainer D, Moody J, Young DR, et al. Physical activity attitudes, preferences, and practices in African American, Hispanic, and Caucasian girls. Health Educ Behav 2006;33(1):40-51.

[17] Dwyer JJ, Allison KR, Goldenberg ER, Fein AJ. Adolescent girls' perceived barriers to participation in physical activity. Adolescence 2006;41(161):75.

[18] Mendonça G, Cheng LA, Mélo EN, de Farias Júnior JC. Physical activity and social support in adolescents: a systematic review. Health Educ Res 2014:29(5):822-39.

[19] Marshall SJ, Biddle SJ, Gorely T, Cameron N, Murdey I. Relationships between media use, body fatness and physical activity in children and youth: a meta-analysis. Int J Obes 2004;28(10):1238-46.

[20] Minges KE, Owen N, Salmon J, Chao A, Dunstan DW, Whittemore R. Reducing youth screen time: qualitative metasynthesis of findings on barriers and facilitators. Health Psychol 2015;34(4):381.

[21] Gordon-Larsen P, Nelson MC, Page P, Popkin BM. Inequality in the built environment underlies key health disparities in physical activity and obesity. Pediatrics 2006;117(2):417-24.

[22] Whitt-Glover MC, Porter AT, Yancey T. Do short physical activity breaks in the classroom work? Research brief. San Diego, CA: Active Living Research. Robert Wood Johnson Foundation, 2013.

[23] Leatherdale ST, Manske S, Faulkner G, Arbour K, Bredin C. A multi-level examination of school programs, policies and resources associated with physical activity among elementary school youth in the PLAY-ON study. Int J Behav Nutr Phys Act 2010;7(1):6.

[24] MIDES (Ministerio de Desarrollo Social de Uruguay). Educacion Fisica en las Escuelas. 2016. [cited 2016 Nov 1]. URL: http://www.mides.gub.uy/innovaportal/v/18634/3/innova.front/educacion_fisica_en_las_escuelas.

[25] Uy.press 41 gimnasios al aire libre en Montevideo. 2016. [cited 2016 Sep 20]. URL: http://www.uypress.net/uc_65612_1.html.

In: Child and Adolescent Health
Editors: A Tenenbaum and J Merrick
ISBN: 978-1-53617-825-8

Chapter 16

CYBERBULLYING IN COLLEGES AND UNIVERSITIES: A SURVEY OF STUDENT EXPERIENCES AND ATTITUDES ABOUT CYBERBULLYING

Salihah Alqahtani[1], PhD, Salman Elbedour[1,*], PhD, Kimberley Freeman[1], PhD, Gregory Reed[1], PhD, Kamilah Woodson Reed[1], PhD and Joav Merrick[2-6], MD, MMedSc, DMSc

[1]Department of Human Development and Psychoeducational Studies, School of Education, Howard University, Washington, DC, United States of America

[2]National Institute of Child Health and Human Development, Jerusalem

[3]Office of the Medical Director, Health Services, Division for Intellectual and Developmental Disabilities, Ministry of Social Affairs and Social Services, Jerusalem

---

* Correspondence: Professor Salman Elbedour, Department of Human Development and Psychoeducational Studies, School of Education, Howard University, 2441 Fourth Street, NW, Washington, DC 20059, United States. E-mail: selbedour@howard.edu.

[4]Division of Pediatrics, Hadassah Hebrew University Medical Center, Mt Scopus Campus, Jerusalem, Israel
[5]Kentucky Children's Hospital, University of Kentucky School of Medicine, Lexington, Kentucky, United States of America
[6]Center for Healthy Development, School of Public Health, Georgia State University, Atlanta, United States of America

Abstract

Many studies have found a decrease in traditional bullying. Yet cyberbullying, while still impacting a fraction of those impacted by traditional bullying, is on the rise and it seems that society is beginning to not only accept, but expect, electronic communication behaviors that are emotionally and physically damaging. It seems that cyberbullying is simply part of the bullying spectrum. The current research relied on a self-reported study to determine the prevalence of the four categories of cyberbullying and victimization: cyberbullies only, victims only, bully/victims, and witnesses of bullying/victimization. The survey population was Howard University graduate and undergraduate students (N=165, aged 19-45 years distributed equally between males and females. Findings included little difference in college level (undergraduate versus graduate) among victims of cyberbullying; significant differences in how male and female students felt about cyberbullying, with females expressing more distress; and the fact that female students were more likely to know the people who were bullying them. Another notable finding was that 49% of students felt that their school could not or would not do anything about cyberbullying, even if it was reported, and 47% felt that university staff would not believe or understand them if they complained. The role of the school psychologist is central to prevention programs. School psychologists can help coordinate the prevention team, help conduct the needs assessment, analyze the results, and set priorities and goals.

Introduction

The first use of the term bully, according to the Oxford English Dictionary, is attributed to Samuel Palmer (1652-1724) in 1710. The act of bullying has appeared in literature since at least the time of Charles Dickens (1812-1870) Oliver Twist, first published as a serial in 1837. Two decades later, Thomas Hughes (1822-1896) wrote "Tom Brown's schooldays" where he tackled the topic of bullying.

Although bullying is clearly an old phenomenon, formal research on bullying did not begin until the 1970s in Scandinavia. In 1983, after the suicide of three Norwegian boys, the Norwegian government hired Dan Olweus to research the problem of bullying. Similarly, school shootings in the United States prompted many professionals to take a look at bullying and its impact on students. Nearly forty years after its introduction as a serious subject for research, the topic was thought important enough for past President and First Lady Obama to host a White House conference on the topic in 2011. Still, the research over the past four decades shows "the complexity of the problem as well as the challenges we face addressing it" (1).

Many of the problems associated with the study of bullying can be attributed to inconsistent definitions. A few high-profile international cases of the sometimes lethal consequences of physical and verbal abuse inflicted on young people by their peers have spotlighted the problem of what Americans call bullying. The fact that some languages, such as German (2), have no equivalents for the English word bullying probably says as much about German and American society as it does about the difficulties of amassing cross-cultural data. In fact, in both the school and the workplace, what Americans might refer to as bullying, Europeans might call mobbing. While the terms at first may appear to be interchangeable, some researchers use the word bullying to refer to aggressive actions taken by management and mobbing as aggressive actions taken by peers; others see bullying as actions taken by one individual and mobbing as actions taken by a group (3). For the most part, however, researchers have come to accept the Swedish scholar Dan Olweus's definition that bullying involves negative actions taken over time by one or more persons against a weaker individual (4).

Researchers also accept that bullying is costly in every sense of the word. Ferris (3) stated that "bullying is associated with negative health outcomes such as anxiety, depression, headache, and musculoskeletal problems" (p. 174). Craig and Pepler (5) agreed that victims are at risk "for anxiety, depression, and somatic complaints," and bullies themselves are at risk "for long-term problems with antisocial behavior and substance use" (p. 87), leading to sexual harassment and dating aggression, and "can extend to workplace harassment, as well as marital, child, and elder abuse" (p. 88). Smith (6) reiterates that bullying in schools can lead to "bullying in the workplace, the home, prisons, and sporting events as well as stalking" (p. 43). Consequently, bullying can cost organizations "billions of dollars through absenteeism, turnover, and legal actions" (3). Because of bullying, society itself will have to bear the burden of increased health care costs, police costs, and court costs (5).

Even more disturbing is the fact that witnesses to bullying can suffer even more. In a study of more than 2,000 students aged 12 to 16 year olds in the United Kingdom, schools found that "observing bullying at school predicted risks to mental health over and above that predicted for those students who were directly involved in bullying behavior as either a perpetrator or a victim" (7). In other words, bullying has seriously negative short- and long-term consequences on the victim, on the bully, on witnesses, and on society as a whole.

Given the measureable deleterious impact of bullying, social scientists and school psychologists have taken a keen interest in curbing its frequency. Many anti-bullying programs have been around for enough time to study their effectiveness. Bradshaw (8) looked at several bullying prevention programs in the United States (US), Canada and Europe. In a study of anti-bullying programs in these locations (the majority of which were outside the US and Canada, with a third of them based on the work of Olweus, the author found that the programs on average reduced perpetration of bullying 20-23% and reduced victimization by 17-20%, although the more rigorously the study was evaluated, the less well it did (p. 323). In general, the programs were more effective in Europe than in either the US or Canada. To be successful, the researchers found, programs must involve more than a single school-wide assembly. They must also involve families and communities, and the efforts must be sustained and integrated (8). Programs that meet those criteria, such as the "Good behavior game" and the "Coping power program," can have an impact on bullying (8).

Bradshaw (8) looked specifically at a Finnish "KiVa program" that provided "classroom materials and discussions between students and teachers, peer support for student victims, disciplinary strategies, and information for parents to combat bullying. Computer games are also used to help students practice bullying prevention skills" (p. 324). The author came away with three observations: First, research is needed to test and isolate the successful critical components of bullying prevention programs (p. 324). Second, like many other researchers, Bradshaw (8) felt that a three-tiered system worked best for all students with some programs, for at-risk students with a more intensive intervention program, and then, for those few students who exhibited consistent negative behavior, the most rigorous intervention was the best. Finally, the author stressed that the biggest problem with evaluating programs was that "most programs lack valid, reliable, and efficient tools for tracking fidelity" (p. 330).

In Canada, which ranks near the bottom of a World Health Organization measure of bullying in 35 countries, Craig and Pepler (5) summarized a program called "Promoting relationships and eliminating violence" (PREVNet), whose aim is "to stop the use of power and aggression in bullying and to promote safe and healthy relationships for children and youth" (p. 86). According to the authors, PREVNet's assumptions are threefold:

- All children have a right to be safe.
- Bullying is a relationship problem. The Surgeon General's report on Youth Violence (9) found that "weak social ties was the most significant risk factor for adolescent violence, well above gang membership, poverty, and drug use."
- Promoting healthy relationships is everyone's responsibility.

To make an impact, the goals of PREVNEet are also threefold:

- Assess prevalence and nature of bullying (collate data from many different sources).
- Develop effective interventions.
- Advocate for policy changes.

To accomplish these goals, teams must draw in community partners and train the trainers. The researchers stress that those who participate need to get over the myths that bullying is "just kids being kids" and that "victims will get over it."

A third program studied was "Expect respect." This program teaches victims how to signal "stop" when they feel bullied, teaches bullies how to stop their negative behavior, and teaches bystanders not to encourage the bullying. It also teaches everyone how to get adult help. In the eyes of the adults taking part in the program, it was successful because they observed fewer bullying behaviors. According to the children involved, however, it was not a success (10).

The rise of cyberbullying

Once cyberbullying is added to the equation, the research becomes less clear. Even the definition of cyberbullying can cause lots of disagreement (6). As a result of varied definitions, "rates of online harassment and cyberbullying are highly varied" (11). The present study relies on the following definitions of cyberbullying: "Cyberbullying is any behavior performed through electronic or digital media by individuals or groups that repeatedly communicates hostile or aggressive messages intended to inflict harm or discomfort to others" (12). Patchin and Hinduja (13) defined cyberbullying as "willful and repeated harm inflicted through the medium of electronic text" (p. 152). Li (14) referred to cyberbullying as "bullying via electronic communication tools such as email, cell phone, personal digital assistant (PDA), instant messaging or the world wide web" (p. 224). Others (15) defined cyberbullying as an intentional and aggressive behavior or act repeatedly carried out by an individual (or a group) against another person(or group) who cannot easily defend himself (or themselves) using electronic tools such as social networks, emails, cellphones.

To avoid the problems caused by varied definition, Jones et al. (11) looked at three surveys of approximately 1,500 youth each at five-year intervals (years 2000, 2005, and 2010) regarding online harassment, defined as threats or other offensive online behavior. While harassment did not meet the standard of bullying (repeated events by more powerful bullies), it can occur as part of bullying. The surveys show clear trends. Internet use increased during the 2000s. Since harassed youth were using the internet more than non-harrassed youth, it should come as no surprise that online harassment increased from 6% in 2000 to 11% in 2010, mostly as indirect harassment. Girls were 48% of victims in 2000, but 69% in 2010.

The relatively good news is that while reporting of harassment dipped from 2000 to 2005, it increased slightly from 2005 to 2010 (9% to 13%). In one of the more recent studies of online harassment, Mitchell et al. (16) surveyed 791 youth aged 10-20 years of age to assess the involvement of technology in harassment in the past year. Of the responders, 34% reported harassment, with 54% of those being off-line; 15% reported online harassment only; and 31% reported both. Once again, the survey was measuring harassment, not bullying, because not all the incidents "involve repetition and power imbalances" (p. 1). In contrast to some studies that show cyberbullying is worse than traditional bullying, the authors found that "technology-only incidents were less likely to involve multiple episodes and power imbalances. They were seen by victims as easier to stop and had significantly less emotional impact. Mixed incidents had the most emotional impact, possibly because they occurred across multiple environments and because perpetrators tended to be more socially connected to victims" (p. 1).

Youth who are victims of multiple types of peer harassment, including technology-based harassment, report depression, injury, and medical concerns at higher rates than traditional victims (16). Identifying the various sub-categories may not be easy considering that Mitchell et al. (16)

found other studies reporting that 95% of cybervictims were also victims of traditional victimization.

Although Bauman and Newman (17) found that programs to address bullying in general were found to reduce cyberbullying as well (p. 35), Jones et al. (11) stated, *"It is currently unclear whether, and to what extent, policies and prevention initiatives that cover traditional bullying are sufficient for technology-related harassment, or whether there are unique features to technology-based harassment that require specialized procedures and policies"* (p. 54). Despite the difficulties of assessing cyberbullying and its consequences, Jones, Mitchell and Finkelhor (11) stressed that schools need to include cyberbullying when working on bullying policies.

Because cyberbullying appears to be a growing problem (18), cyberbullying has now become the focus of many studies (19), including suggestions for online psychological therapy (20). However, the vast majority of these studies deal with cyberbullying among children and adolescents. Only a few have focused on cyberbullying among college students (17,21-023). Because limited research on cyberbullying among adults has been undertaken, adults from Howard University (graduate and undergraduate students) were the focus of this study.

Purpose of the study

The current research relies on a self-reported study to determine the prevalence of the four categories of cyberbullying and victimization: cyberbullies only, victims only, bully/victims, and witnesses of bullying/victimization. The sample consisted of 165 respondents, distributed equally between males and females, selected from undergraduate and graduate students enrolled at Howard University in Washington, DC. A self-reported questionnaire was designed to determine the following research questions:

- During the past 12 months, how often has the student cyberbullied others while using the Internet?
- During the past 12 months, how often has the student been a victim of cyberbullying while using the Internet?
- During the past 12 months, how frequently has the student directly or indirectly witnessed cyberbullying incidents in his or her school?

Additional items on the survey determined 1) the electronic method of delivery of the perpetrator (e.g., Facebook, MySpace, e-mail, text message, instant message, online games, or across multiple venues), 2) whether or not the perpetrator knew the victim or the victim knew the perpetrator, 3) whether or not the victims or perpetrators let others know (peers, instructors, parents, siblings, friends) of their actions, and 4) how the perpetrator felt afterward (very good, good, bad, very bad, neutral).

Research questions pertaining to differences with respect to gender and school level (graduate versus undergraduate), were also tested. These research questions were:

- Research Question 1: Does the prevalence of cyberbullying experiences vary as a function of gender? Hypothesis 1: Like previous research at the high school level (24), this study posits that college female students are more likely than male college students to report being victims of cyberbullying.
- Research Question 2: Does the prevalence of cyberbullying experiences vary as a function of age (undergraduate versus graduate)? Hypothesis 2: This study posits that cyberbullying rates decrease with increased level of educational attainment. More specifically, graduate students were anticipated to be less engaged in cyberbullying as both victims and bullies.

In addition we were interested in examining the possible triggers of cyberbullying. These include individual variables (e.g., gender, age, academic standing), family variables (e.g., parental employment, single-versus two-parent homes), and socioemotional variables (e.g., pride, jealousy of others, anger, alcohol abuse, loneliness). Only those participants who reported a history of being a cyberbully were asked to complete this portion of the scale.

Importance of the study

The end of every calendar always finds the media producing lists, from best restaurants to worst movies. A 2015 list of "ludicrousness" by Washington Post columnist George F Will (31 December 2015) offered at least one mislabeled item. Will included in his column a decision by an Edina, Minnesota, school district to hire "recess consultants." In fact, better monitoring of school playgrounds is frequently on lists of actions to take to improve school climate and reduce bullying, since many bullying episodes take place during play time (25, 26). Like many adults, Will may ridicule what happens at recess because he buys into the myths that bullying is not a large problem, is part of growing up, can build character, does not harm anyone, or will simply be outgrown.

On the contrary, bullying is a significant problem with lasting repercussions, requiring further study as part of a continuum of school violence that can be disruptive to the learning process. In the United States, as many as 21.5% of students aged 12 to 18 years reported being bullied in some fashion during the 2012-2013 school year. Rates around the rest of the world vary, but bullying is a significant problem in other countries as well. A 2012 World Health Organization report from 43 countries indicated rates of bullying from 2-32% (1). These numbers are disturbing because bullying can have long-lasting negative consequences for the bully, the bullied, and witnesses. Finnish longitudinal research has shown a substantial increase in psychopathology two decades after the bullying episodes at age 8 years for both the victim and bullies (27). Liu and Graves (28) agree that bullies and victims have an increased risk for mental health problems, including suicidal ideation. Bullies and victims often underachieve in school and victims may suffer from lower self-esteem, higher rates of depression, and more insecurity than other children (29). You et al. (18) found a dramatic rise in the suicide rate of middle schoolers in Korea from 2000 to 2005, with 54.2% of the victims reportedly being the targets of bullies. Furthermore, even witnesses can be severely depressed by bullying for fear of being a target, once again leading to poor school performance (29).

While bullying may only occasionally involve physical violence, physical violence is clearly one manifestation of bullying that can disrupt the functioning of schools and lead to a school crisis. The Federal Bureau of Investigation has linked school violence and bullying (30). In addition to harassing their peers, bullies can target school staff as well. In what may be an isolated example, an attack on a teacher at Central High School in St. Paul, Minnesota, led the teachers' union there to threaten a strike unless something was done about school climate, including the hiring of more school psychologists (31).

Working to avert a potential school strike is one important aspect of fixing the kind of bullying that can "result in more dangerous and sometimes deadly forms of violence" (29). However, perhaps the most frightening outcome of bullying is that bullies can turn into violent adults. Olweus (4) found that 60% of boys identified as bullies between sixth through ninth grade had at least one criminal conviction by the age of 24, and 40% had more than three arrests. Only 10% of boys who were not bullies in school had criminal records (29). These numbers perhaps more than anything else brought about the anti-bullying movement.

Also helping to spur anti-violence and anti-bullying movements is that fact that certain vulnerable groups are at higher risk for bullying. The 2013 National School Climate Survey by the Gay, Lesbian and Straight Education Network (GLSEN) found that 55.5% of lesbian, gay, bisexual, or transgender (LGBT) students "felt unsafe at school because of their sexual orientation" and "missed at least one entire day of school in the past month because they felt unsafe or uncomfortable."

A 2011 report by the support group for children with special needs, AbilityPath.org, found that children with special needs rank among the highest of any other subgroup experiencing bullying (AbilityPath.org,

2014). Besides non-heterosexual children and children with special needs, another group at significant risk for being bullied are children of low socioeconomic status (30).

With the spread of electronic devices and the proliferation of social media sites, cyberbullying is gaining attention as either an extension of traditional bullying or as a separate area of study with different causes and solutions. Given the lack of a consistent definitions, possible cultural differences in describing bullying, and a scarcity of longitudinal studies, it is difficult to pinpoint whether bullying is increasing, but most data support that traditional bullying is still a larger, although decreasing, problem, while cyberbullying is a smaller, although increasing, problem. In 2008 in the U.K., for example, cyberbullying rates were about half that of traditional bullying (15), but while traditional bullying rates were falling, cyberbullying rates were rising. The decrease in traditional bullying around the world has been attributed to the implementation of anti-bullying programs (32). Given the increasing rates of cyberbullying, it has become an educational concern internationally (33). In fact, some researchers suggest that the potential anonymity of the assault, the potential size of the audience, and the fact that cyberbullying behaviors can occur at any time day or night indicates that cyberbullying has the potential to be far more pervasive and create more emotional harm than traditional bullying (34, 35).

Cyberbullying can include sending mean text messages or emails, spreading rumors via email or social networking sites, setting up fake profiles, or exhibiting embarrassing photos or websites. The problem is exacerbated by the fact that often children are sending (or "sexting") embarrassing photos themselves, giving school-age or adult bullies the opportunity to blackmail the senders, a text-book example of cyberbullying. One Minneapolis police digital media examiner recently called the posting of pornographic images of children on the Internet "out of control" (36).

Predictably, individuals who make extensive use of digital media (cell phones, chat rooms, social media sites, or online gaming sites) are more susceptible to cyberbullying (33). Also, as with traditional bullying, cyberbullying is frequently aimed at students who are different in any way from the mainstream culture (33).

Because of the rapid proliferation of gadgets that can link to the Internet and the potential threat of cyberbullying, even countries like Saudi Arabia have taken an interest in cyberbullying research (37). Because cyberbullying is a relatively new phenomenon, researchers are trying to keep up with its spread and potential for causing harm not only to individuals but to school systems. School psychologists are still seeking to find the best practices to address and prevent cyberbullying.

Results from this study may enable school psychologists and other school personnel to become change agents by creating awareness, assessing the problem, and promoting positive outcomes. According to Adamson and Peacock (38), school mental health professionals, including school psychologists, are best positioned to deal with and counter bullying and cyberbullying in the schools. School psychologists can "educate administrators about the dangers of online victimization, as well as effective preventative measures" (39).

Early on, school mental health professionals can help by determining the nature and types of cyberbullying in their respective schools, as well as the patterns and prevalence of cyberbullying, and share these insights with other staff and administrators. Next, they can create intervention programs. These programs can clearly define cyberbullying so that teachers are aware of the difference between playful behaviors and bullying.

In studies so far, researchers have determined that multi-level approaches are the best to deal with cyberbullying, reaching schools, communities, and individuals. School plans should include activities that involve the entire school, such as hiring more supervisors for playgrounds, bathrooms, cafeterias, and hallways. School plans might also include researching and disseminating information about local laws dealing Internet abuse, including potential laws about cyberbullying. Schools can also implement cyber security software that can help monitor student computer use. Plans need to set clear guidelines for Internet use in the schools, including the regulation of cell phones and other electronic mobile devices. Students can also be taught how to save evidence and report instances of cyberbullying (40). In order to accomplish this, students need to feel that adults will take them seriously and do something about the behavior (29).

Mental health professionals can present school-wide programs about the ethical standards regarding cyberbullying. They can also create programs to promote empathy as well as bullying prevention in the classrooms. Plans should also focus on ways to involve all school personnel in the prevention of cyberbullying, including social workers and parents. School plans should also be put in place to identify students who are deemed at risk because of their status (e.g., non-heterosexual students) or because they spend greater amounts of time on the Internet. Finally, school personnel need to identify bullies and victims and create direct intervention programs for them, including long-term follow-up assistance (41). Teachers and counselors can then instruct potential victims on ways to block unwanted emails, instant messages, and texts from perpetrators.

School psychologists can also research packaged interventions currently being utilized in schools to increase awareness of cyberbullying and prevent it from happening (30). Such curricula include Quality Circle Approach, iSafe Internet Safety Program, Cyber-bullying: A Prevention Curriculum, Sticks and Stones, and Let's Fight It Together.

One of the most important steps school psychologists can take to help eliminate cyberbullying is to work with parents, since much of cyberbullying takes place outside of school. Parents need to be made aware of the dangers of cyberbullying and be instructed in ways to monitor their children's online activities. School psychologists can work with parents to give them the incentive and the skills to talk with their children about what is going on in their lives. Parents can also be given lists of simple things to do, such as putting computers in places that are easily viewed by adults. Parents can be helped with setting filtering and tracking software programs in order to monitor their children's online activities. They should also set clear expectations about the amount of time children spend online, including the playing of online games. Parents should also make their children comfortable about reporting online abuse and learn about the warning signs indicating a child may be the victim of cyberbullies (42).

At a state and national level, school psychologists can work to create policy and laws to address cyberbullying in order to reduce its impact. For example, the National Association of School Psychologists (NASP) recognizes that the kind of relational aggression represented by cyberbullying can jeopardize the psychological and emotional well-being of children and adolescents. Consequently, the organization encourages members to be leaders in the development of programs to prevent this type of school violence.

OUR STUDY

In 1970, after some high profile suicides in Scandinavia, Swedish psychologist Dan Olweus began what is now considered "the first scientific study of bullying problems in the world" (43). Over the intervening 45 years, hundreds if not thousands of studies have been undertaken on bullying around the world (44). While bullying remains a problem, with rates as high as 80% being reported in some cases (45), in what has to be a bright spot in the history of school psychology, bullying rates have actually decreased since efforts were made to reduce the problem. Between 1990 and 2009 a "significant decrease in bullying" was reported in many countries, possibly due to anti-bullying programs (32). Hymel and Swearer (1) also found a decrease in global rates of bullying during a similar period (2000-2010).

Over the past decade, however, a new enemy has arisen with the growth of mobile communication devices and social networking sites: cyberbullying. While Rigby and Smith (32) and Hymnel and Swearer (1) report drops in traditional bullying, both studies picked up indictors that cyberbullying increased during this period. No doubt in an attempt to bring attention to the topic, some researchers have used stories about 13-year-old Vermont resident Ryan Halligan, who committed suicide in 2003 (46), and about the 2010 suicide of Massachusetts teen Phoebe Prince (47) in their journal articles about cyberbullying, without indicating that in both cases the victim had also been a victim of traditional bullying. Nonetheless, because it appears to be a growing problem (18), cyberbullying has now become the focus of many studies (19). The vast majority of these studies deal with cyberbullying among children and adolescents. Only a few have focused on cyberbullying among college students (17, 21-23). Because limited research on cyberbullying among adults has been undertaken, college students (graduates and undergraduates) from Howard University were the focus of this study.

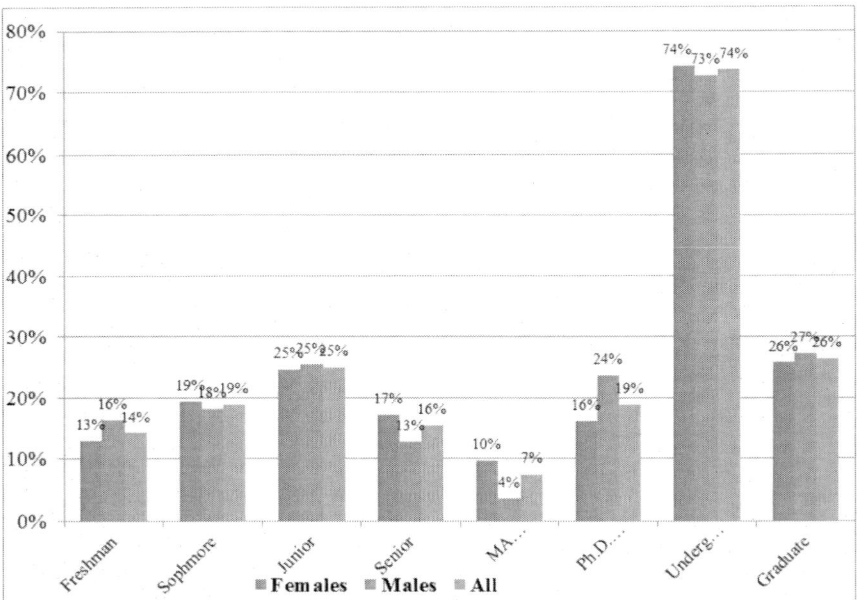

Figure 1. Distribution of school level by gender (in %).

Research sample

The current research relied on a self-reported study to determine the prevalence of the four categories of cyberbullying and victimization: cyberbullies only, victims only, bully/victims, and witnesses of bullying/victimization. The survey population was Howard University graduate and undergraduate students (N = 165). The sample consisted of 165 respondents, distributed equally between males and females. Figure 1 shows the distribution of schooling by gender. As can be seen from the graph, the share of males was not statistically different from that of females, with the exception of MA candidates, where the share of females was more than double that of males: 10% compared to 4%. As shown on the two sets of columns in the right side of the graph, 75% of the students were undergraduates and the other 25% were graduate students distributed equally between males and females.

Measures

This survey was developed by Willard (48), and Li (24). The survey is composed of four components and was modified to capture experiences of Howard University college students. Part I focused on demographics, and Part II focused on direct or indirect exposure and experiences with cyberbullying, beliefs and attitudes pertaining to acts cyberbullying as either participants or bystanders, reaction to cyberbullying, and who has ties to the victim. Part III concerns the witnessing of cyberbullying incidents, and subjects' responses (e.g., join in, watch or look). The fourth part of the survey includes items addressing the triggers of cyberbullying (e.g., it is cool, anger, jealousy), reporting cyberbullying, and students' opinions about online behaviors in general, which will be rated on a 5-point Likert-type scale from 1 (strongly agree) to 5 (strongly disagree).

Recruitment procedure

Founded in 1867, Howard University is a private university consisting of 13 colleges and more than 120 programs from which 120,000 degrees have been awarded in the arts, sciences, and humanities. The university is located in Washington, DC and has a long history of promoting the studies of disadvantaged persons in the US. Established as an academic institution for African-Americans, Howard University has played a critical role in providing opportunities to African-American professionals. Enrollment currently stands at 10,300 undergraduate, graduate, and professional students. Few studies have examined cyberbullying in the context of a university setting, as opposed to studies that have compared students in lower educational levels (including high school and middle school).

After obtaining the Institutional Review Board (IRB) approval from Howard University, the principal researcher contacted the chairs of undergraduate programs currently available at Howard University. The goal of this communication was to provide an overview of the study, its importance, its nature, and its implications for serving the Howard community through program development to help both victims and bullies. In addition to direct communication, the chairs received a letter that described the relevance of the study and ways in which it protects the confidentiality of study participants. From the pool of participant chairs who agreed to help the research team collect data from their departments, seven departments were randomly selected.

Each of the seven departments was contacted once more to arrange the number of classes that could assist in the recruitment of subjects. Five to seven classes were randomly visited in each department at the end of the class session. The departmental chair accompanied the principal investigator to introduce them to the instructor and the class. Upon each meeting with a class, the students were invited to assist with the study and were informed of its importance and the nature of the survey they would be asked to complete for the study. Students were informed about procedures for the maintenance of confidentiality. Students who agreed to participate were given the option to withdraw from the study if they experienced any discomfort.

During this class presentation about the study, students who agreed to participate received an informed consent form to complete confirming their willingness to take part in the research. From the pool of students who agreed to participate, 10 to 15 students were randomly selected and asked to remain after class to complete the survey, which included three sections requiring approximately ten minutes each, for a total of 30 minutes. The PI administered the surveys and collected them from participants. Students were instructed to answer all questions, seal the survey in the envelopes, and keep them on the table. The PI and the student researcher then collected all envelopes at the end of the session.

Collected data from the undergraduate department was coded, and access to this data is limited to the researcher and Howard IRB office. The same procedure was implemented in each of the five graduate programs that agreed to participate in the study.

FINDINGS

This section summarizes the findings in the three categories of cyberbullying under review: cyberbullying when one is a victim, an offender, or a witness.

Cyberbullying as a victim

A chi-square test of association was utilized to examine the association between cyberbullying as a victim, gender, and university level (graduate or undergraduate). Initial frequency tables (observed and expected values) showed that the data met the assumption of sample size and other assumptions. The results of the chi-square are presented below.

The results of the chi-square test showed no significant association between gender and cyberbullying as victim (x2 (df = 2) = 4.147, $p > .05$). When asked if they knew the offender, the results of the chi-square showed that female students tended to know the offender (chi-square (df =1) = 5.492, $p < .05$).

The results of the chi-square test also showed no significant association between school level (undergraduate versus graduate) and cyberbullying as victim (x2 (df = 2) = 2.785, $p > .05$). When asked if they knew the offender, the results of the chi-square showed that both undergraduate and graduate students did not know the offender (chi-square (df = 1) = 1.553, $p > .05$).

Table 1. Frequency of cyberbullying by gender: as victim (N = 155)

			During the past 12 months, how often have you been cyberbullied?			Total
			Never	**Once/Twice**	**3 or more times**	
Gender	1 male	Count	49	4	6	59
		Expected Count	47.2	7.6	4.2	59.0
		% of Total	31.6%	2.6%	3.9%	38.1%
		Residual	1.8	-3.6	1.8	
	2 female	Count	75	16	5	96
		Expected Count	76.8	12.4	6.8	96.0
		% of Total	48.4%	10.3%	3.2%	61.9%
		Residual	-1.8	3.6	-1.8	
Total		Count	124	20	11	155
		Expected Count	124.0	20.0	11.0	155.0
		% of Total	80.0%	12.9%	7.1%	100.0%

Chi- Square(df = 2) = 4.147, $p > .05$.

Table 2. School level by frequency of cyberbullying: as victim (N = 155)

			During the past 12 months, how often have you been cyberbullied?			Total
			Never	Once/Twice	3 or more times	
School Level	1 Undergraduate	Count	94	11	9	114
		Expected Count	91.3	14.2	8.5	114.0
		% of Total	58.4%	6.8%	5.6%	70.8%
		Residual	2.7	-3.2	.5	
	2 Graduate	Count	35	9	3	47
		Expected Count	37.7	5.8	3.5	47.0
		% of Total	21.7%	5.6%	1.9%	29.2%
		Residual	-2.7	3.2	-.5	
Total		Count	129	20	12	161
		Expected Count	129.0	20.0	12.0	161.0
		% of Total	80.1%	12.4%	7.5%	100.0%

Chi-Square (df = 2) = 2.785, $p > .05$.

Table 3. When you are cyberbullied what do you do?

	All		Males		Females	
Do nothing	26	17%	14	24%	12	12%
Tell the cyberbully to stop	20	13%	9	15%	11	11%
Get away	20	13%	11	19%	9	9%
Cyberbully other people	0	0%	0	0%	0	0%
Bully other students	0	0%	0	0%	0	0%
Tell an adult	0	0%	0	0%	0	0%
Tell a friend	1	1%	0	0%	1	1%
Tell instructors	1	1%	1	2%	0	0%
Tell parents	0	0%	0	0%	0	0%
Tell siblings	1	1%	0	0%	1	1%
Other	87	56%	24	41%	63	65%

When asked about their response to cyberbullying, 43% of survey participants were passive: 17% responded by saying they were not going to do anything about it, 13% responded by saying they would ask the cyberbully to stop, and 13% said they will get out. No student, either male or female, was willing to cyberbully other people or bully other students. Of special interest was the unwillingness of both males and female to ask others (student, adult, friend, instructor, or parent) to intervene. Comparing the responses of males and females, the most obvious result is that males were more passive than females, 58% compared to 32%.

Table 4. Methods of electronic harassment: as victim

	How did you receive the electronic harassment?					
	All		Males		Females	
	#	%	#	%	#	%
Via Facebook	14	9%	6	10%	8	8%
Via e-mail	5	3%	3	5%	2	2%
Via text message	12	8%	3	5%	9	9%
Via instant message	3	2%	1	2%	2	2%
Via other electronic method	5	3%	1	2%	4	4%
Combined methods	117	75%	45	76%	72	74%

As shown in Table 4, 75% of females and 76% of males received electronic harassments via multiple electronic methods. The most common methods were Facebook and text messages, which were received by 10% of males and 8% of females. The least-used method was the instant message method, with only 2% of females and 2% of males reporting electronic harassment via instant messaging.

Cyberbullying as an offender

A chi-square test of association was utilized to examine the association between cyberbullying as an offender, gender, and university level (graduate or undergraduate). Initial frequency tables (observed and expected values) showed that the data met the assumption of sample size and other assumptions. The results of the chi-square are presented below.

As shown in Table 5, the results of the chi-square test showed no significant association between gender and cyberbullying as an offender ($x2$ ($df = 2$) $= 5.640$, $p > .05$). When the offender was asked if he or she knew the victim, the results of the chi-square show that both male and female offenders did not know the victim (chi-square ($df = 1$) $= 1.048$, $p > .05$).

The results of the chi-square test also showed no significant association between school level (undergraduate versus graduate) and cyberbullying as an offender ($x2$ ($df = 2$) $= .998$, $p > .05$). When offenders were asked if they knew their victims, the results of the chi-square showed that both graduate and undergraduate offender students did not know their victims (chi-square ($df = 1$) $= .999$, $p > .05$).

Again we can see that both males and females send electronic harassments via multiple electronic methods: 86% of females and 75% of males. Surprisingly, the most common method (other) was not among the four popular methods. Facebook ranked in second place with 5% of males and 3% of females using it to send harassment messages to others. In this study, females did not use either e-mail or instant messages to deliver electronic harassment messages to others.

Table 5. Cyberbullying by gender: as offender (N = 154)

			During the past 12 months, how often have you cyberbullied others?			Total
			Never	Once/Twice	3 or more	
Gender	1 male	Count	48	6	4	58
		Expected Count	52.0	4.1	1.9	58.0
		% of Total	31.2%	3.9%	2.6%	37.7%
		Residual	-4.0	1.9	2.1	
	2 female	Count	90	5	1	96
		Expected Count	86.0	6.9	3.1	96.0
		% of Total	58.4%	3.2%	0.6%	62.3%
		Residual	4.0	-1.9	-2.1	
Total		Count	138	11	5	154
		Expected Count	138.0	11.0	5.0	154.0
		% of Total	89.6%	7.1%	3.2%	100.0%

Chi-Square (df = 2) = 5.640, $p > .05$.

Table 6. Frequency of cyberbullying and school level: as offender (N = 159)

			During the past 12 months, how often have you cyberbullied others?			Total
			Never	**Once/Twice**	**3 or more times**	
School_Level	1 Undergraduate	Count	100	10	3	113
		Expected Count	101.6	8.5	2.8	113.0
		% of Total	62.9%	6.3%	1.9%	71.1%
		Residual	-1.6	1.5	.2	
	2 Graduate	Count	43	2	1	46
		Expected Count	41.4	3.5	1.2	46.0
		% of Total	27.0%	1.3%	0.6%	28.9%
		Residual	1.6	-1.5	-.2	
Total		Count	143	12	4	159
		Expected Count	143.0	12.0	4.0	159.0
		% of Total	89.9%	7.5%	2.5%	100.0%

Chi-Square (df = 2) = .998, $p > .05$.

Table 7. Methods of electronic harassment: as offender

	What method of electronic harassment did you use?					
Facebook	6	4%	3	5%	3	3%
E-mail	0	0%	0	0%	0	0%
Text message	8	5%	4	7%	4	4%
Instant message	1	1%	1	2%	0	0%
Other	14	9%	7	12%	7	7%
Combined methods	127	81%	44	75%	83	86%

Table 8. Why do you cyberbully others?

	All		Males		Females	
	#	%	#	%	#	%
It's cool	3	2%	3	5%	0	0%
Boredom	1	1%	1	2%	0	0%
Dislike for the victim	2	1%	0	0%	2	2%
Bride	0	0%	0	0%	0	0%
My own low self esteem	0	0%	0	0%	0	0%
Revenge	1	1%	1	2%	0	0%
Ability to remain anonymous	1	1%	0	0%	1	1%
Jealousy	0	0%	0	0%	0	0%
Power seeking	0	0%	0	0%	0	0%
Power maintenance	1	1%	0	0%	1	1%
Fear of direct confrontation	0	0%	0	0%	0	0%
Frustration	0	0%	0	0%	0	0%
Anger	2	1%	0	0%	2	2%
depression	0	0%	0	0%	0	0%
alcohol abuse	0	0%	0	0%	0	0%
drug abuse	0	0%	0	0%	0	0%
bear pressure	0	0%	0	0%	0	0%
loneliness	0	0%	0	0%	0	0%
feeling of isolation	1	1%	1	2%	0	0%
Combination of the above reasons	144	92%	53	90%	91	94%

In general, there were no significant differences between the answers of males and females.

In Table 8, we can see that there is no specific reason why students cyberbully others. No single unique answer was significant by itself; no one answer was approved by more than 2% of the respondents, male or female. However, 92% of the students gave more than one reason, and sometimes even ten reasons, for cyberbullying others.

Cyberbullying as direct or indirect witness

This study also questioned participants about their experiences as witnesses to cyberbullying: how often they witnessed it, and whether they were likely to report it to anyone.

Table 9. Gender by frequency of witnessing cyberbullying (N = 155)

			How frequently have you directly or indirectly witnessed cyberbullying incidents in your university?			Total
			1 Never	2 1-2 times	3 3 or more	
Gender	1 male	Count	17	10	32	59
		% of Total	11.0%	6.5%	20.6%	38.1%
		Residual	5.2	-2.9	-2.3	
	2 female	Count	14	24	58	96
		% of Total	9.0%	15.5%	37.4%	61.9%
		Residual	-5.2	2.9	2.3	
Total		Count	31	34	90	155
		% of Total	20.0%	21.9%	58.1%	100.0%

Chi-Square (df =2) = 5.020, $p > .05$.

When asked how often they witnessed a cyberbullying event within the university, both males and female reported equal frequencies. There were no significant difference between males and females on the number of times they witnessed a cyberbullying event (chi-square (df=2) = 5.020, $p > .05$).

When asked how often they witnessed a cyberbullying incident within the university, there was a significant association between the school level and the number of times respondents witnessed cyberbullying (chi-square (df = 2) = 17.578, $p < .001$). Undergraduate students reported significantly higher frequency of witnessing cyberbullying than did graduate students (Spearman's rho = -.33).

Table 10. School level by frequency of witnessing cyberbullying (N = 166)

			How frequently have you directly or indirectly witnessed cyberbullying incidents in your university?			Total
			1 Never	1-2 times	3 or more	
School _Level	1 Undergraduate	Count	15	25	74	114
		% of Total	9.3%	15.5%	46.0%	70.8%
		Residual	-9.1	-1.2	10.3	
	2 Graduate	Count	19	12	16	47
		% of Total	11.8%	7.5%	9.9%	29.2%
		Residual	9.1	1.2	-10.3	
Total		Count	34	37	90	161
		% of Total	21.1%	23.0%	55.9%	100.0%

Chi-Square (df = 2) = 17.578, p < .001.

Table 11. Response to cyberbullying

If you were cyberbullied at school or home would you report it?					
Probably YES		49%		43%	53%
Probably NO		51%		57%	47%
		Frequency	**Percent**	**Valid Percent**	**Cumulative Percent**
Valid	1	82	47.7	49.1	49.1
	2	83	48.3	49.7	98.8
	6	2	.6	.6	99.4
	Total	167	97.1	100.0	
Missing	System	5	2.9		
Total		172	100.0		

Table 11 shows results when students were asked whether they would report being cyberbullied at school or at home. Results were divided equally between "probably yes" and "probably no" without any difference between genders.

When asked the most important reasons why they would probably not report cyberbullying, a substantial percentage of subjects (n = 83, 49.70%) answered, "I don't think the university would/could do anything to stop it." Another 47.7% (n = 82) answered, "I don't think the university staff would understand or believe me."

Table 12 provides additional data on survey respondents' opinions on cyberbullying. For example, the majority either disagreed (29.3%) or strongly disagreed (29.3%) with the statement that there is "nothing you can do to stop it." The remaining 39% strongly agreed (7.85%), agreed (15.6%) or were neutral (18.6%) on this statement.

Table 12. Opinions on cyberbullying

Item	Strongly agree	Agree	Neutral	Disagree	Strongly disagree
Nothing you can do to stop it	7.8	15.0	18.6	29.3	29.3
I know of someone who has been hurt by cyberbullying	13.3	35.8	16.4	15.2	19.4
Things that happened online should stay online	4.8	9.0	17.4	34.1	34.7
It's important to tell somebody about it	43.1	35.9	16.2	4.2	.6
I will report a cyberbullying incident	26.9	31.7	26.3	10.2	4.8
I have the right to say anything I want online even if it hurts someone	3.6	11.4	18.7	23.5	42.8
Students should stay out of this	46.4	32.5	15.7	2.4	3.0
I would like to create a more kind and respectful online world.	48.5	26.1	18.8	2.4	4.2

Results also showed that the majority either strongly agreed (13.3%) or agreed (35.8%) with the statement "I know of someone who has been hurt by cyberbullying," while 16.4% were neutral, 15.2% disagreed, and 19.4% strongly disagreed. Regarding the statement "Things that happened online should stay online," the majority disagreed (34.1) or strongly disagreed (34.7); the majority of subjects either strongly agreed (43.1) or agreed (35.9) that it is important to tell somebody about cyberbullying. In response to the statement "I will report cyberbullying," 26.9% strongly agreed and 31.7% agreed. With respect to the statement "I have the right to say anything I want online even if it hurts someone," 42.8 strongly disagreed or disagreed (32.5%). In addition, 46.4% strongly agreed and

32.5% agreed with the statement "Students should stay out of this." Finally, 48.5% and 26.1% either strongly agreed or agreed with statement "I would like to create a more kind and respectful online world."

Table 13. Gender differences on opinions (Mann-Whitney Test)

Ranks				
	Gender	**N**	**Mean Rank**	**Sum of Ranks**
V51	1 male	56	70.13	3927.00
	2 female	95	79.46	7549.00
	Total	151		
V52	1 male	56	82.73	4633.00
	2 female	93	70.34	6542.00
	Total	149		
V53	1 male	56	63.68	3566.00
	2 female	95	83.26	7910.00
	Total	151		
V54	1 male	56	79.14	4432.00
	2 female	95	74.15	7044.00
	Total	151		
V55	1 male	56	83.16	4657.00
	2 female	95	71.78	6819.00
	Total	151		
V56	1 male	56	71.00	3976.00
	2 female	95	78.95	7500.00
	Total	151		
V57	1 male	56	64.55	3615.00
	2 female	95	82.75	7861.00
	Total	151		
V58	1 male	56	87.15	4880.50
	2 female	94	68.56	6444.50
	Total	150		

Test Statistics[a]								
	V51	**V52**	**V53**	**V54**	**V55**	**V56**	**V57**	**V58**
Mann-Whitney U	2331.000	2171.000	1970.000	2484.000	2259.000	2380.000	2019.000	1979.500
Wilcoxon W	3927.000	6542.000	3566.000	7044.000	6819.000	3976.000	3615.000	6444.500
Z	-1.308	-1.759	-2.790	-.727	-1.608	-1.134	-2.648	-2.735
Asymp. Sig. (2-tailed)	.191	.079	.005	.467	.108	.257	.008	.006
[a.] Grouping Variable: Gender								

The results of the Mann-Whitney U test showed a significant difference between male and female students on three items of their opinions: Things that happened online should stay online; students should stay out of this; and I would like to create more kind and respectful online world. On the first two, females have lower scores than males. On the last item, females had a higher score.

DISCUSSION

The data showed no significant correlation between cyberbullying and gender among college students, although female students tended to know the bullies more often than did male students. On one hand, we can take these data at face value and accept that there is no correlation. On the other hand, this absence of correlation could be a result of males reporting being cyberbullied or perpetrating cyberbullying at lesser rates than females. We have no way of knowing which explanation is correct. It could be that both are, and that in college, reporting of cyberbullying decreases for females as result of culture socialization, and that males in college report cyberbullying at a greater rate than in high school.

If we take these data at face value, the findings would suggest that physical bullying and cyberbullying decrease for female respondents and equalize with male victims and perpetrators. The problem with earlier research on traditional and cyberbullying, however, is that the definitions of both bullying and cyberbullying are different from study to study, and it is difficult to rationalize these various definitions even as they govern the responses of subjects. It could, in fact, be that the different definitions govern the outcomes of the research. Regardless of this difficulty, however, it is clear from Table 12 that female college/university students report being significantly more upset by being bullied than do males.

Because this study examined cyberbullying among both undergraduate and graduate university students, one would expect to see some significant differences from studies of younger (middle school and high school) students. However, among college and university students we found no significant correlation between college/university levels and reports of cyberbullying. These findings did not stand in contrast to studies of high school students. It could be either that college/university students are more subject to cyberbullying than high school students, or that they tend to report cyberbullying more than high school students. Certainly, as is shown in Tables 1 and 2, most Howard University students report they have not been subjected to cyberbullying, and among those who have experienced bullying, most have only been the object of cyberbullying once or twice. This finding indicates that, although being bullied is serious for those experiencing it, most students are not subject to it.

Table 8 shows that there is no single trigger for cyberbullying as a perpetrator. This is not surprising, since people who bully, whether they are males or females, are responding to many factors in their own lives that may be relieved by being mean to other less powerful people.

Among the more important findings of the study is that people witnessing cyberbullying were affected by it. Although there was no correlation between witnessing and gender, there was strong correlation between witnessing and level of education. Undergraduates were more often witnesses to cyberbullying than graduate students. Table 11 suggests that witnesses will not report the cyberbullying. They may not approve of the cyberbullying, but they will avoid dealing with it. This response should not be taken to mean that they approve of it, but only that they will do nothing. The study did not compile data on the effect of witnessing others cyberbullying, but can surmise that it does have some effect on the witnesses. Perhaps some might be sufficiently bothered by witnessing something they believe is wrong, so that they will, in the long term, resolve to report future incidents they witness. Some may prefer the safety of ignoring a wrong and not ever do anything despite believing cyberbullying is wrong.

An important characteristic of cyberbullying that is different from physical bullying is that cyberbullying can be anonymous and is never face-to-face, while physical bullying is necessarily personal and face-to-face (or face to fist). This changes the fundamental nature of bullying. Physical bullying is always about dominance of the bully over the bullied, while cyberbullying may be more about expressing something by the bully and may (or may not) be about the victim. If the victim does not know the bully and may not know even who the bully is, the perpetrator's dominance may not be an issue. Furthermore, physical bullying is almost always same-sex bullying (usually male on male), while cyberbullying may not be. One interesting finding is that although the majority (57%) felt either upset (34%) or very upset (23%) about cyberbullying, and that females were more upset than males about cyberbullying, the vast majority of subjects would not report it, indicating "I don't think the university would/could do anything to stop it." Another 47.7% answered, "I don't think the university staff would understand or believe me."

Limitations

One of the weaknesses of this study is that it was built from self-reported data. In fact, someone may feel cyberbullied for something where the perpetrator does not believe he or she is being a bully at all, but confronting someone with "the truth" of their own behavior. In other words, some of the incidents may be viewed as cyberbullying by the recipient of cyber communication, but not by the sender. This would explain why our data show that victimization is more frequently reported than is perpetration. It could also be that cyberbullies do not care to admit, even in an anonymous survey, that they have cyberbullied others.

Cyberbullying, in Olweus' (4) definition, necessarily puts the victim in a one-down position, since the bullies can be anonymous. On the other hand, a cyberbully remaining anonymous is not likely to be in a one-up position, as in physical bullying. This electronic distance creates a difference in the reaction of the victim. Recently a number of school shooting incidents have been shootings of physical bullies by their victims. On the other hand, many teen suicides have been attributed to being cyberbullied, where the bullies remain anonymous. In other words, physical bullying evokes an externalizing response by the victims, while cyberbullying evokes an internalizing response. In some ways, then, cyberbullying may be even more dangerous than physical bullying.

Another weakness of this study is that it did not explore cyberbullying of faculty (especially teaching assistants) by students. The anonymous character of cyberbullying allows students to bully faculty, and teaching assistants are especially vulnerable. Additionally, because the sample includes Howard University only, it may produce selection bias and will not reflect a true estimate of the problem in other college level institutions. Finally, given the complexity of cyberbullying and its definitions, future studies should also integrate qualitative data to enrich findings. Combinations of data from different school sources (interviews with instructors, students, their peanuts) should also be considered. Although this cross-sectional survey design serves as a preliminary study, the findings have major advantages in terms of implications for practice.

Cyberbullying is a new phenomenon in the past 20 years. Prior to the mid-nineties, in fact, the media for cyberbullying did not even exist. One problem this novelty has created is that we are still having a hard time defining it. For school policy makers and for legislators, the lack of definitions creates a serious problem, in that without an accepted definition of cyberbullying, effective policies and laws cannot be made. For school psychologists, actions cannot be planned or taken, and for researchers, programs cannot be developed or tested.

Given this definitional problem, there has been surprisingly little research conducted. One approach taken in Europe has been to try identifying potential perpetrators and building specific plans to prevent them from acting out. While this approach has some promise, a more promising idea is to build the threat of cyberbullying into school- and district-based actions and crisis management plans. Even this approach, however, presents a problem, since cyberbullying (like physical bullying) often happens away from the school. The results may be a problem for the school district, but the cyberbullying itself may not necessarily happen on school grounds.

Bullying generally has been dealt with in school crisis management plans through bullying prevention programs (49). Raskauskas advocates a comprehensive program involving identifying bullies and victims, including both in face-to-face student "courts," developing an anti-bullying curriculum, and providing counseling and support groups for both bullies and victims. Raskauskas' (49) systematic approach is one of the few comprehensive anti-cyberbullying programs in the literature and presents a thoughtful response and a hopeful direction for school psychologists and policy makers facing the continuing likelihood of cyberbullying among K-12 and university-level student populations.

School psychologists who desire to create anti-cyberbullying programs "are well served to begin" with the issue of bullying (26). The first step is to make stakeholders aware of the consequences of bullying. Larson relates the story of an experienced educator who was surprised at the reactions of his bigger, stronger colleagues to fights that would break out. "They would stand around and watch," he said, "while I weighed in to break them up. I realized later that they had probably been the victors in such altercations when they had been in school and, therefore, were not able to understand what it was like to be on the losing end" (26).

As part of the training in a Canadian anti-bullying program called "Promoting relationships and eliminating violence" relies on three principles:

- Bullying is wrong and hurtful and contravenes the United Nations Convention on the Rights of the Child.
- Bullying as a child can lead to workplace harassment, dating aggression, marital abuse later and requires relationship solutions.
- Promoting healthy relationships is everyone's responsibility (5).

In other words, both the victim and the bully suffer negative consequences and educators, parents, and the entire community need to understand that. Any program needs to confront "cognitive distortions," that bullying is not really that bad, that the bullied person deserved it, that victims need to learn how to take it, etc.

The next step is to create a team that will assess the prevalence and types of bullying in the school. Fears about the reliability of information from surveys of children are unfounded, since "children's aggregated descriptions of peers' social adjustment have been repeatedly found to be consistent, stable over time, and highly predictive of important life outcomes, such as completing school. Adults can be surveyed as well. Since participation in bullying is transmitted across generations surveys must take into consideration "individual, family, peer, school, and community contexts for explanations underlying bullying incidents." Key risk factors include family variables (such as neglect), individual variables (past aggressive behavior), social variables (sibling or peer delinquency or gang membership), and environmental variables (high crime neighborhood). Larson (26) also stresses that the origins of bullying are complex and any anti-bullying programs cannot have a "within-child focus" but must work collaboratively with family, school system, community, and culture (p. 1292). How best to get schools, parents and teachers to comply with any established protocols is clearly one of the fundamental needs that must be met.

Once information on cyberbullying has been gathered, school psychologists can lead a team to design an intervention program from the bottom up, since top-down systems create little lasting change to the overall system.

Nation et al. (50) have come up with a list of nine characteristics of any intervention programs, whether for drug and alcohol abuse, teenage pregnancy, or cyberbullying prevention. They must provide:

- comprehensive, multiple interventions across communities
- varied teaching methods, not relying too much on sharing of information or group discussions.
- sufficient exposure to the program
- a theory-driven program supported by empirical research
- a way to promote strong relationships with adults and peers
- appropriately timed for developmental needs
- activities tailored to the community
- evaluation of the results
- training for the staff

Taking into account these characteristics, many researchers suggest a three-tier approach to bullying or cyberbullying prevention. The first tier involves improving elements that can help all students, such as incorporating architectural design features to discourage criminal behavior, such as good lighting and good sightlines (26). Adult monitoring in areas where bullying behavior takes place, such as playgrounds, can also be part of the first tier. Programs to help teachers improve the classroom climate for every child can also be implemented.

Second-tier programs are aimed at those students who are "at-risk" for cyberbullying behavior based on self-assessments, peer evaluations, teacher recommendations, and any other information gathered during the assessment process. This is approximately 10-15% of the school population. Although some researchers suggest that those students who have already displayed some tendencies toward fighting or bullying should automatically go into the third tier, other researchers (26) think the second tier might be appropriate for some students who have already displayed aggressive behaviors. These second-tier programs can include anger management classes, which, as a general treatment strategy, have been found to be "effective in reducing antisocial behaviors" among second tier students (26).

Those students with the highest risk of offense could be put in the third tier of prevention, which involves about 3-5% of the school population. Larson (26) contends the third tier will require coordination with support groups outside the school to create a proactive plan that is "not purely reactive and punitive" and may include alternate schooling (p. 1301).

By incorporating these attributes, several bullying prevention programs have proven effective, such as the Olweus Bullying Prevention Program, Bully Busters, Steps to Respect, and Bully-Proofing Your School.

Other concerns should be taken into consideration as well. While all prevention programs need to develop clear goals so that everyone knows what is expected, no programs should develop a zero-tolerance approach, which could be too severe and inhibit reporting. That does not mean that intervention should not be consistent, however.

While most of the focus may be on the bully, interventions must be created to help the chronically bullied as well. Counseling for victims should also include teachers who are victims of school violence. The role of the school psychologist is central to prevention programs. School psychologists can help coordinate the prevention team, help conduct the needs assessment, analyze the results, and set priorities and goals (26).

APPENDIX: CYBERBULLYING STUDENT SURVEY

This survey seeks information from students about cyberbullying. Cyberbullying includes, but is not limited to sending angry, rude, vulgar messages about a person to an online group or to that person electronically; or sending harmful, untrue, or cruel statements about a person to other people or posting such material online; or pretending to be someone else and sending or posting material that makes that person look bad; or sending or posting material about a person that contains sensitive, private, or embarrassing information, including forwarding private messages or images, or cruelly excluding someone from an online group. Cyberbullying might occur at home or at school, through the Internet network or a cell phone used.

Your responses to this survey are confidential. You may also choose not to respond to this survey. By completing this survey, you are granting the researcher permission to use this information.

Part 1: About You

1. Gender: M____F
2. Ethnic Background (e.g., Asian): ___________
3. School level:

    ____freshman,

    ____sophomore,

    ____ junior,

____senior,

____Master's student,

____Ph.D. student

4. Your marital status, please specify: ____
5. On the following scale, consider A to be the best and C to be the average, your school grades are usually (circle one):
   A…………B…………C…………D……….F

Part 2: Cyberbullying (Your Experience as a Cybervictim)

1. **During the past 12 months,** how often have you been cyberbullied? (Check one that applies):
   ___ Never
   ___ Once/Twice
   ___ More than three times
2. How did you receive the electronic harassment (check all that apply):
   ___via Facebook,
   ___via e-mail,
   ___via text message,
   ___via instant message,
   ___via Other electronic method, specify: ___
3. Did you know the offender? _______Yes _______No
4. On the following scale, check your reaction to cyberbullying:
   ___No big deal
   ___Live with it
   ___Upset
   ___Very upset
   ___neutral
   ___No opinion
5. When you are cyberbullied, you (check all that apply):
   __Do nothing
   __Tell the cyberbully to stop

__Get away (e.g., log off) from the cyberbully
__Cyberbully other people
__Bully other students
__Tell another adult
__Tell a friend
__Tell instructors,
__Tell parents,
__Tell siblings,

6. If you have been cyberbullied, what happened after you told someone?
   __It got better
   __It got worse
   __Nothing changed
   __I never told anyone.
   __I've never been cyberbullied.
7. If you have been cyberbullied, who has tried to help you? (check all that apply):
   __My parents
   __My sister(s) or brother(s)
   __A instructor or
   __departmental chair
   __ Dean office
   __My friend(s)
   __Nobody
   __I've never been cyberbullied.

Part 3: Cyberbullying (Your Experience as a Cyber offender)

1. **During the past 12 months,** how often have you cyberbullied others? (as offender Check one that applies):
   ___Never
   ___Once/Twice
   ___more than three times

2. What method did you use (check all that apply):
   ___Facebook,
   ___e-mail,
   ___text message,
   ___instant message,
   ___Other, specify: ___
3. Why do you cyberbully others? Because (circle all that apply):
   Because:
   __It is cool
   __Boredom
   __Dislike for the victim
   __Pride
   __My own low self-esteem,
   __Revenge
   __Ability to remain anonymous
   __Jealousy of others
   __Power seeking
   __Power maintenance
   __Fear of direct confrontation
   __Feelings of frustration
   __Anger
   __Depression
   __Alcohol abuse
   __Drug abuse
   __Peer pressure
   __Loneliness
   __Feelings of isolation
   __Other,
   specify____
4. Did you know the victim? _______yes _______No
5. Did you let others know?
   Tell instructors, _______
   Tell Chair, _______
   Tell the Dean office, _______

6. How did you as a perpetrator felt afterward?
   very good, _______
   good, bad, _______
   very bad, _______
   neutral, _______
7. What is your feeling about people being cyberbullied?
   __They deserve it
   __It's too bad, but there is nothing we can do about it.
   __It is a very serious problem and we need to stop it.

Part 4: Cyberbullying (Your Experience as Witness)

1. How frequently have you directly or indirectly witnessed cyberbullying incidents in your university ? ___Never ___Once/Twice ___More than three times
2. If you have been a witness to cyberbullying incidents at the university, what is your normal response (check all that apply)?
   __Join in
   __Cheer the cyberbully on
   __Watch or look, but do not participate
   __Leave the online environment
   __Object to others, but not directly to the cyberbully
   __Object to the cyberbully
   __Try to help or befriend the victim
   __Report the cyberbullying to someone who can help the victim

   __Have not been a witness
   __Other,
   specify____
3. If you were cyberbullied at the university, would you report the cyberbullying to instructors, or administrator?
   ____ Probably yes
   _____ Probably no

• If you answered "probably no," what are the most important reasons why you would probably not report (check all that apply):
__I don't think university staff would understand or believe me
__I don't think the university would or could do anything to stop it
__I could get myself into trouble, because I could also be at fault
__I could get myself into trouble, even if I had done nothing wrong
__The cyberbully could get back at me and make things even worse

__Other students at the university could make fun of me
__I need to learn to deal with cyberbullying by myself
__Cyberbullying is no big deal. People should just ignore it
__Other,
specify____

Your Opinion

1. Please indicate your opinion to the following statements:

• Cyberbullying is a normal part of the online world. There is nothing anyone can do to stop it.

___Strongly agree___ Agree___ Neutral ___ Disagree
___Strongly disagree

• I know of someone who has been really hurt by cyberbullying.

___Strongly agree___ Agree___ Neutral ___ Disagree
___Strongly disagree

• Things that happen online should stay online.

___Strongly agree___ Agree___ Neutral ___ Disagree
___Strongly disagree

• If someone is being hurt by cyberbullying, it is important to tell a responsible adult.

___Strongly agree___ Agree___ Neutral ___ Disagree
___Strongly disagree

• I would report cyberbullying incidents, if I could do so without anyone knowing it was me.

___Strongly agree___ Agree___ Neutral ___ Disagree
___Strongly disagree

• I have the right to say anything I want online, even if what I say hurts someone or violates someone's privacy.

___Strongly agree___ Agree___ Neutral ___ Disagree
___Strongly disagree

• Students should stay out of this.

___Strongly agree___ Agree___ Neutral ___ Disagree
___Strongly disagree

• I would like to create a more kind and respectful online world.

___Strongly agree___ Agree___ Neutral ___ Disagree
___Strongly disagree

REFERENCES

[1] Hymel S, Swearer SM. Four decades of research on school bullying. Am Psychologist 2015;70(4):293-9. doi.org/10.1037/a0038928.

[2] Gradinger P, Strohmeier D, Spiel C. Traditional bullying and cyberbullying: Identification of risk groups for adjustment problems. J Psychology 2009;217(4):205-13. doi.org/10.1027/0044-3409.217.4.205.

[3] Ferris PA. The role of the consulting psychologist in the prevention, detection, and correction of bullying and mobbing in the workplace. Consult Psychol J 2009;61(3):169-89. doi.org/10.1037/a0016783.

[4] Olweus D. Bullying at school. Oxford: Blackwell, 1993.

[5] Craig WM, Pepler DJ. Understanding bullying: From research to practice. Can Psychol 2007;48(2):86-93. doi.org/10.1037/cp2007010.

[6] Smith M. Bullying: Mostly in schools [Review of the book "New perspectives on bullying by K Rigby]. Crisis 2004;25(1):43-4. doi.org/10.1027/0227-5910.25.1.43.

[7] Rivers I, Poteat VP, Noret N, Ashurst N. Observing bullying at school: The mental health implications of witness status. Sch Psychol Quart 2009;24(4):211-23. doi.org/10.1037/a0018164.

[8] Bradshaw CP. Translating research to practice in bullying prevention. Am Psychologist 2015;70(4):322-32. doi.org/10.1037/a0039114.

[9] Office of the Surgeon General. Youth violence: A report of the Surgeon General. Rockville, MD: Office Surgeon General, 2001.

[10] Dickey CR, Stiller B, Tomlanovich A. Decreasing bullying behaviors in middle school: Expect respect. Sch Psychol Quart 2014;29(3):272-86. doi.org/10.1037/spq0000070.

[11] Jones LM, Mitchell KJ, Finkelhor D. Online harassment in context: Trends from three youth internet safety surveys (2000, 2005, 2010). Psychol Violence 2013;3(1):53-69. doi.org/10.1037/a0030309.

[12] Tokunaga RS. Following you home from school: A critical review and synthesis of research on cyberbullying victimization. Comput Hum Behav 2010;26(3):277-87. doi.org/10.1016/j.chb.2009.11.014.

[13] Patchin JW, Hinduja S. Bullies move beyond the schoolyard: A preliminary look at cyberbullying. Youth Violence Juvenile Justice 2006;4(2):148-69.

[14] Li Q. A cross-cultural comparison of adolescents' experience related to cyberbullying. Educ Res 2008;50(3):223-34. doi.org/10.1080/00131880802309333.

[15] Slonje R, Smith PK. Cyberbullying: Another main type of bullying? Scand J Psychology 2008;49:147-54. doi.org/10.1111/j.1467-9450.2007.00611.x.

[16] Mitchell KJ, Jones LM, Turner HA, Shattuck A, Wolak J. The role of technology in peer harassment: Does it amplify harm for youth? Psychol Violence 2016;6(2):193-204. doi.org/10.1037/a0039317.

[17] Bauman S, Newman ML. Testing assumptions about cyberbullying: Perceived distress associated with acts of conventional and cyber bullying. Psychol Violence 2013;3(1):27-38. doi.org/10.1037/a0029867.

[18] You S, Kim E, Kim M. An ecological approach to bullying in Korean adolescents. J Pacific Rim Psychol 2014;8(1):1-10. doi.org/10.1017/prp.2014.1.

[19] Cénat JM, Hébert M, Blais M, Lavoie F, Guerrier M, Derivois D. Cyberbullying, psychological distress and self-esteem among youth in Quebec schools. J Affect Disord 2014;169:7-9. doi.org/10.1016/j.jad.2014.07.019.

[20] Foody M, Samara M, Carlbring P. A review of cyberbullying and suggestions for online psychological therapy. Internet Interventions 2015;2:235-42. doi.org/10.1016/j.invent.2015.05.002.

[21] Goldsmid S, Howie P. Bullying by definition: An examination of definitional components of bullying. Emotional Behavl Diff 2014;19(2):210-25. doi.org/10.1080/13632752.2013.844414.

[22] Barlett CP, Gentile DA. Attacking others online: The formation of cyberbullying in late adolescence. Psychol Popular Media Culture 2012;1(2):123-35. doi.org/10.1037/a0028113.

[23] Barlett CP. Anonymously hurting others online: The effect of anonymity on cyberbullying frequency. Psychol Popular Media Culture 2015;4(2):70-9. doi.org/10.1037/a0034335.

[24] Li Q. Cyberbullying in high schools: A study of students' behaviors, beliefs about this new phenomenon. J Aggress Maltreat Trauma 2010;19:372-92. doi.org/10.1080/10926771003788979.

[25] Duy B. Teachers' attitudes toward different types of bullying and victimization in Turkey. Psychol Sch 2013;50(10):987-1002. doi.org/10.1002/pits.21729.

[26] Larson J. Best practices in school violence prevention. In: Thomas A, Grimes J, eds. Best practices in school psychology V. Bethesda, MD: National Association School Psychologists, 2008:1291-1307.

[27] Nunn KP. Bullying. J Pediatr Child Health 2010;46:140-1. doi.org/10.1111/j.1440-1754.2010.01769.x.

[28] Liu J, Graves N. Childhood bullying: A review of constructs, concepts, and nursing implications. Public Health Nurs 2011;28(6):556-68. doi.org/10.1111/j.1525-1446.2011.00972.x.

[29] Whitted KS, Dupper DR. Best practices for preventing or reducing bullying in schools. Child Sch 2005;27(3):167-75. doi.org/10.1093/cs/27.3.167.

[30] Jones JR, Augustine SM. Creating an anti-bullying culture in secondary schools: Characteristics to consider when constructing appropriate anti-bullying programs. Am Second Educ 2015;43(3):73-83.

[31] Driscoll K. St Paul teachers threaten to strike of problem of school discipline. Villager 2015 Dec 23.

[32] Rigby K, Smith PK. Is school bullying really on the rise? Soc Psychol Educ 2011;14:441-55. doi.org/10.1007/s11218-011-9158-y.

[33] Herrera J, Kupczynski L, Mundy MA. The impact of training on faculty and student perception of cyberbullying in an urban south central Texas middle school. Res Higher Educ J 2015;27(1):1-29.

[34] Hoff DL, Mitchell SN. Cyberbullying: Causes, effects, and remedies. J Educ Adm 2009;47(5):562-5. doi.org/10.1108/09578230910981107.

[35] Sprague J. Integrated approaches to bullying and cyber bullying in schools, 2014. URL: http://www.ibpaworld.org/wp-content/uploads/2014/11/Jeff-Sprague-Integrated-Approaches-1.pdf.

[36] Montemayor S. Metro sees 'out of control' rise in child porn. Star Tribune 2016 Jan 03.

[37] Feinberg T. Bullying prevention and intervention. NASP Principle Leadership Magazine 2003;4(1). URL: http://www.naspcenter.org/principals/nassp_bullying.html.

[38] Adamson AD, Peacock GG. Crisis response in the public schools: A survey of school psychologists' experiences and perceptions. Psychol Sch 2007;44(8):749-64. doi.org/10.1002/pits.20263.

[39] Hase C. Cyberbullying: What school psychologists can do. APA Division 16: From science to practice 2012. URL: http://www.apadivisions.org/division-16/publications/newsletters/science/2012/10/cyberbullying.aspx.

[40] Blake J. Cyberbullying in schools: Invisible bullying with visible effects. Youth Development Initiative 2013. URL: http://ydi.tamu.edu/wp-content/uploads/Research-Brief-22-Bullying-Blake.pdf.

[41] Caplan G. Principles of preventive psychiatry. New York: Basic Books, 1964.

[42] Diamanduros T, Downs T, Jenkins SJ. The role of school psychologists in the assessment, prevention, and intervention or cyberbullying. Psychol Sch 2008;45(8):693-704. doi.org/10.1002/pits.20335.

[43] Olweus Bullying Prevention Program. History. URL: http://www.clemson.edu/olweus/history.html.

[44] Gini G, Pozzoli T. Association between bullying and psychosomatic problems: A meta-analysis. Pediatrics 2009;123:1059-65. doi.org/10.1542/peds.2008-1215.

[45] Perren S, Dooley J, Shaw T, Cross D. Bullying in school and cyberspace: Associations with depressive symptoms in Swiss and Australian adolescents. Child Adolesc Psychiatr Ment Health 2010;4:1-10. doi.org/10.1186/1753-2000-4-28.

[46] Aricak T, Siyahhan S, Uzunhasanoglu A, Saribeyoglu S, Yilmaz N, Memmedov Cl. Cyberbullying among Turkish adolescents. Cyber Psychol Behav 2008;11(3):253-61. doi.org/10.1089/cpb.2007.0016.

[47] Schneider SK, O'Donnell L, Stueve A, Coulter RWS. Cyberbullying, school bullying, and psychological distress: A regional census of high school students. Am J Public Health 2012;102(1):171-77. doi.org/10.2105/AJPH.2011.300308.

[48] Willard N. Educator's guide to cyberbullying: Addressing the harm caused by online social cruelty, 2004. URL: http://www.asdk12.org/MiddleLink/AVB/bully_topics/EducatorsGuide_Cyberbullying.pdf.

[49] Raskauskas J. Bullying: Students hurting students. In: Sandoval JH, ed. Crisis counseling, intervention, and prevention in the schools. New York: Routledge, 2013.

[50] Nation M, Crusto C, Wandersman A, Kumpfer KL, Seybolt D, Morrissey-Kane E, et al. What works in prevention. Principles of effective prevention programs. Am Psychol 2003;58(6-7):449-56.

In: Child and Adolescent Health
Editors: A Tenenbaum and J Merrick
ISBN: 978-1-53617-825-8

Chapter 17

ADOLESCENT CONFIDENTIALITY CONCERNS AND USE OF SENSITIVE HEALTH SERVICES: A RETROSPECTIVE COHORT STUDY OF ADDHEALTH PARTICIPANTS

Kenesha Smith Barber*, PhD
and Larissa R Brunner Huber, PhD
Department of Public Health Sciences, University of North Carolina, Charlotte, North Carolina, United States of America

ABSTRACT

Family planning and sexually transmitted disease (STD) testing are fundamental services to prevent unintended pregnancies and the spread of STDs; however, when adolescents have confidentiality concerns about healthcare providers, they may be deterred from accessing such services. Objective: The purpose of this study was to evaluate if there is an

* Correspondence: Kenesha Smith Barber, Department of Public Health Sciences, 9201 University City Blvd, Charlotte, NC 28223-0001, United States. Email: ksmit392@uncc.edu.

association between confidentiality concerns and use of sensitive health care services among young adults. Study group: Data from 923 participants of AddHealth were used for this analysis. Participation was limited to those who felt they were in need of medical care in the past year, but did not see a health professional. Methods: Information on reasons for not seeing a health care provider and the use of specific services was self-reported. Multivariate logistic regression was used to calculate odds ratios (ORs) and confidence intervals (CIs). Results: After adjustment for confounders, there was no association between forgoing healthcare due to confidentiality concerns and using sensitive health care services (family planning: OR=2.06; 95% CI: 0.51, 8.27; STD testing: OR=0.87; 95% CI: 0.09, 8.77). Conclusions: While the current study did not find any association between confidentiality concerns and use of sensitive health services, more rigorous studies with larger sample sizes are warranted. Understanding the relationship between confidentiality and sensitive health service use may aid health care providers in improving the reproductive health of youth.

INTRODUCTION

Sexually transmitted diseases (STDs) are a serious public health problem, affecting approximately 19 million people each year. Almost half of STD infections are contracted by adolescents and young adults ages 15 to 24 (1). Most STDs may be easily detected and treated; however, because of the asymptomatic nature of most STDs, many people who are infected do not know they need medical care, allowing their disease to worsen and negatively impact their health. Therefore, the use of STD services is important in reducing adverse effects of STDs, especially among adolescents and young adults.

Likewise, family planning clinics are essential in reducing unintended pregnancies among adolescents and young adults. Unintended pregnancy is a serious public health problem; 3.4 million of the 6.6 million pregnancies occurring each year in the US are unintended (2). Approximately 4 out of every 5 pregnancies among those women age 19 and younger are unintended (3). Women who do not know they are pregnant are more likely to delay prenatal care or to practice unsafe habits (3). In 2010, the economic burden of unintended pregnancies totaled approximately 21 billion dollars (4).

While family planning and STD testing are fundamental health services to prevent unintended pregnancies and the spread of STDs, when adolescents feel as though providers will not maintain confidentiality, they may be deterred from accessing those services (5). Surveys indicate that less than 20 percent of adolescents would seek care for sensitive services (i.e., birth control, STDs, or drug use) if parental notice was required (6). Understanding the relationship between confidentiality concerns and the use of sensitive health services, including family planning services and STD testing, is highly valuable, given the low prevalence of adolescents seeking sensitive healthcare services when confidentiality is a concern.

Studies on the relationship between adolescent confidentiality concerns and the use of sensitive healthcare services are limited. One study found adolescent perceptions of lack of confidentiality were associated with decreased use of sensitive healthcare services; however, response rates for the cross-sectional study were low (51%) and there was potential for recall bias (7). More studies have examined barriers causing adolescents to forgo sensitive health care services, finding confidentiality concerns to be one of the most significant barriers (8-12). However, these studies may have limited generalizability due to the fact that they were conducted outside of the US (9-11) and had small sample sizes (8-12). Furthermore, a systematic review examining confidentiality assurance in family planning services and reproductive outcomes found limited evidence suggesting that confidentiality improves reproductive health for young people; however, many of the studies included in the review had high risk of bias and lacked a strong study design (13). Because there are so few studies examining the relationship between confidentiality concerns and the use of sensitive health care services, further research is needed.

The purpose of this study was to evaluate all adolescents who did not see a health care provider when they believed they needed to in order to examine whether young adults with confidentiality concerns are at decreased odds for using sensitive health care services compared to those who do not have confidentiality concerns, using population-based data from the US.

OUR STUDY

Data for this secondary data analysis were obtained from public use files of the National Longitudinal Study of Adolescent to Adult Health (AddHealth), a project initiated to collect data on factors that may influence adolescents' health and risk behaviors (14). In 1994, AddHealth personnel began collecting data from a sample of nationally representative students in grades 7-12, and then followed these same students with a series of in-home interviews until the year 2008. Participants in this analysis are from Wave II of AddHealth data collection, conducted in 1996.

Selected Wave II participants completed 1-2-hour verbal in-home interviews; AddHealth personnel recorded data on laptop computers (15). In Wave II of AddHealth, 4,834 respondents provided data, yielding a response rate of 88.6% (16). Participants in this analysis were limited only to those who felt they were in need of medical care in the past year, but did not see a health professional (N=954) (17). Since the current study was an analysis of de-identified, publicly available data, the UNC Charlotte IRB determines that this study is exempt from IRB review, being that it does not meet the federal definition of human subjects research.

The main exposure in this study was forgoing healthcare due to confidentiality concerns. Participants were asked: "What kept you from seeing a health professional when you really needed to?" (17). Students were given a list of 10 reasons from which to choose. If the student chose "didn't want parents to know" he/she was considered to be exposed; all other answers meant the participant had forgone healthcare for reasons other than confidentiality concerns.

The two outcomes in this analysis were use of family planning services and STD testing. Participants were asked if they had received family planning services, or testing or treatment for STD/AIDS in the past year. The response choices were 'Yes' or 'No.'

Possible confounders of the relationship between confidentiality and sensitive health care services include gender, race/ethnicity, age, grade level, income, insurance type, romantic relationship status, previous sexual intercourse, previous pregnancy, HIV/AIDS status, previous STD diagnoses, and parental closeness (18). All possible confounders were self-reported on the Add Health questionnaire.

Participants' demographic and lifestyle factors were described using frequencies and percentages. Logistic regression was used to obtain a crude association between confidentiality concerns and use of sensitive health services (i.e., family planning and STD testing) and to identify other risk factors for the outcomes. Multivariate logistic regression was used to calculate adjusted odds ratios (ORs) and 95% confidence intervals (CIs) of the association, while controlling for potential confounders. If the potential confounding variable changed the OR estimate by at least 10%, it was considered to be a confounder (19). Due to the complex sampling design used by Add Health, SAS-callable SUDAAN was used in all analyses.

FINDINGS

Participants were excluded from the analysis if they were married (n=15) or missing information regarding previous use of family planning services (n=1), race or ethnicity (n=5), romantic relationship status (n=1), previous sexual intercourse (n=5), previous pregnancy (n=3), or previous STD (n=1). Information regarding alternative reasons participants did not receive health care is not listed in the tables. The main reason participants in this sample did not receive healthcare is because they thought the problem would go away (n=629; 65.9%). The second most common response was that participants were afraid of what the doctor would say or do (n=190; 19.9%). Of the 954 individuals who did not receive healthcare, 2.7% (n=26) did not receive it due to confidentiality concerns. Of the 923 participants remaining for analysis, 2.65% did not receive healthcare due to confidentiality issues (see Table 1). Additionally, 7.43% of participants used family services in the past year and 7.41% received STD or HIV testing in the past year.

Table 1. Characteristics of wave II AddHealth participants who have forgone healthcare in the past year and those who have forgone healthcare due to confidentiality concerns

	Participants who have forgone healthcare (N=923)		Participants who have forgone healthcare due to confidentiality concerns (N=26)	
Variables	**Number N**	**Weighted Percent (%)**	**Number N**	**Weighted Percent (%)**
Forgone Healthcare due to Confidentiality Issues				
Yes	26	2.65	26	100.00
No	897	97.35	0	0.00
Family Planning Service Use Ever				
Yes	65	7.43	4	17.34
No	858	92.57	22	82.66
Previous STD Testing Past 12 Mo.				
Yes	66	7.41	1	7.34
No	857	92.59	25	92.66
Gender				
Male	409	47.98	12	46.54
Female	514	52.02	14	53.46
Race/ethnicity				
Non-Hispanic White	593	70.22	16	68.80
Non-Hispanic Black	225	18.33	8	21.55
Hispanic	53	6.45	0.00	0.00
Other	52	5.00	2	9.65
Age in years				
11-17	714	78.23	21	86.12
≥18	209	21.77	5	13.88
Grade Level				
7-8th	120	15.25	5	16.92
9-12th	673	69.71	18	73.96
Beyond High School	17	2.00	0	0.00
Unavailable/Missing	113	13.04	3	9.13

	Participants who have forgone healthcare (N=923)		**Participants who have forgone healthcare due to confidentiality concerns (N=26)**	
Variables	**Number N**	**Weighted Percent (%)**	**Number N**	**Weighted Percent (%)**
Income				
<$20,000	312	34.31	8	30.77
$20,000-49,999	299	32.71	7	29.52
≥$50,000	312	32.99	11	39.72
Insurance Type				
Medicare	9	0.73	0	0.00
Medicaid	98	11.29	4	12.03
Individual or group private coverage	383	42.01	9	34.71
Prepaid Health Plan	165	17.49	8	38.11
Other	35	2.94	1	0.89
None	112	13.04	2	5.08
Missing	121	12.51	2	9.17
Currently in a Romantic Relationship				
Yes	597	66.62	22	90.09
No	326	33.38	4	9.91
Sexual Intercourse Ever				
Yes	517	55.02	18	77.26
No	406	44.98	8	22.74
Ever Pregnant				
Yes	52	5.48	2	9.65
No	871	94.52	24	90.35
Received Birth Control from Doctor/Clinic				
Yes	107	11.22	3	15.51
No	816	88.78	23	84.49
HIV/AIDS Status				
Yes	7	0.80	0	0.00
No	916	99.20	26	100.00
Previous Chlamydia Diagnosis				
Yes	17	1.61	0	0.00
No	906	98.39	26	100.00
Previous Syphilis Diagnosis				
Yes	8	0.78	0	0.00
No	915	99.22	26	100.00
Previous Gonorrhea Diagnosis				
Yes	6	0.64	0	0.00
No	917	99.36	26	100.00

Table 1. (Continued)

	Participants who have forgone healthcare (N=923)		Participants who have forgone healthcare due to confidentiality concerns (N=26)	
Variables	**Number N**	**Weighted Percent (%)**	**Number N**	**Weighted Percent (%)**
Previous Genital Herpes Diagnosis				
Yes	6	0.44	0	0.00
No	917	99.56	26	100.00
Closeness to Mother (Scale of 1-5)				
1	15	1.16	0	0.00
2	25	2.27	1	4.49
3	118	12.73	5	18.53
4	282	30.35	8	31.82
5	398	44.19	11	44.27
Missing	85	9.31	1	0.89
Closeness to Father (Scale of 1-5)				
1	35	3.57	1	5.18
2	52	5.48	2	10.29
3	145	15.15	5	17.31
4	193	21.43	4	14.94
5	203	22.09	6	15.35
Missing	295	32.28	8	36.92

There were a total of 923 participants; 714 were age 11-17 (78.23%) and the remaining 209 were 18-21 years of age (21.77%). Most participants were Non-Hispanic White (70.22%) and nearly half were female (52.02%). In addition, the majority of participants were in grades 9-12 (69.71%) and less than half reported having individual or group private insurance (42.01%) while 13.04% reported having no health insurance.

Among the 26 individuals with confidentiality concerns, most were female (53.46%), 11-17 years of age (86.12%), and Non-Hispanic White (68.80%). None of the 26 participants with confidentiality concerns reported ever having a previous STD, and 77.26% reported previously having sexual intercourse. Although closeness to father varied, the majority of individuals reported being close with their mother (44.27% indicated a value of 5 on a scale from 1-5 and 31.82% stated a value of 4).

Table 2. Unadjusted odds ratios and 95% confidence intervals for the association between demographic and lifestyle characteristics and family planning service use and STD testing, 1994 AddHealth

Variables	Family Planning (N= 923)		STD Testing (N= 923)	
	OR	95% CI	OR	95% CI
Forgone Healthcare due to Confidentiality Issues				
Yes	2.72	0.81, 9.07	0.99	0.13, 7.54
No	1.00	Referent	1.00	Referent
Gender				
Male	1.00	Referent	1.00	Referent
Female	2.50	1.29, 4.85	1.69	0.96, 2.99
Race/ethnicity				
Non-Hispanic White	1.00	Referent	1.00	Referent
Non-Hispanic Black	1.23	0.64, 2.35	2.10	1.12, 2.92
Hispanic	0.76	0.20, 2.90	2.01	0.81, 4.98
Other	0.95	0.31, 2.90	1.28	0.44, 3.72
Age				
11-17	1.00	Referent	1.00	Referent
≥18	0.98	0.53, 1.83	1.46	0.81, 2.63
Grade Level				
7-8th	0.68	0.28, 1.65	0.17	0.04, 0.73
9-12th	1.00	Referent	1.00	Referent
Beyond High School	-	-	0.76	0.10, 5.99
Unavailable/Missing	1.15	0.52, 2.55	2.32	1.19, 4.55
Income				
<$20,000	0.94	0.46, 1.89	1.72	0.86, 3.46
$20,000-49,999	1.26	0.65, 2.45	1.49	0.74, 3.00
≥$50,000	1.00	Referent	1.00	Referent
Insurance Type				
Medicare	4.55	0.79, 26.08	3.86	0.45, 33.20
Medicaid	1.43	0.61, 3.34	0.89	0.33, 2.33
Individual or group private coverage	1.00	Referent	1.00	Referent
Prepaid Health Plan	1.42	0.66, 3.02	1.82	0.84, 3.95
Other	0.90	0.19, 4.29	1.46	0.38, 5.68
None	1.71	0.71, 4.10	2.96	1.26, 6.99
Missing	0.70	0.23, 2.18	2.24	0.96, 5.20
Currently in a Romantic Relationship				
Yes	1.71	0.91, 3.20	1.99	1.04, 3.81
No	1.00	Referent	1.00	Referent

Table 2. (Continued)

Variables	Family Planning (N= 923)		STD Testing (N= 923)	
	OR	**95% CI**	**OR**	**95% CI**
Sexual Intercourse Ever				
Yes	2.26	1.18, 4.31	4.55	2.09, 9.89
No	1.00	Referent	1.00	Referent
Ever Pregnant				
Yes	1.41	1.01, 1.96	2.68	1.86, 3.85
No	1.00	Referent	1.00	Referent
Received Birth Control from Doctor/Clinic				
Yes	1.98	1.04, 3.75	3.86	2.09, 7.14
No	1.00	Referent	1.00	Referent
HIV/AIDS Status				
Yes	1.03	0.12, 9.12	1.04	0.12, 9.15
No	1.00	Referent	1.00	Referent
Previous Chlamydia Diagnosis				
Yes	3.56	1.00, 12.66	15.88	5.22, 48.27
No	1.00	Referent	1.00	Referent
Previous Syphilis Diagnosis				
Yes	1.05	0.12, 8.98	1.06	0.12, 9.01
No	1.00	Referent	1.00	Referent
Previous Gonorrhea Diagnosis				
Yes	1.31	0.15, 11.76	1.32	0.15, 11.80
No	1.00	Referent	1.00	Referent
Previous Genital Herpes Diagnosis				
Yes	4.32	0.74, 25.27	2.02	0.22, 18.07
No	1.00	Referent	1.00	Referent
Closeness to Mother (Scale of 1-5)				
1	7.19	1.67, 30.90	1.43	0.17, 11.81
2	8.40	2.92, 24.16	2.56	0.76, 8.56
3	1.81	0.71, 4.61	0.67	0.26, 1.72
4	1.64	0.79, 3.40	0.79	0.39, 1.60
5	1.00	Referent	1.00	Referent
Missing	2.17	0.84, 5.58	3.05	1.36, 6.86
Closeness to Father (Scale of 1-5)				
1	3.95	0.39, 39.59	1.51	0.30, 7.61
2	12.99	3.09, 54.49	1.74	0.49, 6.16
3	10.63	2.95, 38.28	2.04	0.77, 5.37
4	3.07	0.79, 12.03	0.43	0.13, 1.42
5	1.00	Referent	1.00	Referent
Missing	6.88	2.01, 23.53	2.20	0.97, 4.97

Participants who chose to forgo healthcare due to confidentiality concerns had increased odds of using family planning services (OR=2.72; 95% CI: 0.81, 9.07; Table 2) compared to participants who omitted healthcare for other reasons; however, these findings were not statistically significant. There was no strong association between forgoing healthcare due to confidentiality issues and STD testing (OR=0.99; 95% CI: 0.13, 7.54). Of all individuals who chose to forego healthcare, females had statistically significant increased odds of using family planning services (OR=2.50; 95% CI: 1.29, 4.85), and Black participants had increased odds of seeking STD testing (OR=2.10; 95% CI: 1.12, 2.92) compared to White participants. In addition, youth who reported being less close to their father had statistically significant increased odds of using family planning services (closeness of 2 on a scale of 1-5 OR=12.99; 95% CI: 3.09, 54.49).

Additionally, those individuals who were in a romantic relationship had statistically significant increased odds of seeking STD testing (OR=1.99; 95% CI: 1.04, 3.81), and those participants who previously had sexual intercourse had increased odds of using both family planning and STD testing services (OR=2.26; 95% CI: 1.18, 4.31 and OR=4.55; 95% CI: 2.09, 9.89, respectively). Participants who had a previous chlamydia diagnosis (OR=15.88; 95% CI: 5.22, 48.27), previous pregnancy (OR=2.68; 95% CI: 1.86, 3.85), and those who were in a romantic relationship (OR=1.99; 95% CI: 1.04, 3.81) had statistically significant increased odds of seeking STD testing.

After adjustment for closeness to father, sexual intercourse, and romantic relationship status, the association between forgone healthcare due to confidentiality issues and use of family planning services was attenuated and remained not statistically significant (OR=2.06; 95% CI: 0.51, 8.27; Table 3). After adjustment for closeness to father, closeness to mother, previous chlamydia diagnosis, previous pregnancy, previous sexual intercourse, and romantic relationship status, those adolescents who had forgone healthcare due to confidentiality issues had slightly decreased odds of seeking STD testing; however, this finding also was not statistically significant (OR=0.87; 95% CI: 0.09, 8.77).

Table 3. Adjusted[a-b] odds ratios and 95% confidence intervals for the association between forgone healthcare due to confidentiality issues and family planning service use and STD testing, 1994 AddHealth

Variables	Family Planning (N=923)		STD Testing (N= 923)	
	OR[a]	95% CI	OR[b]	95% CI
Forgone Healthcare due to Confidentiality Issues				
Yes	2.06	0.51, 8.27	0.87	0.09, 8.77
No	1.00	Referent	1.00	Referent

[a]Model adjusted for closeness to father, sexual intercourse ever, and relationship status.

[b]Model adjusted for closeness to father, closeness to mother, previous chlamydia, ever pregnant, sexual intercourse ever, and romantic relationship status.

DISCUSSION

There was no association between forgoing healthcare due to confidentiality issues and using sensitive health care services (i.e., STD testing and family planning services). The findings of the current study are similar to that of a previous systematic review which included 9 studies addressing confidentiality in family planning services among youth age 10-24 years of age in the US, Canada, Europe, Australia, and New Zealand, and found limited evidence suggesting that confidentiality improves reproductive health for young people (13). However, the findings of the current study differ from other previous studies which found that confidentiality concerns were associated with decreased odds of using sensitive health care services (7-12). For example, Thrall et al. conducted a cross-sectional study in Massachusetts to examine the association between adolescent perceptions of confidentiality with their health care provider and receiving a pelvic exam (7). Researchers found that female adolescents who perceived their provider to be confidential had statistically significantly increased odds of having a pelvic exam in the last two years compared to those who did not perceive their provider to be confidential (OR=3.3; 95% CI: 2.1, 5.5). A randomized control trial conducted in San

Francisco, California examined the influence of assurance of confidentiality by physicians and adolescent willingness to seek healthcare in the future. Adolescents who had physicians assure confidentiality more frequently reported willingness to return to that physician for future healthcare needs compared to those who had physicians who did not mention confidentiality (67%; $p<0.001$) (8). Findings from these studies may differ from the current study because the exposures are slightly different; while the current study examined youth not wanting their parents to find out about sensitive health services, the other studies examined concerns of the physician breaching confidentiality (7-8).

In addition, differences between the 923 participants who did not receive healthcare, and the 26 individuals who did not receive healthcare specifically due to confidentiality concerns may have affected the results of the current study. While the two groups were similar with respect to demographic variables such as gender, race or ethnicity, and age, there were differences in lifestyle characteristics. For example, higher percentages of participants with confidentiality concerns reported being in a romantic relationship or ever having sexual intercourse compared to the total population of individuals who had forgone healthcare.

There are some strengths and limitations to this study. It is possible that nondifferential misclassification may have occurred since the exposure (confidentiality) was self-reported. Participants were asked if they had forgone healthcare in the past year and if so, what their reason was for doing so. It is possible that participants did not remember whether or not they attended health care services, or they may have felt uncomfortable reporting the reason they did not attend health care services. Even so, perceptions of confidentiality may only be measured by self-report, making this an acceptable measure of confidentiality (7, 9-12). The outcome variables, use of family planning and STD testing services in the past year, were also self-reported and may have been inaccurately reported. Any resulting misclassification would most likely bias the results towards the null.

Due to the random sampling procedures used by AddHealth and the high response rate (Wave II response rate: 88.6%), the potential for selection bias is reduced (17). However, it is possible that youth who participated in the study may have differed from those who did not. Because the study takes place within schools, those who are home-schooled or do not attend school are excluded. If selection bias did occur, results would likely be biased away from the null. In addition, the evaluation of possible confounding variables was limited to variables available in AddHealth; failure to control for other known or unknown confounders could have resulted in an over- or under-estimation of the true association. The fairly small sample (N=923) and limited number of participants who reported forgoing healthcare due to confidentiality concerns caused imprecise effect estimates and wide confidence intervals. Thus, generalizability may be limited. Lastly, although the Wave II AddHealth data is older, there is no other recent data available with information concerning adolescent confidentiality concerns. Because so few studies have examined the relationship between confidentiality concerns and the use of sensitive health care services, this study is important to the field of adolescent health.

CONCLUSION

In summary, while the current study did not find any association between confidentiality concerns and forgone sensitive health services, more research is needed. More rigorous studies with larger sample sizes conducted in the US are warranted. Understanding the relationship between confidentiality and sensitive health service use may aid health care providers in improving the reproductive health of youth by decreasing the prevalence of STDs and unintended pregnancies among this population.

ACKNOWLEDGMENTS

The authors have no known conflicts of interest and the contents of this manuscript have not been published elsewhere. As this is a secondary analysis of AddHealth data, there will be no contact with the participants of this study. By signing an informed consent form, AddHealth participants agreed to participate prior to filling out the self-administered questionnaire.

REFERENCES

[1] Office of Disease Prevention and Health Promotion. Healthy people 2020: Sexually transmitted diseases. US Department of Health and Human Services; 2017 Feb 16 [cited 2015 Jun 1]. URL: http://www.healthypeople.gov/2020/topics-objectives/topic/sexually-transmitted-diseases.

[2] Finer LB, Zolna MR. Shifts in unintended pregnancies in the United States, 2001-2008. Am J Public Health. 2014;104(S1):S43-8.

[3] Centers for Disease Control and Prevention. Unintended pregnancy prevention. US Department of Health and Human Services; 2015 Jan 22 [cited 2015 Jun 15]. URL: http://www.cdc.gov/reproductivehealth/UnintendedPregnancy/.

[4] Sonfield A, Kost K. Public costs from unintended pregnancies and the role of public insurance programs in paying for pregnancy-related care: National and state estimates for 2010 [document on the Internet]. Guttmacher Institute, 2015. URL: http://www.guttmacher.org/pubs/public-costs-of-UP-2010.pdf.

[5] Loxterman J. Adolescent access to confidential health services. Washington (DC): Advocates for Youth, 1997. URL: http://www.advocatesforyouth.org/publications/publications-a-z/516-adolescent-access-to-confidential-health-services#2.

[6] Marks A, Malizio J, Hoch J, Brody R, Fisher M. Assessment of health needs and willingness to utilize health care resources of adolescents in a suburban population. J Pediatr 1983;102:456-60.

[7] Thrall JS, McCloskey L, Ettner SL, Rothman E, Tighe JE, Emans J. Confidentiality and adolescents' use of providers for health information and pelvic examinations. Arch Pediatr Adolesc Med 2000;154(9):885-92.

[8] Ford CA, Millstein SG, Halpern-Felsher BL, Irwin CE. Influence of physician confidentiality assurances on adolescents' willingness to disclose information and seek future health care. A randomized controlled trial. JAMA 1997;278(12):1029-34.

[9] Garside R, Ayers R, Owen M, Pearson VA, Roizen J. Anonymity and confidentiality: rural teenagers' concerns when accessing sexual health services. J Fam Plann Reprod Health Care 2002;28(1):23-6.

[10] Thomas N, Murray E, Rogstad KE. Confidentiality is essential if young people are to access sexual health services. Int J STD AIDS 2006;17(8):525-9.

[11] Oppong-Odiseng ACK, Heycock EG. Adolescent health services- through their eyes. Arch Dis Child 1997;77:115-9.

[12] Britto MT, Tivorsak TL, Slap GB. Adolescents' needs for health care privacy. Pediatrics 2010;126(6):1469-76.

[13] Brittain AW, Williams JR, Zapata L, Moskosky S, Weik TS. Confidentiality in family planning services for young people: A systematic review. Am J Prev Med 2015;49(2): S85-95.

[14] Harris KM, Halpern CT, Whitsel E, Hussey J, Tabor J, Entzel, P, et al. The National Longitudinal Study of Adolescent to Adult Health: About. Chapel Hill, NC: UNC Carolina Population Center National Institute of Child Health and Human Development, 2009. URL: http://www.cpc.unc.edu/projects/addhealth/about.

[15] Harris KM, Halpern CT, Whitsel E, Hussey J, Tabor J, Entzel, P, et al. The National Longitudinal Study of Adolescent to Adult Health: Wave II. Chapel Hill, NC: UNC Carolina Population Center National Institute of Child Health and Human Development, 2009. URL: http://www.cpc.unc.edu/projects/addhealth/design/wave2.

[16] Harris KM, Halpern CT, Whitsel E, Hussey J, Tabor J, Entzel, P, et al. The National Longitudinal Study of Adolescent to Adult Health: Public-use dataset descriptions. Chapel Hill, NC: UNC Carolina Population Center National Institute of Child Health and Human Development, 2009. URL: http://www.cpc.unc.edu/projects/addhealth/data/publicdata/public-use-dataset-descriptions.

[17] Harris KM, Udry JR: National Longitudinal Study of Adolescent Health wave II adolescent in-home questionnaire code book. Ann Arbor, MI: Inter-University Consortium for Political and Social Research, 1998.

[18] Lehrer JA, Pantell R, Tebb K, Shafer M. Forgone health care among US adolescents: Associations between risk characteristics and confidentiality concern. J Adolesc Health 2007;40:218-26.

[19] Maldonado G, Greenland S: Simulation study of confounder-selection strategies. Am J Epidemiol 1993;138(11):923-36.

In: Child and Adolescent Health
Editors: A Tenenbaum and J Merrick
ISBN: 978-1-53617-825-8

Chapter 18

SELF-EFFICACY OF OVERWEIGHT AND OBESE YOUTH PARTICIPATING IN A MULTIDISCIPLINARY AFTER-SCHOOL PROGRAM

Victoria N Ivy**, MS, Karen L Gaudreault, PhD and Timothy Baghurst, PhD
Department of Kinesiology, University of Alabama, Tuscaloosa, Alabama, School of Kinesiology and Recreation, Illinois State University, Normal, Illinois and FSU COACH: Interdisciplinary Center for Athletic Coaching, Florida State University, Tallahassee, Florida, United States of America

* Correspondence: Victoria N Ivy, MS, Department of Kinesiology, University of Alabama, 1013 Moore Hall, Box 870312 Tuscaloosa, AL 35487, United States. Email: vnshiver@crimson.ua.edu.

Abstract

Fostering self-efficacy has been shown to positively impact health outcomes among youth, yet little research has considered how self-efficacy is affected across multiple health variables, especially among youth already considered at-risk as overweight or obese. Using Self-Efficacy Theory, the purpose of this chapter was to examine health variables including physical activity, nutrition, and behavioral health and their influence on children's self-efficacy. Participants were 21 boys and girls aged between 8 and 13 years who were classified as overweight or obese and enrolled in a year-long after-school program in the Rocky Mountain region of the United States. Participants completed two interviews and one drawing with narration designed to capture the children's perceptions and feelings. Three major themes emerged: 1) emotions and behavior, 2) impact of modeling, observation, and feedback and 3) being active and eating well feels good. Findings indicate that after-school programming can be effective in fostering self-efficacy among at-risk youth by employing a broad curriculum and high levels of feedback and demonstrations. Finally, results suggest imagery could be an effective tool in such programs and improving mood may lead to enhanced healthful behavior.

Introduction

The most recent information provided by the Centers for Disease Control and Prevention (CDC) (1) states that one third of the adult population and seventeen percent of the child population in the United States are obese and that number has tripled in one generation. Children who are overweight or obese tend to remain obese as adults, and children who are not obese have a much lower percentage of falling into the overweight or obese category later in life. Obesity leads to health consequences that can be life threatening. For example, Type 2 diabetes, which used to be referred to as adult onset diabetes, is being diagnosed in youth. The CDC (1) reported that just under three fourths of obese youth showed at least one cardiovascular disease risk factor and have increased risk for over thirteen different types of cancers. Overweight or obese children may also see a rise in anxiety, sleep disorders, asthma, ADHD, blood pressure, and several other health-related conditions. It is clear that the health of our nation's children is declining as obesity rates continue to rise.

Obesity continues despite physical activity and health focused interventions designed to mitigate this issue. School and community interventions are limited. Further, when they do exist, they tend to provide short-term rather than long-term effects on the prevention of obesity and other diseases (2).

Another factor influencing obesity levels in the United States is the number of overweight or obese children who come from low-income, high-risk living situations. As socioeconomic status increases, overweight and obesity levels decrease (1) while activity levels increase (3). This suggests that low SES youth may need more assistance in developing a proper diet and a physical activity routine compared with children in other SES categories. Children from low SES households may also have higher levels of obesity due to the lack of sidewalks, playgrounds, recreational facilities, access to healthy foods, and additional resources (4), or they are frequently considered unsafe in low-income communities (1). Adolescents from low SES are more defiant and act out based on inattention or impulsivity, particularly between grades six and eight (5), and also exhibit more delinquent behaviors and aggression (6).

Self-efficacy theory

Self-efficacy theory (SET) (7) provided the theoretical underpinning for this study. Self-efficacy has been defined as a strong sense of confidence in an individual's ability to perform a specific behavior. According to Bandura (7):

- Perceived self-efficacy occupies a pivotal role in causal structures because it affects human functioning not only directly, but through its impact on other important classes of determinants. These determinants include goal aspirations, incentives and disincentives

> rooted in outcome expectations, and perceived impediments and opportunity structures in social systems (7).

Bandura suggested that self-efficacy greatly influences every aspect of one's life. It can alter the course of action one takes, the amount of effort put into life's endeavors, the level of perseverance in the face of obstacles or potential failure, the ability to be flexible with change, the way one encourages or discourages themselves, and the stress levels or negative emotions felt when handling high demands. Self-efficacy can be altered via its four primary sources: (a) mastery experience, (b) vicarious experience, (c) verbal persuasion, and (d) physiological and affective states. The most influential of these is mastery experience, because if one succeeds at a task, belief in ability to perform the task again occurs. This is also true for failure, as every time one does not perform a task successfully, belief in ability to do so is reduced. However, if one is regularly successful at tasks that do not provide a challenge, then instant results may be expected and failure results in discouragement. As challenges are faced and overcome by hard work, self-efficacy will increase. For example, if a child is trying to jog more than one lap around a field, self-efficacy will increase every time the child makes it a couple steps beyond a full rotation, and persistence to continue practicing will likely occur.

Vicarious experiences, also referred to as modeling, play a large role in self-efficacy levels. Modeling is useful when performance can be judged based on others' abilities. Having the ability to outperform peers, co-workers, for example, can raise personal self-efficacy beliefs. However, performing below the average can lower it. Seeing someone of equal ability succeed will raise self-efficacy. Likewise, if someone of equal ability fails, self-efficacy is reduced. Modeling is especially important to tasks that are new; if there is no previous experience, there is no judgment of good or poor performance without the help of vicarious experience. Seeing a model fail and continue trying with a positive attitude can also increase one's self-efficacy.

Verbal persuasion (also referred to as behavioral feedback) can significantly impact self-efficacy. Self-efficacy can be altered based on the feedback significant others provide for performance. Providing positive language in reference to one's performance can change self-doubts and reduce time spent thinking about personal deficiencies. However, in order to be effective, the feedback must be accurate and realistic. It is important to build long-lasting self-efficacy as opposed to temporary unrealistic beliefs. Receiving feedback from someone who is considered an expert in the area is the most beneficial for raising self-efficacy. Feedback from someone who is not capable or knowledgeable about the task can actually cause a reduction in self-efficacy.

Several studies have investigated the relationship between imagery and self-efficacy. Imagery has been defined as a way to see oneself or others that are similar performing a task successfully or unsuccessfully without actually doing the task (8). This is visualizing the task in one's mind using all of the senses (sight, smell, hearing, taste, and touch) to make it feel as real as possible. If an individual sees himself or herself or someone similar performing a task successful utilizing imagery, then self-efficacy is likely to rise. If failure is visualized repeatedly, self-efficacy levels are likely to be reduced. Therefore, it is important to picture success in order to be successful. This is a particularly useful way to alter self-efficacy when one does not have the opportunity to perform the task itself. For example, an athlete may visualize running and jumping hurdles while lying in bed before sleep. If successful mentally, it is likely more confidence will be present if the athlete actually runs the hurdles the next day.

As self-efficacy is developed, children are highly dependent on interactions with peers to provide knowledge regarding personal capabilities (9). Due to the organization of school systems, children are paired with other children that are similar in age and experience resulting in ability comparison. Selection of close peers can influence personal interests; the selected peers will likely influence positive self-efficacy in areas of shared interests while self-efficacy in other areas will be reduced or stay stationary. For example, if two friends enjoy skateboarding, they will likely develop high levels of self-efficacy in that area, but they will not develop any self-efficacy in basketball, as they never play it and are not constantly making comparative references in it. When attempting to improve a child's self-efficacy in any area, it is important to identify their peers as either helpful or not in that development.

Self-efficacy and intervention programs

Research has demonstrated a value for self-efficacy and its relation to intervention programs. Scholars have suggested that interventions should be designed with a focus on self-efficacy (10). Further, researchers have concerned themselves with discovering how self-efficacy can be impacted by after-school and intervention activity programs. Research on physical activity programs in schools or after-school have provided evidence that strong predictors of physical activity are enjoyment, social support, and self-efficacy (11, 12).

Many studies have results indicating self-efficacy is highly important for changes in physical activity, yet they all include it as a secondary piece of their research, primarily focusing on physical activity change measurements (11, 13). It is understood that behavioral changes are the top priority in most interventions. However, assuming increased self-efficacy will result in increased physical activity as evidence indicates, it should become a primary focus in the literature to understand what most strongly influences a positive physical activity self-efficacy, which in turn increases activity time.

High levels of self-efficacy result in better healthy behavior choices than low levels (14). Previous research on physical activity and nutrition intervention programs has demonstrated positive changes in self-efficacy. However, it is important to consider several limitations in previous literature. Few studies have examined self-efficacy within intervention programs containing more than one or two health components. The current study provides new insights, as the intervention program in question included physical activity, nutrition, and behavioral health components. The results of this study are applicable in existing intervention programs across the nation and provide those interested in beginning an after-school program with an understanding of how self-efficacy can be enhanced and how a multi-disciplinary program can improve a child's confidence. The present study included several sources of data targeting self-efficacy; this method demonstrates a different approach to investigating self-efficacy and may serve to inform future studies in this area.

The purpose of this study, therefore, was to understand the self-efficacy of youth placed at-risk participating in a multi-disciplinary after-school program. Research questions that guided the study were: (a) How does participation in the program impact children's self-efficacy in engaging in physical activity? (b) How does participation in the program impact children's self-efficacy in making healthy nutritional choices? and (c) How does participation in the program impact children's self-efficacy in engaging in social and emotional healthy behaviors?

OUR STUDY

Participants in this study included 21 children in a rural Rocky Mountain community in the United States who were enrolled in an after-school program (ASP) and met the selection criteria that they: (a) had been identified by local physicians and school district professionals as at-risk and underserved youth; (b) had a BMI in the 85th percentile or higher; (c) were between the ages of 7 and 14 years old (grades 3 – 8); and (d) had been identified by school personnel or their pediatrician as being challenged with behavioral control, other medical conditions, emotional distress, little parental involvement, or take part in sedentary behavior.

Following IRB approval, children meeting the selection criteria were identified by school personnel (school nurse, social worker, and/or principal) and referred to the researcher. The researcher then contacted parents to describe the program and the study, and extend the invitation to participate. Parents provided informed consent and participating children provided assent during the first program session. The participant's parents/guardians provided their demographic information. There were 16 males and 5 females with specific ages of the children being: eight (n=3), nine (n=7), ten (n=4), 11 (n=2), 12 (n=4), and 13 (n=1). The ethnicities of the participants were Caucasian (n=11), Hispanic (n=5), Mixed (n=4), and Not Identified (n=1). The children's socioeconomic status was not provided, but the children were recruited from schools with a large number of lower socioeconomic students.

Program intervention

The ASP program met for 20 weeks each academic year; 10 weeks in the fall and 10 weeks in the spring. The program met twice a week; 11 of the children attended on Tuesdays and the other 10 children attended on Wednesdays. The meeting time lasted for two hours. During these meetings, children engaged in a multidisciplinary intervention program that included a physical activity lesson, a nutrition lesson, a behavioral health lesson, and time spent one-on-one with an assigned college-aged mentor. Table 1 shows an example of how a weekly session was organized.

Table 1. An example of how a weekly after school program session was organized

Afterschool Program (ASP)	
3:45 PM – 4:00 PM	Arrival of mentees and mentor/mentee bonding time, collection of logs for pedometers and activity and review goal sheets with mentors then collect. Give screen time sheets.
4:00 PM – 4:20 PM	Skillastics (FITT Principle: Type)
4:20 PM – 4:45 PM	Nutrition (Reading Labels Activity)
4:45 PM – 5:10 PM	Behavior (Communication with parents, stress with kids)
5:10 PM – 5:25 PM	Noodle Hockey Game
5:25 PM – 5:30 PM	Goal sheets, Closure, mentees exit

It is suggested that children participate in 30-60 min of moderate to vigorous activity per day in order to produce health benefits (15). The physical activity component of ASP was based on this recommendation. Children participated in physical activities while learning activity benefits. Concepts such as the FITT (frequency, intensity, time, type) principle, cardiovascular fitness, and flexibility were taught throughout the program based on the book titled “Physical best activity guide,” which includes detailed lesson plans that teach fitness concepts to children (16). This portion of the weekly sessions lasted approximately 20 minutes and occurred first.

Nutrition lessons were two-fold. First, children were provided the opportunity to make a healthy affordable snack they would easily be able to make at home. For example, they made a parfait with yogurt, granola, and fresh or dried fruit. Then they learned about a nutrition concept while taking part in physical activity. An example included developing an understanding of the difference between a whole grain and a refined grain. In the activity, children were divided into equal teams and ran to plates (hula hoops) across the gym to collect healthy grains (examples printed on pieces of paper and placed in the hula hoops) to bring back to their own plate until they had a full days serving (each paper being equal to one serving). This helped the children learn about the different grains, learn examples of what foods include healthy or unhealthy grains, and learn how many servings they should be consuming each day. The goal was for the children to leave the 20-week program with increased knowledge on nutrition including food groups, healthy portions, and vitamins and minerals. This portion of the weekly sessions lasted approximately 25 minutes and occurred after the physical activity component.

Following the nutrition component of the weekly lesson, behavioral health lessons addressed a child’s internal wellbeing. Research has demonstrated that at-risk youth tend to have low self-esteem, learned helplessness, lack of motivation, and many other issues that need to be addressed (9). During this portion of the lesson, children learned how to set goals, solve problems, address emotions, communicate, and many other social and behavioral health related actions. An example of a behavior lesson involved children drawing an outline of their own bodies and then selecting colors as a group to identify different emotions such as sadness, fear, and happiness. They then filled in the outlines using those colors showing how much of each emotion was being felt at the time. This created discussion opportunities with the mentors and as a group. An explanation for why each color was selected was provided and other children had the opportunity to comment. For example, if one child had a large amount of red to signify anger because they got into trouble at school and that made them angry, then the other children and adults helped figure out how anger could be dealt with replaced with happiness. This portion of the weekly sessions lasted approximately 25 minutes. The final portion of the program was a 15 minute self-selected physically active game or activity that children and mentors participated in together.

Data collection

Following IRB approval and consent acquisition described above, 21 children enrolled in the ASP program participated in this study. Data sources for each child included one initial interview (n=15), one follow-up interview (n=15), one drawing prompt (n=21), and one drawing narration interview (n=21).

Individual interviews

Individual face-to-face interviews were conducted in order to gain a more in-depth understanding of children's self-efficacy in the program curricular areas. Interviews used a semi-structured interview guide which allowed the researcher to ask follow up questions based on the children's initial responses and were used for clarification or to gain a deeper understanding. The interviews also assisted in the development of emergent trends in the data and informed subsequent interview guides so as to dig deeper regarding the children's expressions and self-efficacy. All interviews were conducted by the primary researcher and occurred during weekly sessions in a room located near the activity sessions for privacy. The interviews were performed once two to four weeks into the program and again at seven to nine weeks into the program. The interviews lasted approximately 20-30 minutes, were audio-recorded, and transcribed verbatim for analysis.

Drawings and narration

Drawings were used to triangulate data gathered from individual interviews and served to enrich the entire data set by providing an additional way for children to express their perceived levels of self-efficacy. Following protocol (17), children were asked to create drawings that showed how they felt about the ASP, as well as how they felt outside of the program. Prompts such as, "draw a picture of yourself at the program" were provided and the children were given time to create their own interpretations. While drawing, children described and narrated their drawing to their college student mentor. Their verbal descriptions were audio recorded and transcribed verbatim for analysis. Additionally, college student mentors were provided with written instructions and prompts to utilize in guiding the children's narration in an attempt to enrich these data. "Drawing as a research tool must be complemented by verbal research methods that encourage collaborative meaning making and allow the drawer to give voice to what the drawing was intended to convey" (17). Drawings occurred during weeks 9 and 10. The children's drawing and narration recordings last approximately 25 min.

Trustworthiness

Trustworthiness was ensured through the use of several strategies. Triangulation was accomplished through the use of multiple data sources (interviews and drawings). This provided the ability to cross check the information and ensured that the conclusions made were correct; this also reduced the chance of researcher bias playing a role in the results (18). Bias can also be reduced through peer debriefing. Thus, the data was reviewed by another researcher who worked closely with the ASP. Through peer debriefing, the researchers challenged any inconsistencies related to conclusions or interpretations of the data (19). A rich, thick description increased trustworthiness, as providing full details related to the research process allows the reader to determine transferability.

Data analysis

All data sources were analyzed inductively utilizing elements of grounded theory (20) and following a protocol involving the phases of open coding, axial coding, code categorization, and theme development (21). Open coding (21) was done first, as the first author looked through all of the data at least once and then began to provide codes throughout the documents. Applying codes was the first way themes began to be developed in the data. Once codes had been provided, they were grouped based on commonalities and themes began to emerge. The first author met weekly with an experienced qualitative researcher to engage in peer debriefing, discuss codes, engage in categorization, and identify emerging themes. Finally, the data was returned to for further analysis and constant comparison of ideas within and across themes. Throughout the entire data analysis process, constant comparative strategies (22) were used in which elements of data were constantly compared to one another to fully develop the themes based on the data. In this way, dominant themes and results were 'grounded' in the data (23). Finally, all data were considered relative to "Self-efficacy theory" (9) in order to more fully answer the research questions and fulfill the study's purpose.

Findings

The purpose of this study was to understand the self-efficacy of at-risk youth participating in a multi-disciplinary after-school program. Data analysis revealed three dominant themes: 1) emotions and behavior, 2) impact of modeling, observation, and feedback and 3) being active and eating well feels good. The quotes provided are labeled with pseudonyms for the children's protection and confidentiality purposes. The following section presents each theme in depth including the subthemes within each.

Emotions and behavior

The first and most dominant theme to emerge from the data was that the children's mood impacted their actions and behavior. The children regularly commented on how their emotions changed their performance and thoughts on their ability to make healthy choices. Two subthemes were identified: (a) emotions dictate healthy or unhealthy behaviors, and (b) the influence of peers.

The children described their behaviors as being directly related to their emotions. An overwhelming pattern throughout the interviews was that the children felt they could make a healthy choice if they were happy, but that making this same choice was less likely if they were sad or angry. This was consistent for each portion of the program (physical activity, nutrition, behavioral health). For example, Jared (age 12, grade 6) stated, "When I'm happy I think I'm going to be able to do it. When I'm mad or sad I think I can't" (First Interview). Or Maria (age 11, grade 5) said, "If I'm grumpy or tired or competitive, I'll get frustrated really easily and then it'll be harder to play the game. But when I'm happy and I feel pumped then I play better" (First Interview). A similar pattern was demonstrated when the children described their nutritional choices. Bruce (age 12, grade 7) said:

If I'm mad I don't want to eat vegetables or fruit because, I don't know, that's just the way I am. Like if I get really mad I don't want to want to eat healthy, but if I'm in a good mood and my mom asks me if I want to go to Burger King or somewhere on the weekends, I say no I really want to eat this or that (First Interview).

Another child, Josiah (age 11, grade 5) stated, "When I'm happy, I eat healthy and when I'm sad I don't eat healthy because I just don't care about anything else so I eat what I want" (First Interview).

This theme was consistent through the children's descriptions of their behavioral choices, as well. About this, Harold (age 12, grade 6) said: At school if I'm in a bad mood, I'm a really big jerk or I won't even want to talk to anyone. But if I am in a good mood I'll go hang out with people or I'll introduce students to the school or something like that (Second Interview).

The children continued to discuss their emotions related to their confidence levels while they were drawing. During a discussion about what feelings were present in the drawing and whether or not those feelings change if a healthy behavior can be performed, Josh (age 10, grade 4) said, "Yes because if I'm in a grumpy mood I don't want to do anything. If I have a really good feeling I want to run and do some more stuff. Same if I eat healthy or not healthy" (Drawing Interview).

The second subtheme emerged as children regularly discussed their peers in terms of their positive emotional level and, thus, their opinion on their ability to perform healthy behaviors. When children were in a good mood, they were regularly active with their friends. When they were in a bad mood, they isolated themselves and usually performed more sedentary behaviors. For example, Harold (age 12, grade 6) said, "Uh, well when I'm in a bad mood I don't really want to do anything. I just want to stay home. When I am in a good mood, I want to go outside, go on adventures, or go be with my friends" (First Interview).

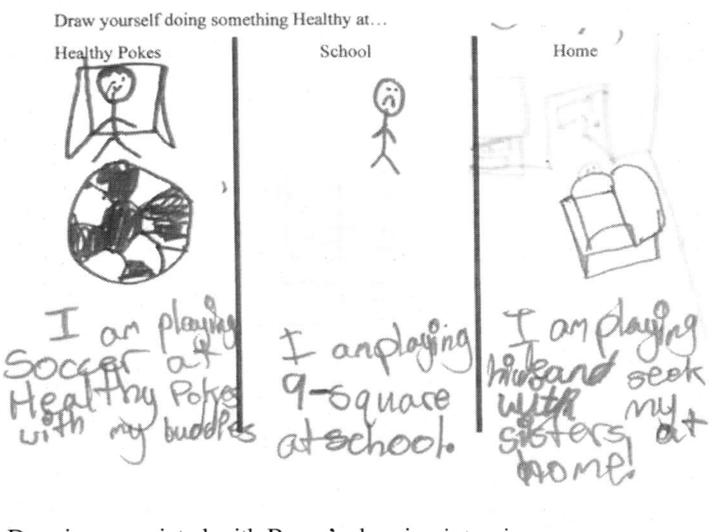
Draw yourself doing something Healthy at…
Healthy Pokes
School
Home
I am playing Soccer at Healthy Pokes with my buddies
I am playing 9-square at school.
I am playing hide and seek with my sisters at home!

Figure 1. Drawing associated with Bruce's drawing interview.

Another child, Jared (age 12, grade 6), spoke about his peer relationships as it relates to emotions in ASP, If I'm here, I'm happy because I get to hang out with friends and play and I'm never sad. But when I get here if I had a bad day at school I get happy because I get to hang out with people (Second Interview).

Peers continued to be present as an influence on healthy behaviors during the drawing data collection. Bruce (age 12, grade 7) talked about his drawing and the presence of others and personal enjoyment, "In the first one I am playing soccer at ASP with my buddies because I like to play soccer. At school I play nine square because it is fun and you still are active" (Drawing Interview; see Figure 1).

Impact of modeling, observation, and feedback

The second theme to emerge from the data was that the children were strongly influenced by modeling, observation, and feedback. They expressed that watching others, picturing themselves, and hearing comments related to healthy behaviors was an important piece of feeling as though they could make healthy choices. Two subthemes emerged within this category: (a) parents influence physical activity and eating, and (b) children are influenced by mental imaging, demonstrations, and feedback.

The children consistently mentioned their parents as a contributor to their health choices, specifically related to physical activity and healthy eating. For example, Miranda (age 10, grade 5) stated:

> My dad [influences me] because usually my dad does sports and that's how I did the sports softball and baseball… my dad said if I work on it more and more each day then I'll get really good at it and I can do a traveling team or something like that (First Interview).

The children felt that feedback provided to them and the demonstrations they saw from their parents played a role in their ability to make healthy choices. Another example was when Bruce said, "My mom cooks a lot of stuff and we have to eat vegetables along with them" (Initial Interview) or when Josh (age 10, grade 4) said, "My mom started eating this salad stuff and it tasted really good but it's really healthy for you. Then me and my brother and sister thought it would be disgusting but she made me try and I liked it." (First Interview).

The children talked about parents' examples of good nutrition and parents selecting food in the house and making meals, which influenced the children's ability to make healthy choices. Often these statements were in combination with their parents' activity levels. Josh said, "My mom eats salad all the time and runs every morning and it inspires me… because I can see she does it every day and I can too" (First Interview). Parents play a vital role in the development of self-efficacy in healthy choices. It is likely that parents also influence social and emotional behavioral health, but it was not discussed as regularly.

The second subtheme emerged as the children consistently discussed the impact their mental image, observation of demonstrations, and receiving feedback had on their belief in their ability to perform healthy behaviors. The importance of mental imaging was mentioned by Josh, when he said, "If I picture myself eating something healthy then I would eat healthy but if I picture myself eating unhealthy then I would probably eat unhealthy" (First Interview). When another child, Harold, was asked if he felt that mentally picturing himself being successful was useful and beneficial in developing self-efficacy in healthy behaviors, he said, "I think that it is because your brain thinks since you pictured it in your head you've already done it so it's no big deal" (First Interview). Similarly, Bruce said, "If, like, I picture it in my head, doing it, like football, I can actually do it in real life" (Second Interview), and Jason said, "When I picture myself doing it really good I feel like I can do it really good" (Second Interview). The children repeatedly discussed the power of demonstration throughout the interviews. About this, Josiah said, "Because when I see someone else eating healthier I want to eat healthy. When I'm not eating healthy and they tell me to eat healthy then I do. If it's someone I trust, I will do it" (First Interview).

Finally, feedback was an essential contributor to confidence related to healthy behaviors. The children often spoke highly of receiving positive feedback and how this encouraged them and made them feel like they could continue their good performance. Contrary to this, a portion of the children regularly said that negative feedback would motivate them as well. For example, Harold stated, "Well if they say I can do it, I have that in mind… like I can do it. I can do it. And I don't give up, because if they believe in me then I should believe in myself. And if they say that I can't, I need to prove them wrong that I can do it" (First Interview).

Several of the children also indicated that receiving negative feedback caused them to feel less like they could do it. An example of this presented itself when Elsa (age 13, grade 6) said, "If someone says something negative I feel bad and, like, I can't do anything. But if it's good I'm like, yeah I can do this" (Second Interview). The drawings and narrations continued to develop this subtheme. For example, Rhonda (age 10, grade 5) said, "[I drew] my coach for gym class telling me some tips on how to score points in basketball… now I know how to do something better and it'll help me be healthier." (Drawing Interview; see Figure 2).

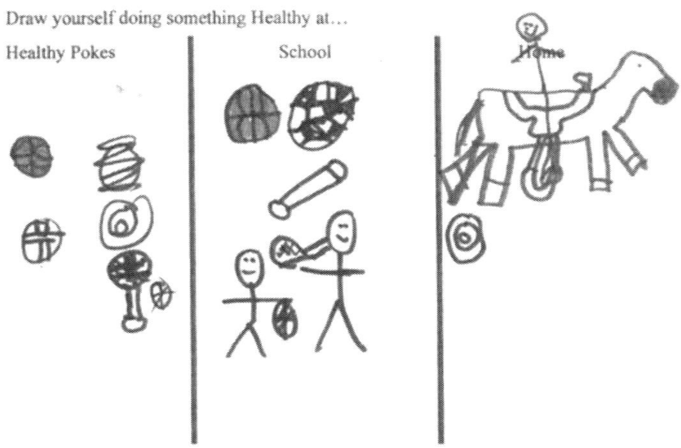
Draw yourself doing something Healthy at…
Healthy Pokes
School
Home

Figure 2. Drawing associated with Rhonda's drawing interview.

Being active and eating well feels good

The last theme that emerged from the data was that being active and eating well made the children feel good. The children talked about how specific healthy behaviors were influenced by the way it made their body feel, if they made positive or negative choices. Physical activity can have several different bodily influences, such as, sweating, rapid heart rate, tensed muscles, and so on. These have been known to either motivate or limit one's confidence (9). The children that were interviewed frequently said that it was a positive influence that kept them going. Bruce discussed his body's response to physical activity by saying, "I know that I am exercising and its good for me so I want to keep going" (Second Interview); he also said, "So if I'm like really sweaty or I went out to like ride my bike or play soccer with my dad I feel good because I know I'm being healthier" (Initial Interview). Another child, Harold said, "When I'm exercising, I'm sometimes tired. But it feels like I have a lot of energy and I could just run and climb an entire mountain." (First Interview). Josh also said, "If I get sweaty or my heart beat rises or yeah one of those then I feel like I can do it again and I challenge myself" (Drawing Interview).

The children consistently talked about how their bodies felt better after eating healthy than they did after eating poorly. Harold said, "Well if I choose something really unhealthy, my stomach feels like really bad like I have 500 rocks in it. I feel like throwing up, so I know that I shouldn't eat it all time" (Second Interview). Another child, Josh said, "My body responds if I eat healthy because I have more energy and I can go faster and do more things" (Second Interview). During Keith's (age 11, grade 4) drawing reflection, he said, "When I eat some of this yogurt my body feels really good because I ate something healthy for the day. And when I'm eating at school my tummy feels really good when I eat my strawberries and blueberries" (Drawing Interview).

DISCUSSION

Self-efficacy theory guided the process of making meaning on how children's experiences at home, school, and ASP fostered their confidence in their ability to know and perform healthy choices in physical activity, nutrition, and behavioral health. Findings from this study extend previous literature regarding each component of SET as it pertains to health-related choices.

Emotional and physiological states

Bandura (9) suggested that emotional and physiological states are important factors within self-efficacy development. Connected to this is the influence of mood: excitement, joy, and other positive emotions will likely increase self-efficacy while sadness, anger, or any other negative emotion will likely decrease self-efficacy. Bandura stated that elevated heart rate, sweaty palms, and/or muscular tension can all cause the feeling of inability and reduce confidence levels (9), but this was not necessarily the case with the children in this study.

Overwhelmingly, the children believed their moods had a large impact on whether or not they felt they could perform healthy behaviors. Their responses confirmed the idea that happiness is directly related to self-confidence. It is interesting to note that this was the most powerful influence of self-confidence to emerge from the data, as opposed to mastery experience, which is commonly considered the most influential (9). Findings presented here are consistent with (12), as self-efficacy and enjoyment were listed as strong predictors of physical activity, and the present study indicates that enjoyment fosters self-efficacy. This was the case with respect to physical activity in general, the intervention program, and across disciplines. For example, a good mood would often result in healthy eating whereas a bad mood made the children eat poorly. Similarly, a positive mood would increase the children's likelihood to choose positive behavioral health, and vice versa. The ASP program focused on fostering a safe and positive environment for the participants. When this occurred, results indicate that the children experienced high levels of self-efficacy in their ability to make healthy choices (though this has not been quantified).

The role of peers within the development of self-efficacy (9) was also shown to be significant for children in the current study. Studies have indicated that an individual's closest peers impact interest and self-belief by developing positive interactions and experiences, thus improving one's emotional state. Consistent with this, the children in the current study said their peers played a role in creating a positive mood as well as keeping them active. Thus, the peer interaction within ASP may improve the children's moods causing them to have more confidence in their health choice abilities.

Findings presented here seem to differ from (9) description of the factors of self-efficacy; Bandura suggested that the common response to the body's physiological reaction to physical activity would be to discontinue movement. The children in the present study reported experiencing the effects exercise can have on the body (e.g., increased heart rate, sweating), but they tended to be motivated by it and felt it was a sign they could do the activity and continue to work hard. The ASP program provided activities specifically designed to promote moderate to vigorous physical activity. Our results seem to indicate that the children were increasing their self-efficacy towards challenging physical activity each time they had this opportunity. This leads us to offer that the more active the children were, the higher their self-efficacy, which resulted in a continuous growth of self-efficacy and physical activity.

Mastery experiences

Bandura (9) posited that mastery experiences are the most influential source of self-efficacy. While not the most dominant theme presented here, our findings support this notion. Mastery experiences are powerful because if a task is performed successfully, there is an instant belief in one's ability to perform that task. If one fails, there is instant disbelief. Setting goals and creating challenges allows for self-efficacy to grow through personal experiences. The children in this study talked about mastery experience differently between physical activity, nutrition, and behavioral health. When they discussed physical activity, they primarily spoke about either traditional sports (e.g., basketball, soccer, volleyball) or lifetime activities (e.g., walking, jogging, bike riding). They described feeling confident in these activities and felt they had the most experience successfully performing in these areas at home, school, and at ASP, which was why they felt they could do them. Other activities such as adventurer cooperative learning were not mentioned. The children did not have regular experience in these other activities, which may explain why they did not emerge as areas of confidence.

When discussing nutrition, the children's expressions were limited to the identification of food groups. Previous research (24) suggested that self-efficacy related to nutrition has been associated with improvements in nutrition behavior. Our findings support this, as the children felt they could select the appropriate group for the food on their plate and that they could select the correct food in order to fulfill each category throughout the day. The ASP program curriculum included MyPlate food groups throughout its weekly curriculum, providing the children experience interacting with this content by listening to small lectures and then engaging in kinesthetic learning via a physical activity to reinforce that content.

With respect to confidence within behavioral health, the children largely characterized this as positive interactions with others. They expressed that talking, listening, and respect were the three core pieces of positive interactions. The ASP curriculum had a specific focus on positive interactions and respect for self and others. This leads us to conclude that a connection exists between the children's experience in the program and their confidence in the area of behavioral health. This is important with this group of participants in particular, because previous research has indicated that elevated behavior issues are seen among children with a lower SES (4, 6). Findings presented here are consistent with (9) suggestion that mastery experience is an important influence and is powerful when children are regularly performing a healthy behavior. The children in this study were specific in their descriptions of self-efficacy in each discipline. In order to further develop the children's self-efficacy, ASP curricula should be adjusted in order to provide children with broader experiences in each area.

Vicarious experiences

Vicarious experiences (or modeling) have been documented as influential in the development of self-efficacy, as observing someone of equal ability perform a task successfully has been shown to result in enhanced self-efficacy (9). Findings from this study are consistent with this, as the children described being frequently influenced by observing their parents successfully performing healthy behaviors. Seeing their parents being active by running, playing baseball, for example, and seeing them buying healthy food, making it, and eating it made the children feel more like they could perform those behaviors. Given this, it is important to note the significance of parents' healthful behavior within the home environment, as our findings indicate this can influence self-efficacy for at-risk youth. For those without a positive influence at home, the ASPs may provide an opportunity to witness modeling of positive behaviors. The ASP leadership, therefore, would benefit from ensuring that the ASP staff and mentors consistently demonstrate positive healthy behaviors in the areas of physical activity, nutrition, and behavioral health.

The children in this study also spoke about the impact observing peers had on their self-efficacy. The idea that if their peer could do it meant that they could do it was important in determining how confident they were when performing different tasks. The children rarely spoke about observing healthy behaviors that provided them with confidence at school, but they frequently spoke about this within the ASP. The ASP group maintained a relatively small number of children, which resulted in frequent interaction with one another as well as with mentors in the program. Consistent with previous literature, the children also spoke about the influence of mentors on their self-efficacy through vicarious experience. Scholars have suggested that mentors are positive role models that can influence positive changes in children's lives (25). These studies illustrate positive results relative to the effect a mentor can have on a child experiencing positive change and increased self-efficacy, and are related to the current study's results. In this study, seeing their mentor be successful and make good choices was influential on the ASP participants.

Imagery

Results indicated the children felt picturing themselves or someone performing a task in their mind without actually doing the task was another factor that influenced their self-efficacy. According to (8), imagery is a component of confidence building. The children discussed picturing themselves performing a task, like successfully running a mile or performing an act of kindness, and stated that if they pictured themselves being successful in this way, they felt they could perform that in a real-life context. They were often aware of the influence mental image had on their performance. They explained that if they pictured themselves eating unhealthily, they would feel less like they could make a healthy eating choice when it came time to actually do it. If they became aware of their thought process, they could attempt to picture themselves in a different way, like switch to picturing themselves eating healthily. This correlates with (7) description of imagery as a positive influence on the SET in explaining that a mental image of success is a way to develop outside of actually performing the task. This can be extremely valuable when the appropriate resources or situation to perform the task is unavailable.

The ASP program curriculum asked the children to "picture" themselves doing specific activities, and use their imagination to role play different scenarios. This provided an opportunity for them to practice taking control of their mental image to enhance the positive health-enhancing thoughts they have, thus increasing their self-efficacy in the areas present in their minds. This is particularly important with this population, as there is a documented lack of resources (e.g., safe locations to be active, healthy food access) to make healthy choices (3). Given this, mental imaging could provide one alternative to enhancing self-efficacy when actual performance is not possible.

LIMITATIONS

It is important to note that the context of the ASP provided a limitation to this study. Set in a rural Rocky Mountain state, it may not be representative of programs in other environments. This program was contextually unique in several ways. First, the ratio of mentors to children was high, with a one-to-one match up of children with adults. This may be challenging in other areas. The program focused on a small group of children to provide full attention, whereas other programs may have a larger number of participants. The present program had many resources such as transportation provided to and from the program for the participants, the use of a university gymnasium, and a large collection of equipment and supplies. Other programs may not have these resources, and some may not have any of them. Any further studies of this nature should expand to other locations, if possible, to provide results that are applicable in a larger variety of sites.

Implications for ASPs

The results of this study provide possible implications for other after-school and wellness programs. First, findings from this study suggest that programs should place emphasis on children's emotions, as it had the most meaningful impact on self-efficacy development. Creating a positive and safe environment will result in children developing higher levels of confidence in program areas. It is important for programs to provide a setting where relationship development is of great significance, as peers and mentors alike had a strong impact on positive emotions and thoughts related to healthy behaviors. Thus, fostering positive relationships is a powerful way for children to increase self-efficacy based on observation of others and verbal exchanges. Providing positive feedback is important in all health areas; any time a participant shows any level of success, praise and positive feedback will increase their confidence levels, likely resulting in increased amounts of the behavior being addressed. Regular opportunities to observe others successfully demonstrating a task will also increase the children's confidence. Mentors could play a strong role in feedback and demonstrations by consistently showing the children how to perform tasks and then providing verbal feedback in the form of praise and encouragement.

When developing program curriculum, it is important to consider what is desired for participant learning and performance. The activities in which children engage will have a direct impact on their level of self-efficacy, as they will become more confident in activities they have previously been successful with, Therefore, providing a variety of lessons and activities will increase the diversity of healthy behaviors in which they feel comfortable performing. Providing children with maximal opportunities to be successful in many activities allows for further development and confidence.

Children develop self-efficacy based on actions and practice, but our findings suggest that it can also be increased through imagery. Programs could dedicate a small portion of their time to describing the importance of having positive thoughts, as they often result in positive actions. Children could learn how to picture themselves making healthy choices, which will likely increase their confidence to actually make that choice in the future. Finally, ASP's could benefit from bringing children's attention to the body's response to healthy choices. The children of the present study stated that their physiological response had an impact on their confidence levels. Regular discussion about the way participants feel after taking part in healthy behavior will support children in interpreting their body's responses and assist them in feeling like they can regularly make healthy choices.

Acknowledgments

This work was supported by funds received from the SHAPE America Research Grant Program.

REFERENCES

[1] Centers for Disease Control and Prevention. Childhood and adult overweight and obesity, 2013. URL: http://www.cdc.gov/obesity/childhood/index.html.

[2] Flynn MT, McNeil DA, Maloff B, Mutasingwa D, Wu M, Ford C, et al. Reducing obesity and related chronic disease risk in children and youth: a synthesis of evidence with 'best practice' recommendations. Obes Rev 2006;7 Suppl 1):7-66.

[3] Drenowatz C, Eisenmann JC, Pfeiffer KA, Welk G, Heelan K, Gentile D, et al. Influence of socioeconomic status on habitual physical activity and sedentary behavior in 8- to 11-year old children. BMC Public Health 2010;10:214.

[4] Singh GK, Siahpush M, Kogan MD. Neighborhood socioeconomic conditions, built environments, and childhood obesity. Health Aff 2010;29:503-12.

[5] Olson SL, Sameroff AJ, Lansford JE, Sexton H, Davis-Kean P, Bates JE, et al. Deconstructing the externalizing spectrum: Growth patterns of overt aggression, covert aggression, oppositional behavior, impulsivity/inattention, and emotion dysregulation between school entry and early adolescence. Dev Psychopathol 2013;25:817-42.

[6] Amone-P'Olak K, Burger H, Ormel J, Huisman M, Verhulst FC, Oldehinkel, AJ. Socioeconomic position and mental health problems in pre- and early-adolescents. Soc Psychiatry Psychiatr Epidemiol 2009;44:231-8.

[7] Bandura A. Cultivate self-efficacy for personal and organizational effectiveness. In: Locke EA, ed. Handbook of principles of organization behavior, 2nd edition. West Sussex, UK: John Wiley, 2009:179-200.

[8] Blankenship BT. The psychology of teaching physical education: From theory to practice. London: Taylor Francis, 2017.

[9] Bandura A. Self-efficacy: The exercise of control. New York: WH Freeman, 1997.

[10] Dishman RK, Motl RW, Saunders R, Felton G, Ward DS, Dowda M, et al. Self-efficacy partially mediates the effect of a school-based physical-activity intervention among adolescent girls. J Prev med 2004;38:628-36.

[11] Huberty JL, Dinkel DM, Beets MW. Evaluation of GoGirlGo!; A practitioner based program to improve physical activity. BMC Public Health 2013;14:118.

[12] Branscum P, Sharma M. After-school based obesity prevention interventions: a comprehensive review of the literature. Int J Environ Res Public Health 2012;9:1438-57.

[13] Werner D, Teufel J, Holtgrave PL, Brown SL. Active generations: an intergenerational approach to preventing childhood obesity. J Sch Health 2012;82:380-6.

[14] Hausenblas HA, Carron AV, Mack DE. Application of the theories of reasoned action and planned behaviour to exercise behaviour: A meta-analysis. J Sport Exerc Psychol 1998;19:36–51.

[15] Sallis JF, Prochaska JJ, Taylor WC. A review of correlates of physical activity of children and adolescents. Med Sci Sports Exerc 2000;32:963-75.

[16] Borsdorf L, Boeyink L. Physical best activity guide: Elementary level. Champaign, IL: Human Kinetics, 2011.

[17] Theron L, Mitchell C, Smith AL, Stuart J. Picturing research. Dordrecht: Springer, 2011.

[18] Krefting L. Rigor in qualitative research: The assessment of trustworthiness. Am J Occupat Ther 1991;45:214-22.

[19] Houghton C, Casey D, Shaw D, Murphy K. Rigour in qualitative case-study research. Nurse Res 2013;20:12-7.

[20] Glaser BG, Strauss AL. The discovery of grounded theory: Strategies for qualitative research. New Brunswick, NJ: Transaction Publishers, 2009.

[21] Merriam SB. Qualitative research: A guide to design and implementation: Revised and expanded from qualitative research and case study applications in education. San Franscisco, CA: Jossey-Bass, 2009.

[22] Glaser BG, Strauss AL. The constant comparative method of qualitative analysis. Soc Problems 1965;12:436-45.

[23] Strauss A, Corbin JM. Grounded theory in practice. Thousand Oaks, CA: Sage, 1997.

[24] Rinderknecht K, Smith C. Social cognitive theory in an after-school nutrition intervention for urban Native American youth. J Nutr Educ Behav 2004;36:298-304.

[25] Jackson Y. Mentoring for delinquent children: An outcome study with young adolescent children. J Youth Adolesc 2002;31:115-22.

In: Child and Adolescent Health
Editors: A Tenenbaum and J Merrick
ISBN: 978-1-53617-825-8

Chapter 19

ANTI-DOPING KNOWLEDGE OF JUNIOR INTERNATIONAL RACQUETBALL ATHLETES

Timothy Baghurst*, PhD
FSU COACH: Interdisciplinary Center for Athletic Coaching,
Florida State University, Tallahassee, Florida, United States of America

ABSTRACT

Anti-doping education is a growing area of importance for the World Anti-Doping Agency (WADA), yet little research has evaluated anti-doping knowledge, especially among youth athletes. Therefore, the purpose of this study was to evaluate anti-doping knowledge of junior international racquetball athletes. Participants were 153 junior athletes (*Mage* = 14.69) from 15 countries who completed WADA's True Sport quiz. Participants scored on average 7.11 out of 10 where a score of 8 was the most frequently occurring score. There were no significant difference by sex [t (151) = .73, p = .47], but the youngest group of participants scored significantly lower than the oldest group [F (2,150), = 9.51, p = .001]. Findings indicate that while international junior racquetball athletes

* Correspondence: Timothy Baghurst, PhD, FSU COACH: Interdisciplinary Center for Athletic Coaching, Florida State University, Tallahassee, FL 32306, United States. Email: tbaghurst@fsu.edu.

possess some knowledge of anti-doping, further education is needed in order to reduce the likelihood of an accidental positive. Given the mediocre scores, it is possible that these athletes will erroneously fail a doping test, not through choice, but through a lack of knowledge.

INTRODUCTION

The implementation of the 2015 World Anti-Doping Code [WADC] (1) highlighted the importance of anti-doping education. This is particularly relevant given the numerous times in which the Code identifies the athlete as the primary individual responsible for a violation. Therefore, it is important to evaluate whether athletes are knowledgeable about anti-doping, as a positive test may be due to a lack of knowledge rather than a deliberate attempt to cheat.

Studies on doping focus primarily on investigating why athletes take prohibited substances and what strategies exist to eliminate their use, yet many athletes are simply unaware of what ergogenic aids are prohibited (2, 3) and doping regulations in general (4). As a consequence, athletes may take a banned substance purely by accident, for there are banned substances in many everyday products such as allergy medications, cold medications, and nutritional supplements (4). Accidental positives can be stressful and costly, and are sometimes caused by a lack of education and knowledge.

The Court of Arbitration for Sport (CAS) has investigated multiple situations of athletes testing positive whereby the athlete had taken a substance in error (5-7). For example, of the 40 positive cases in tennis between the years of 2003-2007, 19 were found to have resulted from no intent to enhance performance and an additional 8 through no significant fault or negligence (8). Only 13 were found to have been deliberately seeking to enhance performance. There are multiple examples of how an athlete can inadvertently cause a positive test (9).

Testing positive for a prohibited substance is caused by two distinct reasons: the athlete deliberately took a substance he or she knew to enhance athletic performance or it was accidental. Inadvertent positive tests can occur from ignorance, naiveté, and carelessness, or they can be caused by a lack of knowledge or education. In investigating knowledge and education levels, Somerville and Lewis (4) surveyed 74 Olympic-level sportspeople from British track and field, cycling, rowing, and sailing. Lack of knowledge was the joint highest reason given for accidental breaches. Four of the participants (5%) admitted to accidentally consuming an illegal substance with no intention to cheat. In concluding, Somerville and Lewis suggested that, "part of the doping problem stems from inadequate information and education" (p.516).

In a recent study, Ćorluka et al. (10) asked 181 Bosnian and Herzegovinian soccer players a variety of questions pertaining to doping. Most concerning was the reported 31% who had no learned knowledge about doping. Some sports and athletes receive regular education (4), but many athletes worldwide are not privy to such support; thus, they must rely on their own efforts to ensure that they remain drug free. As evidenced, even with the best intentions, this is not always successful. Amatya (2) found that 61% of Nepalese international athletes surveyed were not aware that cough medicines might contain banned substances. This is important to note, as the responsibility of a positive test is almost always – except in very unusual circumstances – that of the athlete. That the athlete is responsible has been recognized by athletes themselves (11).

Need for education

Several studies have supported the need for better education. For example, Sas-Nowosielski and Świątkowska (12) investigated the knowledge of WADA code among Polish athletes. Using the responses from 830 athletes, they found that with respect to athletes' knowledge, only 42% had correct scores. Thus, 58% of participants demonstrated inaccurate knowledge of banned substances. Interestingly, when asked where their knowledge of doping and doping control was acquired, the primary source cited was television (68%) followed by the internet (54%). It was concluded that in order for doping control to be successful, reactive measures such as testing and punishments must be matched by proactive efforts, and in particular effective education.

Other studies have reported similar poor levels of knowledge concerning WADA categories and methods of doping in sport (e.g., 13, 14). According to Parr et al. (15), failed doping tests can occur from an athlete's "poor knowledge of banned substances indicated on the label." (p.153) Wanjek and colleagues (16) found that of the 2319 adolescents surveyed on knowledge of doping, only 1% had substantial knowledge compared with 56% who had a poor knowledge. Competitive athletes scored only marginally better than recreational athletes and non-athletes.

Study purpose

It is apparent that while athletes recognize that they are responsible for a positive doping test, they frequently lack the education necessary to make informed decisions. Although in some sporting organizations a system is in place whereby doping education and a well-informed medical team can provide advice, for many athletes this is not the case (2). Thus, athletes are required to rely on the recommendations from others such as coaches or personal doctors, who lack sufficient knowledge themselves (17-20). Therefore, the purpose of this study was to evaluate anti-doping knowledge of junior racquetball athletes, and to determine whether differences in knowledge existed by sex and age. It was hypothesized there would be no statistical difference by sex, but that scores would significantly improve by age.

OUR STUDY

Participants were 153 junior athletes from 15 countries who attended a Racquetball Junior World Championships. This total equated to 84.53% of all athletes at the event. Participants were 62.7% male and 27.3% female, and mean age was 14.69 years (*Range* = 9-19). Participants were from

Argentina [two], Bolivia [15], Canada [12], Chile [six], Colombia [four], Costa Rica [15], Dominican Republic [six], Ecuador [16], Guatemala [11], Honduras [five], Ireland [seven], South Korea [three], Mexico [21], Puerto Rico [three] and the United States [27]. Participants had no anti-doping education or knowledge acquired from international participation.

Instruments

During the week of the tournament, participants were asked to complete a True Sport quiz, which is an anti-doping survey designed and hosted by the World Anti-Doping Agency (21). For the purposes of this study, the youth version of the quiz was selected. The quiz asks participants to complete 10 multiple choice or true/false questions that are randomly selected from a pool of 40 questions. Questions reflect anti-doping policies, procedures, behaviors, and other areas that are pertinent to knowledge and education of doping. Participants were able to complete the quiz in their preferred language.

Procedure

During the tournament, coaches or parents scheduled a time to bring their athlete to complete the survey. Once participants confirmed their name, nationality, and age, they were provided with a personal computer on which the survey was presented. The survey took approximately 15 minutes to complete.

FINDINGS

Participants scored on average out of 7.11 (SD = 1.76) out of 10 where a score of 8 was the most frequently occurring score (Figure 1). An independent samples t-test revealed no significant difference by sex [t

(151) = .73, p = .47] where boys (M = 7.19; SD = 1.71) scored only slightly higher than girls (M = 6.98; SD = 1.85).

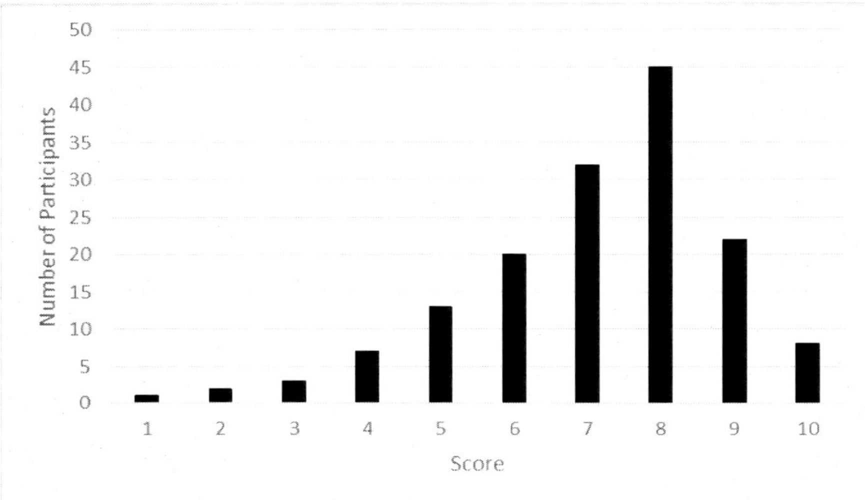

Figure 1. Frequency of scores on the True Sport Quiz.

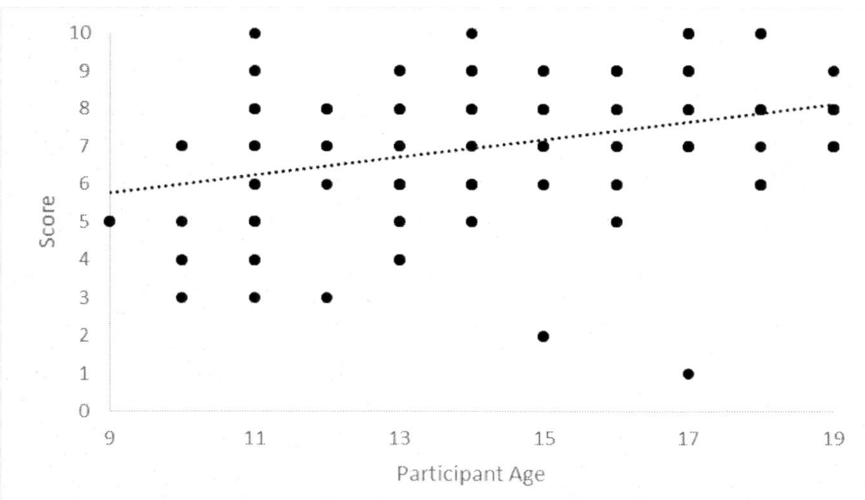

Figure 2. Participant scores relative to their age on the True Sport Quiz.

Participants were grouped according to age to determine whether scores improved by age. Three groups were formed: ages 9-12 ($n = 35$), 13-15 ($n = 56$), and 16-19 ($n = 63$). A one-way analysis of variance found significant differences [F (2,150), = 9.51, $p = .001$], and a post-hoc Tukey HSD test revealed a significant difference between the youngest group ($M = 6.18$; $SD = 1.88$) and oldest group ($M = 7.71$; $SD = 1.46$). There were no other significant differences, although the middle aged group ($M = 7.02$; $SD = 1.75$) approached significance with both the younger ($p = .057$) and older ($p = .063$) groups (see Figure 2).

Discussion

The primary purpose of this study was to assess the knowledge of anti-doping among a group of international junior athletes. A secondary purpose was to determine whether knowledge was mediated by sex and age. Results indicate that participants had a good knowledge of anti-doping, scoring on average 7.11 out of 10 on the Play True quiz, but it could be improved; only eight participants (5.2%) scored a perfect 10.

It is encouraging that there were no significant score differences by sex, and that older participants scored higher than those in the youngest age bracket. However, the 1.5 score improvement is not large, and suggests that over the course of several years, these athletes are not greatly improving their knowledge of anti-doping. These findings reflect scores presented by Moston, Engelberg, and Skinner (22), who reported an average score of 7.5 acquired from 415 adult athletes across several sports. Therefore, those in the present study were only slightly less knowledgeable than adults. Future research may wish to investigate comparisons by age and experience to determine whether knowledge increases over time in sport and whether anti-doping education is successful in increasing knowledge.

These findings provide opportunities for funders of anti-doping education and policies to consider how best to educate youth athletes. A recent release by the Association of Summer Olympic International

Federations [ASOIF] (23) noted that on average, international governing bodies for sports have decreased the amount of funding toward anti-doping education programming from 4.1% to 2.9% of annual expenditure during 2009 to 2015. This is "despite [anti-doping education] being one of the central recommendations of the 2010 report, and being an explicit item in the 2015 WADA Code" (p. 5). Based on the current findings, where participants score approximately 70% on a multiple choice and true/false test, more funding and support is necessary to educate young athletes on anti-doping knowledge, policies, and procedures.

These findings should be considered in light of the study's limitations, which create opportunities for future research. First, participants completed a series of questions that have not been evaluated for their reliability or validity, and future studies should consider evaluating each item. Second, participants were from one sport, which may not reflect the knowledge of anti-doping in other sports, particularly those with greater financial support to provide educational programming. For example, ASOIF (23) reported that 6 of the 28 international federations contributed 80% of the total anti-doping expenditure, suggesting a very disproportionate financial commitment among sports organizations to anti-doping. Third, it should be recognized that as junior athletes, some may have more international experience than others, having represented their country more than others. Therefore, future research should investigate the length or frequency of international participation to evaluate its mediation on knowledge.

Conclusion

In sum, this study determined that while international junior racquetball athletes possess some knowledge of anti-doping, further education is needed in order to reduce the likelihood of an accidental positive. Given the mediocre scores, it is possible that these athletes may erroneously fail an doping test or positive, not through choice, but through a lack of knowledge. Further measures need to be developed to help assess adolscent knowledge of doping and perceptions of doping (24).

References

[1] World Anti-Doping Agency. World Anti-Doping Code (WADC). Canada: World Anti-Doping Agency, 2015.

[2] Amatya D. Anti-doping education for Nepalese national and international athletes. ICSSPE Bull 2009;56:32.

[3] Laure PP, Reinsberger HH. Doping and high-level endurance walkers. Knowledge and representation of a prohibited practice. J Sports Med Phys Fitness 1995;35(3):228-31.

[4] Somerville SJ, Lewis MM. Accidental breaches of the doping regulations in sport: Is there a need to improve the education of sportspeople?. Br J Sports Med 2005;39(8):512-6.

[5] Court of Arbitration for Sport. CAS OG 12/07. Accessed 2017 Feb 22. URL: http://www.tas-cas.org/d2wfiles/document/6212/5048/0/Award2007.PDF.

[6] Court of Arbitration for Sport. CAS 2012/A/2804. Accessed 2017 Feb 22. URL: http://www.tas-cas.org/d2wfiles/document/6318/5048/0/Award20280420 INTERNET.pdf.

[7] Court of Arbitration for Sport. CAS 2012/A/2756. Accessed 2017 Feb 22. URL: http://www.tas-cas.org/d2wfiles/document/6319/5048/0/Award20275620 INTERNET.pdf.

[8] Pluim B. A doping sinner is not always a cheat. Br J Sports Med 2008;42(7):549-50.

[9] Yonamine M, Garcia P, de Moraes Moreau R. Non-intentional doping in sports. Sports Med 2004;34(11):697-704.

[10] Ćorluka M, Gabrilo G, Blažević M. Doping factors, knowledge and attitudes among Bosnian and Herzegovinian football players. Kinesiologia Slovenica 2011;17(3):49-59.

[11] Mroczkowska H. Responsibility for "doping slip-up" in the perception of young athletes. Polish J Sport Tour 2009;16(2):93-6.

[12] Sas-Nowosielski K, Świątkowska L. The knowledge of the world anti-doping code among Polish athletes and their attitudes toward doping and anti-doping policy. Hum Mov 2007;8(1):57-64.

[13] Bielec G. The swimmers' knowledge and attitudes towards doping. Sport Wyczynowy 2005;43(1/2):52-9.

[14] Gawroński W, Smoleń R, Szyguła Z. Assessment of knowledge on performance enhancing drugs and doping in Polish slalom canoeists. Med Sport, 1999;9:16-7.

[15] Parr MK, Pokrywka AA, Kwiatkowska DD, Schänzer WW. Ingestion of designer supplements produced positive doping cases unexpected by the athletes. Biol Sport 2011;28(3):153-7.

[16] Wanjek BB, Rosendahl JJ, Strauss BB, Gabriel HH. Doping, drugs and drug abuse among adolescents in the state of Thuringia (Germany): Prevalence, knowledge and attitudes. Int J Sports Med 2007;28(4):346-53.

[17] Bhagirathi SE. Knowledge and awareness towards doping in sports: A survey study. ICSSPE Bull 2009;(56):31.

[18] Greenway PP, Greenway MM. General practitioner knowledge of prohibited substances in sport. Br J Sports Med 1997;31(2):129-31.

[19] Laure PP, Thouvenin FF, Lecerf TT. Attitudes of coaches towards doping. J Sports Med Phys Fit 2001;41(1):132-6.

[20] Weithers HH, Gregory PL, White JJ, Lorde AA. Knowledge of banned substances in sports. (Abstract). Br J Sports Med 2003;37(5):469.

[21] World Anti-Doping Agency. WADA quiz. Accessed 2017 Feb 22. URL: http://quiz.wada-ama.org/youth/.

[22] Moston S, Engelberg T, Skinner J. Athletes' and coaches' attitudes about drugs in sport. Report prepared for the Department of Health and Ageing. Gold Coast, Australia: Griffith University, 2011.

[23] Association of Summer Olympic International Federations. International federation anti-doping processes and expenditure report. Lausanne, Switzerland: ASOIF, 2016.

[24] Nicholls, AR, Perry JL, Levy AR, Meir R, Jones L, Baghurst T, Sanctuary C, Thompson MA. Coach perceptions of performance enhancement in adolescence: The sport drug control model for adolescent athletes. Perform Enhanc Health 2015;3(2):93-101.

SECTION FOUR: ACKNOWLEDGMENTS

In: Child and Adolescent Health
Editors: A Tenenbaum and J Merrick
ISBN: 978-1-53617-825-8

Chapter 20

ABOUT THE EDITORS

Ariel Tenenbaum, MD is the director of the Center for Children with Chronic Diseases at the Hadassah-Hebrew University Medical Center at the Mount Scopus Campus, Jerusalem, Israel. He graduated the Hadassah-Hebrew University Medical School and after pediatric residency at the Department of Pediatrics at Mount Scopus Campus, he continued his work at the hospital as a senior pediatric consultant and teacher of medical students. In 2004 he was appointed the head of the new Israeli Down syndrome program in the hospital. In 2005 he started the pre-adoption clinic together with Professor Isaiah D. Wexler. In 2012 he opened the Hadassah Intellectual and Developmental Disability Multidisciplinary Evaluation Center in collaboration with the Ministry of Social Affairs. He co-founded the Disability Studies Center at the Hebrew University, where he teaches students from humanities and social studies. He was recently appointed as a child development consultant. In 2019 he was elected to the Israeli Pediatric Association Committee and serves as its scientific secretary. His main research topics are disabilities, adoption, chronic diseases and general pediatrics. He has published numerous book chapters, edited several books, and published dozens of scientific articles in international journals. Email: tene@hadassah.org.il

Joav Merrick, MD, MMedSci, DMSc, born and educated in Denmark is professor of pediatrics, Division of Pediatrics, Hadassah Hebrew University Medical Center, Mt Scopus Campus, Jerusalem, Israel and Kentucky Children's Hospital, University of Kentucky, Lexington, Kentucky United States and professor of public health at the Center for Healthy Development, School of Public Health, Georgia State University, Atlanta, United States, the former medical director of the Health Services, Division for Intellectual and Developmental Disabilities, Ministry of Social Affairs and Social Services, Jerusalem, the founder and director of the National Institute of Child Health and Human Development in Israel. Numerous publications in the field of pediatrics, child health and human development, rehabilitation, intellectual disability, disability, health, welfare, abuse, advocacy, quality of life and prevention. Received the Peter Sabroe Child Award for outstanding work on behalf of Danish Children in 1985 and the International LEGO-Prize ("The Children's Nobel Prize") for an extraordinary contribution towards improvement in child welfare and well-being in 1987. In 2017 appointed a Kentucky Colonel by the Commonwealth of Kentucky, the highest honor the governor can bestow to a person. Email: jmerrick@zahav.net.il

In: Child and Adolescent Health
Editors: A Tenenbaum and J Merrick
ISBN: 978-1-53617-825-8

Chapter 21

About the Center for Children with Chronic Diseases and Down Syndrome Center Jerusalem, Israel, Department of Pediatrics, Mt Scopus Campus, Hadassah Hebrew University Medical Center, Jerusalem, Israel

Chronic illnesses are common among children. These conditions last longer than a year and require continuous medical care and special needs. It is estimated that 10-20% of children in developed countries have one or more chronic condition. Advances in medicine and technology lead to an increase in the survival rate and longevity of children with chronic diseases and special needs. The severity of different chronic illnesses is variable, but there are many similarities. The child with a chronic illness faces physical, social, and emotional challenges. Therefore, medical care is not sufficient without rehabilitative service and emotional care for the child and his family.

Chronic illnesses are time and energy consuming. These children go through treatments, procedures and many healthcare visits. At home they often continue treatments as well, e.g., physiotherapy, breathing support machines and medications. This lifestyle may have detrimental effect on the child's social and emotional well-being, and similarly affect his parents and siblings.

Center for Children with Chronic Diseases

The aim of the Center for Children with Chronic Diseases at the Hadassah-Hebrew University Medical Center at the Mount Scopus Campus, Jerusalem, is to enhance medical care, comfort and well-being of patients and their families in the hospital and beyond. The center provides integrated and comprehensive care for these patients. This includes extensive support services and helping their families cope with the burden of care.

Numerous pediatric specialty programs and medical divisions have been established in the center to care for specific chronic conditions; among them are cystic fibrosis, Down syndrome, diabetes mellitus, familial dysautonomia, neuromuscular diseases, rheumatic diseases, feeding disorders and metabolic diseases. All these programs include evaluation and support from common services in the center: Nursing, nutrition, psycho-social care, speech therapy, physiotherapy and more.

The center works as a "one stop shop" for these children; As many services as possible, under one roof, on the same visit. Centralizing the care enables parents to come to one location to receive care. The physicians and nurses coordinate the care of the children thereby alleviating some of the burden of care off the families.

Children who are included in the programs of the center usually need returning visits to various medical specialists, consultations by multidisciplinary health professionals and performing diagnostic tests e.g., blood work, x-rays and respiratory functions. Some children may need hospitalization or palliative care. The center can concentrate all diagnostic and follow-up testing, medical surveillance and treatment in the hands of an experienced staff who knows the child and his unique situation.

The center is situated close to the entrance of the hospital and the families can access it without going through the main hospital building. In the center there are ten rooms for consultations. In addition, there are dedicated rooms for tests, e.g., respiratory functions, blood tests, sweat test and more. There is a large space with eight beds for continuous treatments, for example intravenous immunoglobulins and biological medications. In this space several unique tests are performed as well, for example growth hormone test and allergy challenge tests. There is also a special room for procedures, in which children can go through painful treatments with appropriate anesthetics and surveillance.

A special classroom in the center is operated by the ministry of education. In the classroom, children can continue their studies or play and interact with other children, in arts and crafts and many other programs.

The center is surrounded by a large healing garden that is partially maintained by the children themselves.

Conclusion

In conclusion, we believe that the "all inclusive" model of a center for children with chronic conditions is beneficial for the children and their families in terms of health and quality of life, and that this model is currently the best service for them.

Contact

Ariel Tenenbaum, MD, Isaiah D Wexler, MD, PhD
Center for Children with Chronic Diseases, Department of Pediatrics,
Mt Scopus Campus, Hadassah Hebrew University Medical Center,
Jerusalem, Israel
Email: TENE@hadassah.org.il

In: Child and Adolescent Health
Editors: A Tenenbaum and J Merrick
ISBN: 978-1-53617-825-8

Chapter 22

About the National Institute of Child Health and Human Development in Israel

The National Institute of Child Health and Human Development (NICHD) in Israel was established in 1998 as a virtual institute under the auspices of the Medical Director, Ministry of Social Affairs and Social Services in order to function as the research arm for the Office of the Medical Director. In 1998 the National Council for Child Health and Pediatrics, Ministry of Health and in 1999 the Director General and Deputy Director General of the Ministry of Health endorsed the establishment of the NICHD.

Mission

The mission of a National Institute for Child Health and Human Development in Israel is to provide an academic focal point for the scholarly interdisciplinary study of child life, health, public health, welfare, disability, rehabilitation, intellectual disability and related aspects of human development. This mission includes research, teaching, clinical work, information and public service activities in the field of child health and human development.

Service and academic activities

Over the years many activities became focused in the south of Israel due to collaboration with various professionals at the Faculty of Health Sciences (FOHS) at the Ben Gurion University of the Negev (BGU). Since 2000 an affiliation with the Zusman Child Development Center at the Pediatric Division of Soroka University Medical Center has resulted in collaboration around the establishment of the Down Syndrome Clinic at that center. In 2002 a full course on "Disability" was established at the Recanati School for Allied Professions in the Community, FOHS, BGU and in 2005 collaboration was started with the Primary Care Unit of the faculty and disability became part of the master of public health course on "Children and society". In the academic year 2005-2006 a one semester course on "Aging with disability" was started as part of the master of science program in gerontology in our collaboration with the Center for Multidisciplinary Research in Aging. In 2010 collaborations with the Division of Pediatrics, Hadassah Hebrew University Medical Center, Jerusalem, Israel around the National Down Syndrome Center and teaching students and residents about intellectual and developmental disabilities as part of their training at this campus.

Research activities

The affiliated staff have over the years published work from projects and research activities in this national and international collaboration. In the year 2000 the International Journal of Adolescent Medicine and Health and in 2005 the International Journal on Disability and Human Development of De Gruyter Publishing House (Berlin and New York) were affiliated with the National Institute of Child Health and Human Development. From

2008 also the International Journal of Child Health and Human Development (Nova Science, New York), the International Journal of Child and Adolescent Health (Nova Science) and the Journal of Pain Management (Nova Science) affiliated and from 2009 the International Public Health Journal (Nova Science) and Journal of Alternative Medicine Research (Nova Science). All peer-reviewed international journals.

National collaborations

Nationally the NICHD works in collaboration with the Faculty of Health Sciences, Ben Gurion University of the Negev; Department of Physical Therapy, Sackler School of Medicine, Tel Aviv University; Autism Center, Assaf HaRofeh Medical Center; National Rett and PKU Centers at Chaim Sheba Medical Center, Tel HaShomer; Department of Physiotherapy, Haifa University; Department of Education, Bar Ilan University, Ramat Gan, Faculty of Social Sciences and Health Sciences; College of Judea and Samaria in Ariel and in 2011 affiliation with Center for Pediatric Chronic Diseases and National Center for Down Syndrome, Department of Pediatrics, Hadassah Hebrew University Medical Center, Mount Scopus Campus, Jerusalem.

International collaborations

Internationally with the Department of Disability and Human Development, College of Applied Health Sciences, University of Illinois at Chicago; Strong Center for Developmental Disabilities, Golisano Children's Hospital at Strong, University of Rochester School of Medicine and Dentistry, New York; Centre on Intellectual Disabilities, University of Albany, New York; Centre for Chronic Disease Prevention and Control, Health Canada, Ottawa; Chandler Medical Center and Children's Hospital, Kentucky Children's Hospital, Section of Adolescent Medicine, University of Kentucky, Lexington; Chronic Disease Prevention and Control Research

Center, Baylor College of Medicine, Houston, Texas; Division of Neuroscience, Department of Psychiatry, Columbia University, New York; Institute for the Study of Disadvantage and Disability, Atlanta; Center for Autism and Related Disorders, Department Psychiatry, Children's Hospital Boston, Boston; Department of Pediatric and Adolescent Medicine, Western Michigan University Homer Stryker MD School of Medicine, Kalamazoo, Michigan, United States; Department of Paediatrics, Child Health and Adolescent Medicine, Children's Hospital at Westmead, Westmead, Australia; International Centre for the Study of Occupational and Mental Health, Düsseldorf, Germany; Centre for Advanced Studies in Nursing, Department of General Practice and Primary Care, University of Aberdeen, Aberdeen, United Kingdom; Quality of Life Research Center, Copenhagen, Denmark; Nordic School of Public Health, Gottenburg, Sweden, Scandinavian Institute of Quality of Working Life, Oslo, Norway; The Department of Applied Social Sciences (APSS) of The Hong Kong Polytechnic University Hong Kong.

Targets

Our focus is on research, international collaborations, clinical work, teaching and policy in health, disability and human development and to establish the NICHD as a permanent institute in Israel in order to conduct model research.

Contact

Professor Joav Merrick, MD, MMedSci, DMSc
National Institute of Child Health and Human Development, Jerusalem, Israel.
Email: jmerrick@zahav.net.il

SECTION FIVE: INDEX

INDEX

A

abuse, 169, 315, 316, 325, 326, 347, 353, 418
academic performance, 201, 311
AddHealth, xx, 361, 362, 364, 366, 369, 372, 374, 375
additives, xix, 229, 230, 231, 232, 234, 235, 237, 238, 239, 240, 241, 242
ADHD, 63, 378
adolescence, v, vii, viii, ix, x, xi, xii, 3, 6, 311, 357, 402, 414
adolescent female, 67
adolescent health, vi, viii, x, xiii, xv, xvi, 4, 6, 152, 374, 376, 425
adolescents, v, vi, ix, xii, xiii, xvii, xviii, 45, 46, 50, 55, 56, 57, 59, 60, 64, 70, 71, 72, 77, 88, 90, 93, 103, 199, 201, 203, 204, 205, 208, 210, 211, 213, 238, 268, 294, 295, 296, 299, 305, 306, 308, 309, 311, 312, 320, 327, 328, 357, 359, 361, 362, 363, 364, 371, 372, 375, 376, 402, 403, 408, 413
Africa, 47, 53, 58, 60, 65, 81, 91, 96, 100, 190, 200, 216
African Americans, 207, 329
aggressive behavior, 318, 348, 349
AIDS, x, 212, 365, 376
Alaska, 4, 5, 207
alcohol, xvii, 3, 5, 6, 16, 19, 112, 115, 118, 121, 123, 124, 125, 137, 138, 145, 322, 338, 348, 353
alcohol abuse, 112, 115, 118, 121, 124, 322, 338, 348
alcohol consumption, 123
anemia, 173, 178, 180, 185, 186, 187, 191, 196
anorexia, 80, 81, 219
antibiotic, 216, 218, 221, 225
antibody, 73, 76, 83, 84, 86, 87, 92, 98, 101, 102, 179, 188, 196
anti-doping, 405, 406, 408, 409, 411, 412, 413, 414
anti-doping policy, 413
antiepileptic drugs, 165
antisocial behavior, 316, 349
anxiety, 130, 132, 139, 140, 141, 142, 146, 151, 202, 211, 277, 282, 316, 378
anxiety disorder, 130, 139, 146
Argentina, 50, 92, 96, 294, 310, 409

Asia, 47, 53, 75, 82, 187, 197, 216
athletes, xx, 405, 406, 407, 408, 411, 412, 413, 414
autism, xviii, 49, 61, 63, 64, 91, 94, 95, 129, 146, 150, 152, 153, 154, 155
autoimmune disease, 81
autosomal dominant, 36, 42, 43

B

Bangladesh, 22, 83, 187, 220, 269
behaviors, 5, 130, 295, 306, 314, 318, 324, 325, 329, 357, 358, 364, 383, 389, 390, 391, 392, 394, 395, 398, 400, 401, 409
bilingualism, xix, 245, 246, 247, 248, 249, 258, 259, 260, 261, 262
birth weight (birthweight), 21, 114, 126, 135, 140, 144, 146, 153, 178, 187, 203
births, 10, 21, 36, 114, 117, 118
body mass index (BMI), xviii, 126, 132, 135, 144, 146, 150, 199, 201, 203, 205, 208, 209, 210, 211, 212, 213, 383
bullying, 203, 205, 314, 315, 316, 317, 318, 319, 320, 322, 323, 324, 325, 326, 327, 328, 343, 344, 345, 346, 347, 349, 356, 357, 358, 359

C

cannabinoids, xviii, 4, 159, 160, 161, 164, 165, 167, 168, 169
cannabis, xvii, xviii, 3, 4, 5, 6, 157, 160, 161, 162, 165, 167, 168, 169
cardiovascular disease, 294, 295, 378
cardiovascular disorders, 73
Caribbean countries, 55
CBD, 159, 161, 162, 163, 164, 165, 166, 167, 169
CDC, 47, 48, 50, 57, 58, 60, 61, 62, 66, 69, 71, 77, 78, 82, 83, 84, 90, 91, 92, 96, 97, 98, 103, 130, 147, 294, 378
Central African Republic, 100
childhood, xvii, 7, 19, 48, 57, 58, 69, 89, 91, 92, 94, 100, 101, 104, 105, 106, 129, 130, 131, 132, 133, 134, 142, 146, 147, 148, 149, 150, 151, 159, 165, 167, 168, 201, 203, 212, 213, 223, 227, 246, 289, 295, 311, 402
China, 46, 75, 104, 223, 248, 269, 285
cleft lip, 44
cleft palate, 35, 37, 39
cognitive ability(ies), 246, 247, 248, 249, 259, 261, 262
cognitive development, xix, 39, 124, 245, 247, 248, 249, 250, 260, 261, 262
cognitive flexibility, 246
cognitive impairment, 160, 167
cognitive performance, 258, 295
college students, 50, 61, 95, 96, 287, 320, 321, 328, 329, 343
colleges, xix, 270, 271, 275, 287, 313, 329
counseling psychology, 264, 275, 276
craniofacial complex, xvii, 23, 25, 26, 28, 34
cyberbullying, xix, 4, 6, 313, 314, 318, 319, 320, 321, 324, 325, 326, 327, 328, 329, 330, 331, 332, 333, 334, 335, 336, 337, 339, 340, 341, 343, 344, 345, 346, 347, 348, 349, 350, 351, 352, 354, 355, 356, 357, 358, 359
cytomegalovirus, 52, 85, 103

D

delinquency, 278, 279, 280, 281, 282, 348
Democratic Republic of Congo, 269
Denmark, 418, 426
Department of Agriculture, 213, 230, 235, 241
Department of Labor, 289
dependent variable, 114, 208

depression, 151, 212, 277, 278, 280, 281, 282, 316, 319, 323, 338
developed countries, 45, 64, 88, 90, 249, 419
developed nations, 219
developing countries, 22, 53, 54, 79, 80, 86, 249
developmental disorder, 42, 94
developmental milestones, 106
diabetes, vii, 71, 73, 74, 77, 112, 113, 115, 118, 121, 122, 132, 136, 199, 201, 203, 212, 223, 227, 294, 378, 420
disability, v, vi, vii, viii, ix, xi, 418, 423, 424, 426
diseases, 45, 46, 47, 49, 51, 52, 57, 58, 59, 62, 79, 81, 82, 88, 89, 93, 96, 97, 98, 99, 101, 103, 114, 125, 193, 218, 221, 222, 294, 362, 375, 379, 420
doping, xx, 405, 406, 407, 408, 409, 411, 412, 413, 414
drug abuse, 132, 338, 413
drug interaction, 160, 167, 170
drug therapy, 222
drugs, 5, 19, 20, 70, 71, 138, 160, 167, 169, 222, 225, 235, 413, 414

E

education, 12, 13, 14, 15, 16, 17, 19, 22, 48, 80, 148, 246, 247, 248, 249, 259, 260, 261, 264, 265, 266, 269, 270, 274, 275, 276, 283, 286, 287, 288, 290, 403, 405, 406, 407, 408, 409, 411, 412, 413, 421
embryogenesis, 26, 27, 30
emotional distress, 383
emotional health, 383
emotional state, 396
emotional well-being, 327, 420
employment status, 124
encephalitis, 51, 61, 62, 82, 100
encephalopathy, 56, 93
endothelial cells, 27, 172, 175, 178, 182, 183, 186
epidemiology, 93, 95, 197, 218, 230
erythrocytes, 172, 175, 178, 179, 180, 181, 182, 183, 185, 193, 194, 195, 196, 197
Europe, 63, 81, 95, 241, 316, 346, 372

F

Facebook, 13, 165, 321, 334, 335, 338, 351, 353
falciparum malaria, 193, 196, 197, 222, 227
familial dysautonomia, 420
FDA approval, 57, 238
focus groups, 294, 296, 297, 298, 307
food, xviii, 4, 6, 17, 80, 105, 157, 199, 200, 201, 202, 203, 204, 205, 207, 208, 209, 210, 211, 212, 213, 218, 219, 220, 226, 229, 230, 231, 232, 233, 234, 235, 236, 237, 238, 239, 240, 241, 242, 385, 392, 397, 398, 399
food additives, 4, 6, 230, 231, 232, 234, 235, 236, 237, 238, 239, 240, 241
Food Additives Amendment, 235, 237
Food and Drug Administration (FDA), 57, 59, 66, 68, 83, 230, 231, 234, 235, 236, 237, 238, 240, 241
food industry, 230, 234, 239, 241
food insecurity, 4, 6, 199, 200, 201, 202, 203, 204, 205, 207, 208, 209, 210, 211, 212, 213
food security, 202, 204, 205, 207, 208, 209, 212

G

Georgia, 3, 50, 129, 264, 314, 418
Germany, 413, 426
gestational age, 112, 113, 116, 118, 119, 120, 121, 122, 124, 146, 153
gestational diabetes, 126

good manufacturing practices (GMP), 237
graduate students, 320, 321, 329, 331, 339, 344
gymnastics, 304, 305

H

health care, 15, 16, 17, 19, 50, 57, 61, 69, 72, 76, 83, 89, 212, 220, 316, 362, 363, 365, 372, 373, 374, 375, 376
health care costs, 69, 212, 316
health care professionals, 19, 220
health care system, 50, 89
health condition, 4, 129, 130, 132, 146, 205
health education, 20, 311
health effects, 227, 237, 238, 239
health information, 19, 90, 375
health insurance, 129, 131, 132, 141, 142, 146, 148, 368
health problems, 4, 20, 112, 203, 204, 215, 216, 217
health services, xx, 148, 154, 268, 361, 362, 363, 365, 373, 374, 375, 376
health status, 131, 132, 146, 224
hemoglobin, 172, 173, 176, 179, 180, 183, 184, 185, 188, 191, 192, 194, 196, 197
hemoglobinopathies, 77, 172, 180, 185, 187, 190, 192, 193
hemolytic anemia, 173
hemophilus influenza, 54
hepatitis, 48, 50, 52, 54, 69, 70, 71, 82, 85, 90, 97, 98, 101
herpes simplex, 52, 69, 85, 103
herpes zoster, 72
heterozygote, 185
high school, 17, 210, 246, 251, 253, 254, 256, 257, 258, 287, 321, 330, 343, 358, 359
higher education, 268, 288, 290, 291
Hispanics, 70, 122, 207
histidine, 175, 176, 180
HIV/AIDS, 51, 52, 66, 69, 73, 74, 77, 85, 89, 92, 97, 101, 104, 216, 222, 225, 227, 365, 366, 367, 370
Hong Kong, ix, xii, 426
HPV, 51, 67, 68, 69, 90, 96, 97
hypersensitivity, 79, 238, 239
hypertension, 77, 199, 201, 203, 224, 295
hypoglycemia, xviii, 111, 112, 113, 114, 117, 118, 120, 121, 122, 125, 126
hypoplasia, 30, 35, 36, 37, 39
hypothermia, 112, 115
hypoxia, 178
hysteria, 46, 64, 104

I

immune response, 66, 84, 92, 183, 197
immune system, 186, 217, 218, 221
immunity, 46, 50, 51, 56, 57, 59, 61, 62, 65, 71, 72, 73, 76, 81, 83, 86, 92, 93, 179
immunization(s) , xvii, 4, 6, 45, 46, 47, 48, 49, 50, 53, 54, 55, 57, 58, 59, 64, 65, 67, 69, 70, 72, 74, 77, 79, 81, 83, 85, 86, 87, 88, 89, 90, 91, 94, 97, 98, 100, 101, 102, 103, 189
immunocompromised, 66, 76
immunodeficiency, 79, 217, 218, 224
immunogenicity, 68, 101
immunoglobulin, 84, 85
immunosuppression, 74
India, 46, 53, 60, 71, 90, 91, 94, 104, 172, 187, 241, 247, 248, 269
Indiana, xvii, 4, 6, 9, 10, 11, 12, 13, 14, 15, 16, 17, 18, 19, 20, 21, 22, 94
indirect additives, 237
infant mortality, 4, 6, 9, 10, 11, 12, 13, 15, 16, 18, 19, 20, 21
infants, 9, 11, 16, 19, 22, 38, 40, 48, 49, 56, 57, 64, 71, 76, 77, 79, 80, 83, 84, 85, 86, 87, 88, 94, 96, 100, 101, 102, 106, 111, 112, 122, 124, 126, 153, 173

infection, 53, 55, 56, 57, 61, 63, 65, 67, 70, 71, 72, 73, 74, 75, 77, 79, 81, 82, 85, 86, 87, 88, 93, 95, 97, 99, 101, 102, 103, 172, 177, 178, 188, 189, 190, 192, 217, 218, 227
infectious agents, 90
influenza, 48, 51, 52, 54, 59, 74, 75, 76, 77, 78, 83, 86, 90, 99, 101, 102, 104
influenza a, 52, 83, 90
influenza vaccine, 74, 76, 77, 78, 83, 99, 104
influenza virus, 75, 99
injury, xvi, 126, 132, 140, 150, 154, 319
intervention, 36, 122, 123, 131, 147, 202, 210, 211, 212, 215, 217, 252, 264, 266, 268, 272, 273, 277, 281, 282, 283, 286, 288, 289, 294, 295, 296, 306, 307, 308, 309, 317, 325, 326, 348, 349, 358, 359, 382, 384, 395, 402, 403
intervention strategies, 212, 309
IQ scores, 248, 259
IQR, 164, 165, 166
Iran, 269
Ireland, 130, 409
Islam, 286, 290
isolation, 284, 338, 353
Israel, xii, xx, 3, 263, 314, 417, 418, 419, 421, 423, 424, 426

J

Japan, 269, 283
Jordan, 171, 245
juvenile delinquency, 200

K

Kenya, 47
Korea, 323
Kuwait, 261

L

language acquisition, 246, 250, 254, 255, 256, 258, 259, 262
language skills, 130
languages, 247, 248, 249, 250, 252, 259, 260, 315
Latin America, 55, 103, 295, 310
level of education, 321, 344
lifestyle behaviors, 206
lifetime, 58, 75, 130, 238, 396
liver disease, 70, 71, 97
low birthweight, 123, 146

M

macrophages, 178, 183, 191
malaria, xviii, 52, 85, 89, 92, 101, 171, 172, 174, 175, 178, 179, 180, 181, 182, 184, 185, 186, 187, 188, 189, 190, 191, 192, 193, 194, 195, 196, 197, 222
malignancy, 74, 83, 101
malnutrition, xviii, 204, 215, 216, 218, 219, 221, 222, 223, 224, 226, 227
marijuana, 3, 4, 5, 6, 161, 162, 168, 169
measles, 48, 49, 59, 60, 61, 62, 63, 64, 72, 89, 94, 95
Medicaid, 112, 115, 117, 118, 119, 120, 148, 367, 369
medical cannabinoids, 160
medical care, 123, 362, 364, 419, 420
Medicare, 115, 117, 119, 120, 123, 127, 367, 369
meningitis, 48, 54, 62, 64, 65, 66, 96
mental health, 132, 136, 137, 140, 143, 145, 146, 148, 151, 154, 264, 266, 267, 268, 269, 288, 301, 316, 322, 325, 357, 402
mental health professionals, 325
mental illness, 267
mental image, 392, 399
mental retardation, 61, 64, 267, 279

mercury, 63, 64
mesenchyme, 26, 27, 28, 29, 31, 33, 34
mesoderm, 25, 27, 28
meta-analysis, 97, 127, 153, 197, 312, 359, 402
methamphetamine, 4, 20
Middle East, vii, 172, 248, 249, 261, 290
morbidity, 46, 52, 69, 71, 75, 77, 79, 83, 89, 112, 118, 121, 195, 215, 216
morphology, 28, 44, 177, 182, 183
mortality, xvii, 4, 9, 10, 11, 12, 13, 15, 16, 18, 19, 20, 21, 46, 47, 52, 54, 55, 64, 71, 75, 77, 78, 79, 83, 87, 89, 94, 114, 123, 127, 179, 184, 185, 189, 193, 195, 216, 217, 218, 220, 221, 222, 227
mortality rate, 10, 15, 54, 55, 64, 87, 123, 185, 189, 217, 218, 220, 221
mortality risk, 184

N

National Health and Nutrition Examination Survey, 97
National Health Service, 130, 153
National Institute of Mental Health, 152
National Institutes of Health, 310
National Survey, 129, 131, 132, 151, 152, 154, 212
Native Americans, 118, 121, 207
Nigeria, 47, 60, 93, 94, 269
Nissen fundoplication, 40
nitric oxide, 178, 195
nitric oxide synthase, 179
North Africa, 261
Norway, 78, 426
nutrition, 17, 150, 200, 203, 204, 212, 213, 227, 236, 378, 382, 384, 385, 389, 392, 394, 396, 397, 398, 403, 420
nutritional deficiencies, 229
nutritional state, 216, 219, 224
nutritional status, 220, 221, 222, 223

O

obesity, 10, 143, 150, 155, 199, 200, 201, 203, 204, 205, 210, 211, 212, 213, 294, 295, 301, 306, 311, 312, 379, 402
oral health, 132, 140, 149
oral polio vaccine, 53
orthodontic treatment, 37
ossicles, 31, 36
overweight, xx, 139, 150, 155, 201, 203, 204, 206, 211, 213, 295, 377, 378, 379, 402
oxidative stress, 180, 183, 196

P

parents, 16, 18, 19, 49, 56, 90, 91, 129, 131, 132, 133, 138, 139, 141, 142, 146, 148, 149, 151, 165, 202, 212, 249, 252, 262, 266, 302, 305, 317, 321, 326, 334, 347, 348, 352, 364, 373, 383, 384, 391, 392, 398, 409, 420
pertussis, 48, 55, 56, 57, 58, 63, 82, 83, 84, 89, 91, 92, 93, 101
phagocytosis, 184, 190, 196
physical activity, xix, 293, 294, 295, 296, 297, 298, 299, 300, 301, 302, 303, 305, 306, 307, 308, 309, 310, 311, 312, 378, 379, 382, 383, 384, 385, 389, 391, 394, 395, 396, 397, 398, 402, 403
physical education, 303, 308, 402
physical health, 136, 138, 140, 143, 144, 151, 295
physiological psychology, 271
plasma membrane, 176, 182
plasmodium, 175, 179, 193, 194, 195, 196, 197
polysaccharide, 51, 66, 74, 85, 86, 87, 98, 102, 233
positive behaviors, 398
positive emotions, 395, 400

positive feedback, 392, 400
positive interactions, 396, 397
positive mood, 395, 396
positive relationship, 400
pregnancy, 10, 16, 17, 18, 19, 51, 61, 72, 73, 74, 77, 78, 83, 84, 85, 87, 91, 101, 102, 195, 348, 362, 365, 371, 375
premature infant, 85, 123
prematurity, 112, 114, 118, 121, 122
preschool children, 154, 201, 210, 211, 213, 239, 242
prevention, 3, 6, 17, 78, 91, 93, 97, 98, 99, 101, 102, 103, 104, 113, 202, 211, 212, 266, 268, 288, 295, 314, 316, 317, 320, 326, 346, 348, 349, 350, 356, 357, 358, 359, 375, 379, 418
prevention strategies, 3, 6
preventive programs, 266
prophylactic, 69, 220
prophylaxis, 71, 101, 218
protection, xvii, xviii, 45, 46, 57, 59, 60, 65, 66, 68, 71, 73, 79, 82, 89, 101, 103, 171, 172, 174, 182, 184, 188, 189, 190, 191, 192, 193, 194, 196, 197, 248, 265, 388
protective factors, 295
protective mechanisms, 192
protective role, 172, 190
protein family, 178
protein synthesis, 175, 217
proteins, 66, 75, 175, 176, 180, 182, 183, 187, 189, 191, 194, 233
proteoglycans, 178
proteome, 176, 177
psychological distress, 357, 359
psychologist, 63, 265, 267, 271, 275, 283, 290, 314, 327, 350, 356
psychology, xix, 263, 264, 265, 266, 267, 268, 269, 270, 271, 274, 275, 276, 282, 284, 285, 288, 289, 290, 402
psychopathology, 322
public health, viii, ix, xii, xiii, 3, 5, 6, 9, 16, 50, 53, 91, 92, 93, 94, 99, 101, 103, 104, 124, 127, 129, 142, 171, 200, 213, 216, 226, 236, 264, 293, 294, 297, 310, 311, 314, 358, 359, 361, 362, 375, 402, 418, 423, 424, 425, 426

Q

qualitative research, 295, 307, 388, 403
quality of life, 19, 43, 160, 418, 421

R

regression model, 129, 133, 134, 139, 141
regulations, 230, 235, 237, 406, 413
regulatory agencies, 241
regulatory requirements, 236
rehabilitation, 114, 124, 227, 418, 423
Republic of the Congo, 217
respiratory syncytial virus, 82, 85, 88, 103
retardation, 174, 278, 279, 280, 281
rheumatic diseases, 420
rubella, 47, 48, 59, 60, 61, 62, 64, 72, 85, 94, 95

S

Saudi Arabia, xix, 171, 245, 246, 247, 248, 249, 250, 251, 253, 258, 259, 260, 263, 264, 265, 270, 271, 272, 274, 275, 276, 282, 283, 284, 285, 286, 287, 288, 290, 291, 325
school psychology, 264, 265, 267, 268, 269, 270, 272, 273, 275, 276, 277, 282, 284, 285, 286, 288, 289, 290, 327, 358
second language, 246, 247, 248, 249, 250, 254, 255, 259
secondary school students, xix, 213, 293, 294, 296, 298, 306, 308
secondhand smoke, 21
sedentary behavior, 383, 390, 402

sedentary lifestyle, 123
seizure, 159, 161, 162, 163, 164, 165, 166, 167
self-efficacy, 309, 378, 379, 380, 381, 382, 383, 386, 387, 388, 392, 395, 396, 397, 398, 399, 400, 401, 402
sex differences, 154
sexual behavior, 67, 68, 70
sexual contact, 67
sexual harassment, 316
sexual orientation, 323
sexually transmitted diseases, 70
siblings, 5, 147, 153, 262, 307, 321, 334, 352, 420
sickle cell, 74, 171, 172, 174, 179, 180, 181, 182, 190, 191, 192, 195, 197
sickle cell anemia, 172
signaling pathway, 42, 178
sleep disorders, 378
smallpox, 46, 47, 49, 53, 63, 83, 90, 91
smoking, 5, 10, 18, 65, 123, 132, 138, 169, 213
soccer, 299, 300, 303, 304, 305, 391, 394, 396, 407
social network, 123, 309, 319, 324, 327
socioeconomic status, 18, 122, 123, 248, 295, 296, 311, 324, 379, 384, 402
South Africa, 47, 74, 79, 98, 100
South America, 81, 307
South Korea, 409
Southeast Asia, 173
special education, 269, 271, 275, 276, 283, 288
stress, 103, 132, 137, 139, 140, 141, 142, 144, 146, 147, 149, 151, 154, 186, 196, 318, 380, 384
sub-Saharan Africa, 64, 172, 222
substance use, 230, 316
sudden infant death syndrome (SIDS), 10
Switzerland, 48, 50, 103, 414

T

tetanus, 48, 51, 54, 56, 57, 58, 59, 82, 83, 85, 86, 89, 91, 92, 93, 101, 102
thalassemia, xviii, 171, 173, 174, 181, 182, 183, 185, 187, 188, 189, 190, 191, 192, 193, 194, 196, 197
tobacco, 3, 6, 16, 19, 21, 137, 140, 296
trafficking, 175, 176, 182, 189, 191, 194
Treacher Collins syndrome, 36

U

United Kingdom, 49, 96, 130, 200, 316, 426
United Nations, 226, 265, 269, 285, 347
United Stated Food and Drug Administration (FDA), 57, 59, 66, 68, 230, 231, 234, 235, 236, 237, 238, 240, 241
United States, xix, 4, 9, 10, 19, 20, 21, 23, 45, 47, 49, 50, 53, 54, 55, 56, 58, 59, 60, 63, 64, 67, 69, 70, 72, 73, 76, 77, 79, 82, 86, 91, 92, 93, 94, 96, 97, 98, 99, 103, 105, 109, 111, 112, 129, 130, 131, 152, 171, 199, 200, 201, 206, 212, 213, 215, 229, 230, 233,234, 235, 236, 241, 245, 247, 260, 261, 263, 264, 265, 266, 283, 293, 296, 310, 313, 314, 315, 316, 322, 361, 375, 377, 378, 379, 383, 405, 409, 418, 426
universities, xix, 264, 270, 271, 274, 275, 283, 287, 288, 313
upper respiratory infection, 51
Uruguay, xix, 293, 294, 295, 296, 297, 306, 307, 308, 309, 310, 311, 312
US Department of Health and Human Services, 213, 311, 375
US FDA, 83, 236
USDA, 202, 205, 207, 210, 212, 237

V

vaccinations, 50, 52, 56, 60, 62, 63, 84, 89, 90, 92, 104
vaccine, 46, 47, 48, 49, 50, 51, 52, 53, 54, 55, 56, 57, 58, 59, 60, 61, 62, 63, 64, 65, 66, 68, 69, 71, 72, 73, 74, 75, 76, 78, 79, 80, 81, 82, 83, 84, 85, 86, 87, 88, 89, 90, 91, 92, 93, 94, 95, 96, 97, 98, 99, 100, 101, 102, 103, 104, 187
vegetables, 204, 231, 232, 233, 389, 391
victimization, 203, 314, 316, 320, 325, 328, 345, 357, 358
victims, 277, 278, 279, 280, 281, 282, 314, 316, 317, 318, 319, 320, 321, 322, 326, 328, 330, 335, 343, 345, 347, 350
video games, 294, 299, 302, 308, 310
violence, xi, 137, 138, 140, 145, 317, 322, 323, 327, 347, 350, 357, 358
viral gastroenteritis, 79
viral infection, 59, 79
vitamins, 230, 232, 385
vocabulary, 259
volleyball, 300, 304, 305, 396

W

Washington, 4, 5, 6, 56, 93, 95, 99, 101, 171, 245, 260, 263, 290, 311, 313, 320, 322, 329, 375
Wechsler Intelligence Scale (WIC), 17, 246, 250, 261
weight gain, 40, 205, 211, 221
weight loss, 223
weight status, 203
West Africa, 65, 172
Western countries, 248
WISC subtest, 253
World Anti-Doping Agency, 405, 409, 413, 414
World Health Organization (WHO), 47, 50, 153, 200, 206, 216, 221, 226, 227, 295, 310, 311, 317, 322

Y

yellow fever, 48, 81, 100
young adults, 64, 65, 70, 362, 363
young people, 208, 294, 295, 306, 307, 309, 315, 363, 372, 376
young women, 97

Z

zinc, 80
zygomatic arch, 36